EDUCATION PSYCHOLOGY

T0383581

Founded by C. K. Ogden

The International Library of Psychology

DEVELOPMENTAL PSYCHOLOGY
In 32 Volumes

I	The Child's Discovery of Death	*Anthony*
II	The Psychology of the Infant	*Bernfeld*
III	The Psychology of Special Abilities and Disabilities	*Bronner*
IV	The Child and His Family	*Bühler*
V	From Birth to Maturity	*Bühler*
VI	The Mental Development of the Child	*Bühler*
VII	The Psychology of Children's Drawings	*Eng*
VIII	Educational Psychology	*Fox*
IX	A Study of Imagination in Early Childhood	*Griffiths*
X	Understanding Children's Play	*Hartley et al*
XI	Intellectual Growth in Young Children	*Isaacs*
XII	Conversations with Children	*Katz*
XIII	The Growth of the Mind	*Koffka*
XIV	The Child's Unconscious Mind	*Lay*
XV	Infant Speech	*Lewis*
XVI	The Growth of Reason	*Lorimer*
XVII	The Growing Child and its Problems	*Miller*
XVIII	The Child's Conception of Physical Causality	*Piaget*
XIX	The Child's Conception of Geometry	*Piaget et al*
XX	The Construction of Reality in the Child	*Piaget*
XXI	The Early Growth of Logic in the Child	*Inhelder et al*
XXII	The Growth of Logical Thinking from Childhood to Adolescence	*Inhelder et al*
XXIII	Judgement and Reasoning in the Child	*Piaget*
XXIV	The Moral Judgment of the Child	*Piaget*
XXV	Play, Dreams and Imitation in Childhood	*Piaget*
XXVI	The Psychology of Intelligence	*Piaget*
XXVII	Mental Health and Infant Development, V1	*Soddy*
XXVIII	Mental Health and Infant Development, V2	*Soddy*
XXIX	Modern Psychology and Education	*Sturt*
XXX	The Dynamics of Education	*Taba*
XXXI	Education Psychology	*Thorndike*
XXXII	The Principles of Teaching	*Thorndike*

EDUCATION PSYCHOLOGY

Briefer Course

EDWARD L THORNDIKE

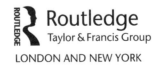

Routledge
Taylor & Francis Group

LONDON AND NEW YORK

First published in 1923
by Routledge
2 Park Square, Milton Park, Abingdon, Oxfordshire OX14 4RN
711 Third Avenue, New York, NY 10017

First issued in paperback 2014

Routledge is an imprint of the Taylor and Francis Group, an informa business

British Library Cataloguing in Publication Data
A CIP catalogue record for this book
is available from the British Library

Education Psychology
ISBN 0415-21011-9
Developmental Psychology: 32 Volumes
ISBN 0415-21128-X
The International Library of Psychology: 204 Volumes
ISBN 0415-19132-7

ISBN 13: 978-1-138-87519-7 (pbk)
ISBN 13: 978-0-415-21011-9 (hbk)

PREFACE

Our knowledge of human instincts and capacities, of the processes of learning and remembering, of mental work and fatigue, and of individual differences and their causes has been much increased in the past score of years. This knowledge I have organized for advanced students in separate volumes on *The Original Nature of Man, The Psychology of Learning, Work and Fatigue and Individual Differences.* This *Briefer Course* represents a simpler treatment of the more fundamental subject matter of these volumes, organized as a text-book in Educational Psychology for students in colleges and normal schools.

Its scope is sufficiently indicated by the table of contents. Its method is that of straightforward and systematic presentation of principles. The wise teacher will introduce students to these principles through problems made real and intelligible by the students' own experiences and will assist students to verify them by observation and experiment and to apply them to appropriate matters of educational theory and practice.

Certain topics are included which are a little beyond the interests and capacities of the lowest third of college students, notably the anatomy and physiology of original tendencies, the causes of changes in the rate of improvement, the effect of equal amounts of practice upon individual differences, and the quantitative treatment of learning, fatigue and individual differences. These facts and principles, however, if mastered, will simplify and economize thought about important educational problems, and I make no apology for including them. If education is to be a serious profession, preparation for it should not avoid matters which require study and are beyond the interests of dull minds.

Teachers College,
April, 1914

CONTENTS

PART I

The Original Nature of Man

CHAPTER   PAGE

I. GENERAL CHARACTERISTICS OF ORIGINAL TEN-
DENCIES 1
Original *versus* Learned Tendencies
The Problems of Original Nature
Names for Original Tendencies
The Components of an Original Tendency
The Action of Original Tendencies

II. MAN'S EQUIPMENT OF INSTINCTS AND CAPA-
CITIES 11
Sensory Capacities
Original Attentiveness
Gross Bodily Control
Food-getting, Protective Responses and Anger

III. MAN'S EQUIPMENT OF INSTINCTS AND CAPA-
CITIES: RESPONSES TO THE BEHAVIOR OF OTHER
HUMAN BEINGS 27
Motherly Behavior
Responses to the Presence, Approval and
Scorn of Men
Mastering and Submissive Behavior
Other Social Instincts
Imitation
General Imitativeness
The Imitation of Particular Forms of Behavior

IV. ORIGINAL SATISFIERS AND ANNOYERS.......... 50
The Original Nature of Wants, Interests and
Motives

vii

Chapter   Page

The Principle of Readiness
The Explanation of 'Multiple Response' or
'Varied Reaction'

V. Tendencies to Minor Bodily Movements and
Cerebral Connections 59
Vocalization, Visual Exploration and Manipula-
tion
Other Possible Specializations
Play

VI. The Capacity to Learn .... ˙69
The Laws of Learning
Limitations to Modifiability
The Supposed Formation of Connections by
'Faculties'
The Supposed Formation of Connections by
the Perception of Their Action in Another
The Supposed Formation of Connections by
the Power of an Idea to Produce the Act
which It Represents

VII. The Anatomy and Physiology of Original
Tendencies 84
The Structure of the Neurones
The Arrangement of the Neurones
Sensitivity and Conductivity
The Physiology of the Capacity to Learn and
of Readiness

VIII. Order and Dates of Appearance and Disap-
pearance of Original Tendencies........ 100
The Recapitulation Theory
The Utility Theory
The Gradual Waxing of Delayed Instincts
and Capacities

CHAPTER   PAGE

The Probable Frequency of Transitoriness in
  Original Tendencies

IX. THE VALUE AND USE OF ORIGINAL TENDENCIES 116
The Doctrine of Nature's Infallibility
Defects in Man's Original Nature

PART II

The Psychology of Learning

X. THE LAWS OF LEARNING IN ANIMALS.......... 125
Samples of Animal Learning
Characteristics of Animal Learning

XI. ASSOCIATIVE LEARNING IN MAN.............. 138
Varieties of Learning
The Laws of Habit

XII. LEARNING BY ANALYSIS AND SELECTION........ 153
Analysis and Selection in General
The Subtler Forms of Analysis
The Higher Forms of Selection

XIII. MENTAL FUNCTIONS 173
The Organization of Connections
Characteristics of Mental Functions
The Concepts of Efficiency and Improvement

XIV. THE AMOUNT, RATE AND LIMIT OF IMPROVEMENT 186
Practice Curves
The Frequency and Rapidity of Improvement
  under Experimental Conditions
Differences amongst Individuals in the Rate
  of Improvement in the Same Function
The Limit of Improvement

CHAPTER   PAGE
XV. THE FACTORS AND CONDITIONS OF IMPROVEMENT 202
        The Elements in Improvement
        External Conditions of Improvement
        Psychological Conditions of Improvement
        Educational Conditions of Improvement

XVI. CHANGES IN RATE OF IMPROVEMENT........... 225
        Illustrative Cases
        The Causes Determining Changes in the Rate
           of Improvement

XVII. THE PERMANENCE OF IMPROVEMENT.......... 243
        Deterioration by Disuse
        Results of Experimental Studies
        General Conclusions

XVIII. THE INFLUENCE OF IMPROVEMENT IN ONE MEN-
           TAL FUNCTION UPON THE EFFICIENCY OF
           OTHER FUNCTIONS 259
        Facilitation and Inhibition
        Changes in Expectation of Mental Discipline
        The General Rationale of Mental Discipline

XIX. MENTAL FATIGUE 283
        The Decrease in Efficiency of a Single Func-
           tion under Continuous Exercise
        The Curve of Work
        The Curve of Satisfyingness

XX. MENTAL FATIGUE (continued) 305
        The Influence of Continuous Mental Work,
           Special or General, upon General Ability
        Experimental Results
        General Theories of Mental Work and Fatigue
        The Hygiene of Mental Work

PART III

Individual Differences and Their Causes

XXI. INTRODUCTION 331
The Problems of Individual Differences

XXII. THE CAUSES OF INDIVIDUAL DIFFERENCES: SEX
AND RACE 340
Sex Differences in Ability
Sex Differences in Traits Not Measured
Objectively
A Sample Study of Racial Differences

XXIII. THE INFLUENCE OF IMMEDIATE ANCESTRY OR
FAMILY 354

The Variability of Individuals of the Same
Sex and Ancestry
Measurements of Resemblances in Related
Individuals

XXIV. THE INFLUENCE OF MATURITY................ 369

XXV. THE INFLUENCE OF THE ENVIRONMENT........ 376
Difficulties in Estimating the Amount of Influence of the Environment
Measurements of the Influence of the Environment
The Method of Action of Differences in Environment
The Relative Importance of Original Nature
and Environment

XXVI. THE NATURE AND AMOUNT OF INDIVIDUAL DIF-
FERENCES IN SINGLE TRAITS............... 402
The Continuity of Mental Variations
The Relative Frequency of Different Amounts
of Difference

CHAPTER   PAGE
XXVII. THE NATURE AND AMOUNT OF INDIVIDUAL DIF-
        FERENCES IN COMBINATIONS OF TRAITS: TYPES
        OF INTELLECT AND CHARACTER.............. 411
        A Sample Problem: Individual Differences in
            Imagery
        The Theory of Multiple Types and the Single-
            Type Theory
        Individual Differences in the Average Amount
            of a Combination of Traits

BIBLIOGRAPHY OF REFERENCES MADE IN THE TEXT........ 423

INDEX 431

Educational Psychology

Briefer Course

PART I

The Original Nature of Man

CHAPTER I

GENERAL CHARACTERISTICS OF ORIGINAL TENDENCIES

The arts and sciences serve human welfare by helping man to change the world, including man himself, for the better. The word education refers especially to those elements of science and art which are concerned with changes in man himself. Wisdom and economy in improving man's wants and in making him better able to satisfy them depend upon knowledge—first, of what his nature is, apart from education, and second, of the laws which govern changes in it. It is the province of educational psychology to give such knowledge of the original nature of man and of the laws of modifiability or learning, in the case of intellect, character and skill.

A man's nature and the changes that take place in it may be described in terms of the responses—of thought, feeling, action and attitude—which he makes, and of the bonds by which these are connected with the situations which life offers. Any fact of intellect, character or skill means a tendency to respond in a certain way to a certain situation—involves a *situation* or state of affairs influencing the man, a *response* or state of affairs in the man, and a *connection* or bond whereby the latter is the result of the former.

ORIGINAL *versus* LEARNED TENDENCIES

Any man possesses at the very start of his life—that is, at the moment when the ovum and spermatozoon which are to produce him have united—numerous well-defined tendencies to future behavior.* Between the situations which he will meet and the responses which he will make to them, pre-formed bonds exist. It is already determined by the constitution of these two germs, that under certain circumstances he will see and hear and feel and act in certain ways. His intellect and morals, as well as his bodily organs and movements, are in part the consequence of the nature of the embryo in the first moment of its life. What a man is and does throughout life is a result of whatever constitution he has at the start and of all the forces that act upon it before and after birth. I shall use the term 'original nature' for the former and 'environment' for the latter.

THE PROBLEMS OF ORIGINAL NATURE

Elementary psychology acquaints us with the fact that men are, apart from education, equipped with tendencies to feel and act in certain ways in certain circumstances—that the response to be made to a situation may be determined by man's inborn organization. It is, in fact, a general law that, other things being equal, the response to any situation will be that which

*Since the term, *behavior*, has acquired certain technical meanings in its use by psychologists, and since it will be frequently used in this book, the meaning which will be attached to it here should perhaps be stated. I use it to refer to those activities of thought, feeling, and conduct in the broadest sense which an animal—here, man—exhibits, which are omitted from discussion by the physics, chemistry and ordinary physiology of today, and which are referred by popular usage to intellect, character, skill and temperament. Behavior, then, is not contrasted with, but inclusive of, conscious life.

is by original nature connected with that situation, or with some situation like it. Any neurone will, when stimulated, transmit the stimulus, other things being equal, to the neurone with which it is by inborn organization most closely connected. The basis of intellect and character is this fund of unlearned tendencies, this original arrangement of the neurones in the brain.

The original connections may develop at various dates and may exist for only limited times; their waxing and waning may be sudden or gradual. They are the starting point for all education or other human control. The aim of education is to perpetuate some of them, to eliminate some, and to modify or redirect others. They are perpetuated by providing the stimuli adeqûate to arouse them and give them exercise, and by associating satisfaction with their action. They are eliminated by withholding these stimuli so that they abort through disuse, or by associating discomfort with their action. They are redirected by substituting, in the *situation-connection-response* series, another response instead of the undesirable original one; or by attaching the response to another situation in connection with which it works less or no harm, or even positive good.

It is a first principle of education to utilize any individual's original nature as a means to changing him for the better— to produce in him the information, habits, powers, interests and ideals which are desirable.

The behavior of man in the family, in business, in the state, in religion and in every other affair of life is rooted in his unlearned, original equipment of instincts and capacities. All schemes of improving human life must take account of man's original nature, most of all when their aim is to reverse or counteract it.

NAMES FOR ORIGINAL TENDENCIES

Three terms, reflexes, instincts, and inborn capacities, divide the work of naming these unlearned tendencies. When the tendency concerns a very definite and uniform response to a very simple sensory situation, and when the connection between the situation and the response is very hard to modify and is also very strong so that it is almost inevitable, the connection or response to which it leads is called a reflex. Thus the knee-jerk is a very definite and uniform response to the simple sense-stimulus of sudden hard pressure against a certain spot. It is hard to lessen, to increase, or otherwise control the movement, and, given the situation, the response almost always comes. When the response is more indefinite, the situation more complex, and the connection more modifiable, instinct becomes the customary term. Thus one's misery at being scorned is too indefinite a response to too complex a situation and is too easily modifiable to be called a reflex. When the tendency is to an extremely indefinite response or set of responses to a very complex situation, and when the connection's final degree of strength is commonly due to very large contributions from training, it has seemed more appropriate to replace reflex and instinct by some term like capacity, or tendency, or potentiality. Thus an original tendency to respond to the circumstances of school education by achievement in learning the arts and sciences is called the capacity for scholarship.

There is, of course, no gap between reflexes and instincts, or between instincts and the still less easily describable original tendencies. The fact is that original tendencies range with respect to the nature of the responses from such as are single, simple, definite, uniform within the individual and only slightly variable amongst individuals, to responses that are highly compound, complex, vague, and variable within one individual's life and amongst individuals. They range with respect to the nature of the situation from simple facts like temperature, oxygen or humidity, to very complex facts like 'meeting suddenly and unexpectedly a large animal when in the dark without human companions,' and include extra-bodily, bodily, and what would be commonly called purely mental, situations. They range with respect to the bond or connection from slight modifiability to great modifiability, and from very close likeness amongst individuals to fairly wide variability.

Much labor has been spent in trying to make hard and fast distinctions between reflexes and instincts and between instincts and these vaguer predispositions which are here called capacities. It is more useful and more scientific to avoid such distinctions in thought, since in fact there is a continuous gradation.

THE COMPONENTS OF AN ORIGINAL TENDENCY

A typical reflex, or instinct, or capacity, as a whole, includes the ability to be sensitive to a certain situation, the ability to make a certain response, and the existence of a bond or connection whereby that response is made to that situation. For instance, the young chick is sensitive to the absence of other members of his species, is able to peep, and is so organized that the absence of other members of the species makes him peep. But the tendency to be sensitive to a certain situation may exist without the existence of a connection therewith of any further exclusive response, and the tendency to make a certain response may exist without the existence of a connection limiting that response exclusively to any single situation. The three-year-old child is by inborn nature markedly sensitive to the presence and acts of other human beings, but the exact nature of his response varies. The original tendency to cry is very strong, but there is no one situation to which it is exclusively bound.

Original nature seems to decide that the individual will respond somehow to certain situations more often than it decides just what he will do, and to decide that he will make certain responses more often than it decides just when he will make them. So, for convenience in thinking about man's unlearned equipment, this appearance of *multiple response* to one same situation and multiple *causation* of one same response may be taken roughly as the fact.

It must not, however, be taken to mean that the result of an action set up in the sensory neurones by a situation is essentially unpredictable—that, for instance, exactly the same neurone-action (paralleling, let us say, the sight of a dog by a certain two-year-old child) may lead, in the two-year-old, now to the act of crying, at another time to shy retreat, at another to effusive joy, and at still another to curious examination of the newcomer, all regardless of any modification by experience. On the contrary, *in the same organism the same neurone-action will always produce the same result—in the same individual the really same situation will always produce the same response.* The apparent existence of an original sensitivity unconnected with any one particular response, so that apparently the same cause produces different results, is to be explained in one of two ways. First, the apparently same situations may really be different. Thus, the sight of a dog to an infant in its mother's arms is not the same situation as the sight of a dog to an infant alone on the doorstep. Being held in its mother's arms is a part of the situation that may account for the response of mild curiosity in the former case and fear in the latter. Second, if the situations are really identical, the apparently same organism really differs. Thus a dog seen by a child, healthy, rested and calm, may lead to only curiosity, whereas, if seen by the same child, ill, fatigued, and nervously irritable, it may lead to fear.

Similarly, the really same response is never made to different situations by the same organism. When the same response seems to be made to different situations, closer inspection will show that the responses do differ; or that the situations were, in respect to the element that determined the response, identical; or that the organism is itself different. Thus, though 'a ball seen,' 'a tin soldier seen,' and 'a rattle seen' alike provoke 'reaching for,' the *total* responses do differ, the central nervous system being provoked to three different responses manifested as three different sense-impressions—of a ball, of a tin soldier, and of a rattle. Thus, if 'ball grasped,' 'tin soldier grasped,' and 'rattle grasped' alike provoke 'throwing,' it is because only one particular component, common to the three situations, is effective in determining the act. Thus, if a child now weeps whenever spoken to, whereas before he wept only when hurt or scolded, it is because he is now exhausted, excited, or otherwise changed.

The original connections between situation and response are never due to chance in its true sense, but there are many minor coöperating forces by which a current of conduction in the same sensory neurones or receptors may, on different occasions, diverge to produce different results in behavior, and by which very different sensory stimulations may converge to a substantially common consequence.

One may use several useful abstract schemes by which to think of man's original equipment of reflexes, instincts and capacities. Perhaps the most convenient is a series of S-R connections of three types. Some are of the type—S_1 leads to R_1, its peculiar sequent; some are of the type—S_1 leads to R_1 or R_2

or R_3 or R_4 or R_5, etc., according to very minor casual contributory causes; some are of the type—S_1 leads to $R+r_1$, S_2 leads to $R+r_2$, S_3 leads to $R+r_3$ etc., where r_1, r_2 and r_3 are minor results.

Graphically this scheme is represented by Figs. 1, 2 and 3.

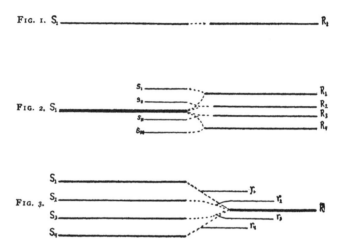

FIG. 1. S_1 ———————— .... ———————— R_1

FIG. 2. S_1

FIG. 3.

Besides such a system of tendencies deciding which response any given situation will produce, there are certain tendencies that decide the status of features common to all situation-response connections. There is, for example, in man an original tendency whereby any connection once made tends, other things being equal, to persist. There is also a tendency whereby any connection or response may or may not be in readiness to be made—may be excited to action easily or with difficulty. These tendencies toward the presence or absence of a certain feature in all connections or responses will be examined by themselves in due time.

THE ACTION OF ORIGINAL TENDENCIES

We can imagine a man's life so arranged that one after another original tendency should be called into play, each by itself. Let him be in a certain status, and let, successively, the light grow five times as intense, snuff be blown up his nostrils, a dear friend approach, and the earth quake, without in any case any other changes whatever either in the surroundings or in his internal status. Then the pupils of his eyes would contract, he would sneeze, he would smile, and he would start. The original tendencies of man, however, rarely act one at a time in isolation one from another. Life apart from learning would not be a simple serial arrangement, over and over, of a hundred or so situations, each a dynamic unit; and of a hundred or so responses, fitted to these situations by a one-to-one correspondence. On the contrary, they coöperate in multitudinous combinations. Their combination may be apparent in behavior, as when the tendencies to look at a bright moving object, to reach for a small object passing a foot away, and to smile at a smiling familiar face combine to make a baby smilingly fixate and reach for the watch which his father swings. Or the combination may take place unobserved in the nervous system, as when a large animal suddenly approaching a solitary child makes him run and hide, though the child in question would neither run nor hide at solitude, at the presence of the animal, or at the sudden approach of objects in general.

It is also the case that any given situation does not act absolutely as a unit, producing either one total response or none at all. Its effect is the total effect of its elements, of which now one, now another may predominate in determining response, according to coöperating forces without and within the man. The action of the situations which move man's original nature is not that of some thousands of keys each of which unlocks one door and does nothing else whatever. Any situation is a complex, producing a complex effect; and so, if attendant circumstances vary, a variable effect. In any case it does, so to speak, what it can.

CHAPTER II

MAN'S EQUIPMENT OF INSTINCTS AND CAPACITIES

I shall not give a complete inventory of human original tendencies, much less a full description of each one of them. Some of them, such as the tendencies directly concerned in food-getting, are of little consequence to school education. Concerning some, science can give us little information beyond what common-sense observation already reveals. Some, such as the tendencies to respond to water in its common forms, to wind, to thunder, to strange men, to large animals approaching one suddenly, to the dark, to various sorts of blows, clutches and restraints, to enclosure, to slimy things, creeping things, snakes, blood, pus, entrails and the like, are not well enough known to be safely made the basis for educational practice.

The account given here will serve two purposes. First, it will list and describe some of the unlearned tendencies in man which education has oftenest to work with; and, second, it will form the habit of seeking to replace the vague facts that man has instincts of 'pugnacity,' 'gregariousness,' 'cruelty,' 'curiosity,' 'constructiveness,' 'play,' and the like, by definite descriptions of what the responses are in each of such cases, and what the situations are to which they are bound.

SENSORY CAPACITIES

To certain situations man responds originally by special changes in the first sensory neurones and, through these, by special changes in other neurones. He is thus affected by the situation 'a certain substance in touch with the olfactory membrane' as he is not by the situation 'that substance in touch with his fingers.' To the general pressure, absorption of heat and what not that the substance causes in both cases, there are added, in the former case, special effects, notably the excitement of certain neurones giving the sensation of smell. Well-known illustrations of original tendencies to sensitivity are the capacities to receive special impressions *via* the cones of the retina from light waves of 450 to 750 million million vibrations per second, that are not received from those of 350 million million vibrations (the infra-red) ; and to be influenced by air waves of 30 to 30,000 vibrations per second as one is not by air waves of 50,000 and over per second, and the like. All the remaining original tendencies hang by these tendencies to be sensitive to certain situations in ways in which a stone, a drop of water, or a potato-plant is not. Sensitivity, or impressibility, or receptivity, is the necessary preliminary to attention, approach, flight, and all other features of original intellect and character.

It must not be supposed that the neurone-action which is set up by a given stimulus in touch with a given sense-organ in a trained adult can fairly be taken as that by which he would have responded to the same situation originally. Even in sensory capacities original and eventual nature differ. The states of consciousness which vibrations of the ether of a given rate, or the air-vibrations caused by a given tuning fork, or the presence on the tip of the tongue of a tiny drop of saturated salt-solution, and the like, provoke by their original connections are probably very unlike the states of consciousness which the trained analytical psychologist knows. The latter does not, by attending to one after another feature of the sensed world, eliminate the results of acquired connections. On the contrary, his analysis itself occurs precisely by acquiring new connections. The overtone which one hears along with the fundamental, after training in getting it separately and in listening for it in the complex, is created by forming, with a part of the stimulus, connections which that part originally lacked and so letting it produce a consciousness which it did not originally produce. The original capacities of sensation do not give us the clear sounds, colors, pressures, degrees of heat and cold, and the like, in which long experience has taught us to feel the world. To get an idea of the way the world would be sensed apart from training, we must subtract all that we know *about* it, and all the definite 'things,' 'qualities' and 'relations' which have, in the course of training, been analyzed out of the flux of gross sensations. We must take as types, the sensations which an adult psychologist gets from suffocation, heart-burn, itching or nausea rather than those which he gets from a black dot, a 100-vibration tuning fork, or a band of spectral light.

For educational theory and practice, indeed, it is often more instructive to consider what is *not* original in human sensitiveness to events than what is. That 'dead' and 'bead' are *seen* by an adult reader as they are not by the beginner; that ∴ does not *look* the same to one who cannot add or count as it does to us; that the separate tones in a chord may not be *heard* by original nature—such facts as these are the most significant results which a student of education gets from surveying sensory capacities. Just as the training of the expert musician makes him hear a symphony as the beginner does not, or as the expert tea-taster has acquired tastes which the same objects once did not give,—so training in reading, mathematics and geography makes a pupil see letters, words, geometrical forms, magnitudes, collections, maps and photographs anew; and so the general training of infancy changes the original perceptions in response to the different vibration-rates of light, degrees of temperature, or amplitudes of sound waves.

ORIGINAL ATTENTIVENESS

Of the situations to which man is sensitive some originally excite the further responses—of disposing him, especially his sense organs and central nervous system, to be more emphatically impressed thereby—which we call responses of attention to the situations in question. Thus, he moves his head and eyes so that the light rays from a bright-colored object moving across the visual field are kept upon or near the spot of clear vision. The features which are so selected for special influence upon man vary with sex and age, but are substantially covered by the rule that man is originally attentive (1) to *sudden change and sharp contrasts* and (2) to *all the situations to which he has further tendencies to respond,* as by flight, pursuit, repulsion, play and the like.

Since, as will be seen in the following chapters, man has tendencies to respond to an enormous range of situations by visual exploration, manipulation, curiosity and experimentation, his attentiveness is omnivorous to an extent not approached by any other animals save the monkeys, and far from equalled by them. Very early the human infant devotes a large fraction of his waking hours to watching what is and happens in his neighborhood. When he gains control of reaching and grasping he examines what he can move. When he gains power to move about, he attends to almost every object that he can get to until its possibilities as a stimulus to manipulation and experimentation are exhausted. In the meantime, parts of his own body and the sounds that he and the persons

and things about him make have been selected from the total
medleys in which they inhere by the preparation of the sense-
organs, and perhaps of the neurones associated therewith, to be
stimulated by this or that sight or sound or touch.
One is tempted to assert that man is originally attentive to
everything until its novelty wears off. But certain notable
lacks show that original attentiveness is the sum of many particular tendencies and not an indifferent general capacity.
For example, man lacks the attentiveness to small differences
in smells, or small intrusions of new smells into a familiar
medley, which is so characteristic of many mammals.

GROSS BODILY CONTROL

How far man's management of his body in holding up his
head, sitting, standing, walking, running, stooping, jumping
up, jumping down, leaping at, crouching, lying down, rolling
over, climbing, dodging, stooping to pick up, raising oneself
again, balancing, clinging, pushing with arms and with legs,
pulling with arms, and in such other movements of position,
locomotion and the displacement of large objects as man has in
common with the primates in general, is unlearned, is still a
disputed question. Reputable opinion can be cited in support
of remote extremes.

It appears to the writer that the contribution from training
is slight, that these accomplishments are in origin much more
like breathing, winking or sucking, than like playing tennis,
dancing or swimming. The case of walking is instructive.
Here, although, under the conditions of civilized family life,
children appear to learn, or even to be taught, to walk, it has
been shown that the appearance is illusory.* The baby's trials

*See, for example, Kirkpatrick ['03], pp. 79-81 ; Trettien ['00], p. 42 ;
Woodworth ['03], p. 315.

with varying and increasing success are not the causes of a habit, but the symptoms of a waxing instinct. The parent's tuition does not create a tendency, but only stimulates or rewards it.

It must be remembered further that gradualness in appearing and imperfections in early manifestations are entirely consistent with unlearnedness. The 'perfecting' of a tendency may come from the mere inner growth that time implies as well as from exercise and tuition. Thus the reactions of running, crouching and chirring by chicks when a large object is thrown at them are surely unlearned but develop gradually. The reactions of roosters in combat are surely unlearned but are at the start so 'imperfect' that unless one traces their behavior continuously he will hardly even recognize the early manifestations. (These are that two chicks, as young even as six days, will suddenly rush at each other, face each other for a moment and then go about their previous business.) 'Imperfection' at the start and gradualness in development are the rule rather than the exception with all original tendencies.

I judge therefore that children gain power to manage their bodies in connection with the movements listed above, as required by the ordinary exigencies of an animal-like life in the woods, largely by the inner development of original tendencies.* Just how largely cannot be said. I do not assert that man, or any of the mammals, would manage his body as well without experience as with it, or that all the gross bodily manipulations listed are as well developed by original nature as walking is. But the notion that these activities develop by trial and success and imitation wholly, or with slight assistance from

*If this is the fact, the customary incitements of the nursery are largely useless and possibly harmful. So also with many of the maternal precautions against childish adventures in locomotion.

some very indefinite 'predispositions,' does seem indefensible as an account of their causation in the children whom I have had opportunity to observe. The 'predispositions' can, on the contrary, be relied on to produce the behavior with a very small amount of assistance from the pains of stumbling, falling, going in the wrong direction and the like, and with no assistance at all from imitation.

FOOD-GETTING, PROTECTIVE RESPONSES AND ANGER

The original tendencies concerned with food-getting, habitation, fear, fighting and anger may be described here only in part and very briefly.

Acquisition and Possession.—To any not too large object which attracts attention and does not possess repelling or frightening features the original response is approach or, if the child is within reaching distance, reaching, touching and grasping. An object having been grasped, its possession may provoke the response of putting it in the mouth, or of general manipulation, or both. The sight of another human being going for the object or busied with it strengthens the tendencies toward possession. To resistance the response is pulling and twisting the object and pushing away whoever or whatever is in touch with it. Failure to get nearer, when one has moved toward such an object of attention, and failure to grasp it when one reaches for it, provoke annoyance, more vigorous responses of the same sort as before and the neural action which produces an emotion which is the primitive form of desire.

To the situation, 'a person or animal grabbing or making off with an object which one holds or has near him as a result of recent action of the responses of acquisition,' the responses

s

are:—the neural action paralleling the primitive emotion of anger, a tight clutch on the object, and pushing, striking and screaming at the intruder.

Hunting.—It is not hard to show that man's original nature somehow leads to activities which justify us in speaking of a hunting instinct. But it is hard to discover just what the hunting instinct is. It is, for instance, doubtful whether James is right in assuming the 'hunting' response toward "all living beasts, great and small," and toward "all human beings in whom we perceive a certain *intent* toward *us,* and a large number of human beings who offend us peremptorily, either by their look, or gait, or by some circumstance in their lives which we dislike." Is there perhaps, on the contrary, so specialized a tendency as that to rob birds' nests, as Schneider maintains? Just what, in any case, are the situations and the responses, referred to by the hunting instinct?

In the writer's opinion they are as follows:

To 'a small escaping object,' man, especially if hungry, responds, apart from training, by pursuit, being satisfied when he draws nearer to it. When within pouncing distance, he pounces upon it, grasping at it. If it is not seized he is annoyed. If it is seized, he examines, manipulates and dismembers it, unless some contrary tendency is brought into action by its sliminess, sting or the like. To 'an object of moderate size and not of offensive mien moving away from or past him' man originally responds much as noted above, save that in seizing the object chased, he is likely to throw himself upon it, bear it to the ground, choke and maul it until it is completely subdued, giving then a cry of triumph.

With both small and larger 'game,' there is, I think, a tendency to bring the captured animal to some familiar human being.

The responses of cautious approach, ot fighting, of avoidance and of protective behavior may be mingled in all sorts of ways with the hunting responses in accordance with variations in the size of the animal, the offensiveness of its mien, and the struggle it makes when seized, and in accordance with its alternations from flight to resistance or attack.

The presence of this tendency in man's nature under the conditions of civilized life gets him little food and much trouble. There being no wild animals to pursue, catch and torment into submission or death, household pets, young and timid children, or even aunts, governesses or nurse-maids, if sufficiently yielding, provoke the responses from the young. The older indulge the propensity at great cost of time and money in hunting beasts, or at still greater cost of manhood in hounding Quakers, abolitionists, Jews, Chinamen, scabs, prophets, or suffragettes of the non-militant variety. Teasing, bullying, cruelty, are thus in part the results of one of nature's means of providing self and family with food: and what grew up as a pillar of human self-support has become so extravagant a luxury as to be almost a vice.

Possible Specialized Tendencies.—It is possible that tendencies to seek particular objects as food and to capture them by specialized sets of movements may also be original in man. Thus Schneider ['82] thinks that bird's nests and eggs are situations of particular potency to attract attention and possession, and Acher ['10] seems to think that throwing stones, hitting with a club, and cutting with pointed objects are responses apart from learning. It has been asserted that there is a special instinct to insert the fingers into crannies (to dislodge small animals hidden there)! There is some evidence to show that a small object held out or tossed to a young human is more readily seized and tasted than one otherwise encountered, and that he will eat food that he himself picks up more readily than the same food when put in his mouth by another.

Collecting and Hoarding.—There is originally a blind tendency to take portable objects which attract attention, and carry them to one's habitation. There is the further response of satisfaction at contemplating and fingering them there. These tendencies commonly crystallize into habits of collecting and storing certain sorts of objects whose possession has additional advantages, and abort as responses to other objects whose possession brings secondary annoyances. Thus, money, marbles, strings, shells, cigar-tags and picture-postals become favored objects by their power in exchange, convenience of carriage, permanent attractiveness and utility in play. But clear evidences of the original tendency may remain, as in those who feel a craving to gather objects which they know will be a nuisance to them or who cannot bear to diminish hoards which serve no purpose save that of being a hoard. So of the man who stole utensils from his own kitchen to increase his hoard, and bought substitutes!

Fear.—The inner perturbation which we call the emotion of fear, running, crouching, clinging, starting, trembling, remaining stock-still, screaming, covering the eyes, opening the mouth and eyes, a temporary cessation followed by an acceleration of the heart-beat, difficulty in breathing and paleness, sweating and erection of the hair are responses of which certain ones seem bound, apart from training, to certain situations, such as sudden loud noises or clutches, the sudden appearance of strange objects, thunder and lightning, loneliness, and the dark.

Since the responses and the situations provoking them which are involved in what men call instinctive fear are both so numerous, there should be, in an account of original nature, a section telling just which of the responses are bound to each of the situations, and how firmly. As yet this has not been done, or even attempted.

Surely, however, the sciences of human nature cannot rest content with the fact that by original nature strange men and animals advancing toward us with threatening mien, thunder and lightning, reptiles, darkness, solitude, dark holes and corners, rats, spiders and other creeping things, sudden noises, contacts and clutches unprepared for tend to produce more or less an indeterminate assortment of discomfort, running, crouching, screaming, clinging, trembling, and so on. They need to know just what the effect of each of these situation-elements is. Practically, it makes a great difference whether a man responds only with discomfort, palpitations and the inner subjective fear, still shooting at the enemy, or also runs and hides. Theoretically, it makes a great difference whether the situations involved are regarded as producing indiscriminately a vague X, fear, which then may at random produce any assortment of its various 'expressions,' or are regarded as each producing, under the same conditions, an effect proper to it and to nothing but it. In the latter case we are encouraged to study the exact details of human behavior in fear, tho we may never know them, while in the former case we are told beforehand that they are unknowable.

As a sample of such inquiries, let us ask whether each of the situations tends equally to provoke each of the responses and in the same degree, so that one or another, or one after another, and more or less of it, will come according to accidental physiological conditions in the animal. Surely not. The 'fear' due to a large animal coming toward one rapidly is not the same as the 'fear' due to thunder and lightning. The large animal is much more likely to be responded to by running than by hiding. With thunder and lightning the reverse is true. Still surer is the specialization of the intensity of the response. One can vary the amount of a child's 'starting' from a contraction hardly perceptible up to one approaching a convulsion, by varying the stimulus. Can anyone doubt that each degree of strangeness or suddenness has a determinate effect?

Consider the specialized effects of solitude, of sounds compared with sights, and of seeing a large animal approaching one rapidly compared with grasping a cold clammy reptile. In my opinion at least, the clutching, clinging and nestling responses are relatively rare in solitude, tho occasionally a human being, so frightened, will clutch at trees or even at nothing. Fearful sounds rarely provoke turning the head away and covering the eyes, but fearful sights often do. A large animal approaching one rapidly and distant, say, forty feet, is often responded to by turning and running, but very rarely by jumping backwards. The reverse is true of the response to the same animal met suddenly at a distance of three feet, or to a clutch (from in front) in the dark.

It is probable further that an impartial survey of human behavior, unprejudiced by the superstition that a magic state of consciousness, 'fear,' is aroused by 'danger,' and then creates flight and other symptoms of itself, would show that pursuit and capture may produce distinctive responses whether or no the peculiar inner trepidation which introspection knows is present. A large object coming rapidly toward one seems often to provoke instinctive turning, fleeing, seeking cover (and the human horde, if that is present) without necessarily doing more. Being pounced on or grasped by a large object seems often to be responded to by instinctive dodging, writhing and pulling, without anything that deserves the name of the inner emotion of fear.

Fighting.—Tendencies to fight are certainly inherent in man's nature, the situations, responses and bonds concerned being apparently the following:

(1) To the situation, 'being interfered with in any bodily movements which the individual is impelled by its own constitution to make, the interference consisting in holding the individual,' the little child makes instinctively responses of stiffening, writhing and throwing back the head and shoulders. These are supplemented or replaced by kicking, pushing, slapping, scratching and biting in the older. This tendency, if it exists, may be called the instinct of *escape from restraint.*

(2) To a similar situation, with the difference that the interference is by getting in the way or shoving, the responses are:—dodging around, pushing with hands or body, hitting, pulling and (though, I think, much less often) slapping, kicking and biting. This may be called the instinct of *overcoming a moving obstacle.*

Parents who are scientific observers will admit the existence and unlearnedness of these two tendencies, and, I think, will by close observation find that they are fairly distinguishable one from the other, and both from the forms of anger and fighting whose description follows. The angry behavior in these two cases usually ceases when the confinement or obstruction ceases, and rarely leads to more violent behavior thereafter, whereas in some other cases it is maintained and may arouse the hunting instinct, teasing, bullying and cruelty after its own immediate end has been attained.

(3) To the situation 'being seized, slapped, chased or bitten (by any object), the escape-movements having been ineffective or inhibited for any reason,' the fighting movements or the paralysis of terror may be the response. When the former occurs, the total complex may be called the instinct of *counter-attack.*

To the particular situations that arise when attack provokes counter-attack, there are, I believe, particular responses. If A clings to B, trying to throw him down or bite him, B will, by original nature, more often try to push A away or throw him down than to hit or bite him. If A rushes at B, slapping, scratching and kicking, B will, by original nature, more often hit and kick at A than try to push him away or throw him down. I believe that there is a basis in original nature for the distinction in sport between the fight with fists, which I judge to be a refinement (inappropriate as the word may seem) of the 'slap-scratch-poke' fighting, and the wrestling match, which I judge to be a refinement of the 'push-pull-throw down-jump upon' fighting. When A and B are both down, the response is an effort to get on top. When A is beaten, it is originally satisfying to B to sit on him (or it), to stand exulting beside him (or it), and to remain unsatisfied (if A is a human being) until A has given signs of general submissiveness. Many other specialized original tendencies, such as to remove things from different parts of the body in different ways, and to duck the head and lift up the arm, bent at the elbow, in response to the situation, 'an object coming toward the head rapidly,' appear in the course of a fight.

(4) To the situation 'sudden pain' the response is attack upon any moving object near at hand. This may be called the instinct of *irrational response to pain*. This fact, common in everyone's experience, may of course be interpreted as an acquired habit of response by analogy, but it seems to the writer that it is a true and beautiful case of nature's very vague, imperfect adaptations, which only on the whole and in a state of nature are useful. When a loving child with indigestion beats its mother who is trying to rock it to sleep (though it would protest still more if not rocked), or when a benevolent

master punches the servant who is lifting his gouty foot, the contrary habits seem too strong to be overcome by the force of mere analogy with an acquired habit of hitting in response to the pain of conflict. Indeed the existence of the latter habit is in such cases only a matter of speculation.

(5) To the situation, 'an animal of the same species toward whom one has not taken the attitude of submission and who does not take it toward him' the human male responds by threatening movements, shoving the person away, and, if these fail to produce the attitude of submission, by either submission or further attack. The encounter is closed by the submission of either party, which may take place at any point. This tendency may be called the instinct of *combat in rivalry*.

(6) To the situation, 'the mere presence of a male of the same species during acts of courtship,' the human male tends to respond by threatening or attacking movements until the intruder is driven away or the disturbed one himself flees.

(7) Either as habits of analogy developing from these specialized tendencies, or as an equally original but vaguer tendency in addition to them, the following behavior occurs:—

To the situation—being for some length of time thwarted in any instinctive response by any thing, especially if the thwarting continues after one has done various things to evade it, the response-group of pushing, kicking, hitting, etc., is made, the attack continuing until the situation is so altered as to produce instinctively other responses, such as fulfilling the original activity, hunting, mangling, triumphing over, or fleeing from, the thwarting thing.

The state of affairs, angry and pugnacious behavior, is apparently satisfying. Of course, some of the situations that provoke it are far from satisfying intrinsically, but the responses made to them *are*, and often are enough so to make one rather seek than avoid the situation itself. The misery reported in connection with anger seems to be an after-effect, the accompaniment of shame, grief, or rational deprecation of one's past behavior, or of the exhaustion due to it.

CHAPTER III

MAN'S EQUIPMENT OF INSTINCTS AND CAPACITIES *(continued)*: RESPONSES TO THE BEHAVIOR OF OTHER HUMAN BEINGS

Human intercourse and institutions are as surely rooted and grounded in original nature as man's struggles with the rest of nature for food and safety. The first, and all in all the greatest, social bond and condition is the original behavior of mother to young.

MOTHERLY BEHAVIOR

All women possess originally, from early childhood to death, some interest in human babies, and a responsiveness to the instinctive looks, calls, gestures and cries of infancy and childhood, being satisfied by childish gurglings, smiles and affectionate gestures, and moved to instinctive comforting acts by childish signs of pain, grief and misery. Brutal habits may destroy, or competing habits overgrow, or the lack of exercise weaken, these tendencies, but they are none the less as original as any fact in human nature.

With the changes in the woman's nature and life that conception and child-birth bring, these tendencies gain new power and special attachments. To a woman who has given birth to a child, a baby to see and hold and suckle is perhaps the most potent satisfaction life can offer, its loss the cause of saddest yearning. To a woman who has given birth to a child, the baby she sees, holds and nurses appeals almost irresistibly when it gives the cry of hunger, pain or distress, the start of surprise,

27

the scream of fear, the smiles of comfort, the cooing and gurgling and shouting of vocal play. She cuddles it when it cries, smiles when it smiles, fondles and coos to it in turn. As the first human face it sees and turns to follow, as the familiar form which it nestles against in comfort and clutches in fear, she wins its tokens of affection. When it later points at objects, she looks and shares its interest. And later still, every signal of joy, or grief, or pain by this being whom she has held and nursed and fondled, has its quick response. In all this, original nature is the prime mover and essential continuing force.

This series of situations and responses constitutes the 'maternal instinct' in its most typical form. But, as do all original tendencies, it acts somehow, though its ordinary situations be complicated or deformed. To have given birth to a child, though ordinarily an enormous intensifier of maternal care, is not a *sine qua non*. The sequence may, though less surely, begin with holding and nursing. Similarly, suckling the child, though ordinarily an enormous intensifier of maternal care, may be absent but still leave the situation potent enough to arouse the later sequences. So childless women, who lack also the stimuli of care of early infancy, may yet manifest the later tendencies toward the children they adopt.

Boys and men share more in the instinctive good will toward children than traditional opinion would admit, though the tendencies are not so strong, and the responses are different. Very weak in the specific tendencies to clasp and carry an infant (the proverbial distress and awkwardness of the male when an infant is thrust into his arms, as contrasted with the typical woman's 'Let me hold him,' is at bottom instinctive) and to fondle and prattle to it, and lacking also the special incitement of the tendency due to the inner changes of child-birth and lactation, they yet in their own way respond to many of its appeals. To offer a little child scraps of food and see it eat, to snatch it from peril by animals, and to smile approvingly at its more vigorous antics, seem to me to be truly original tendencies of the human male.

Male thoughtlessness and brutality toward children, and whatever living being or thing makes a similar appeal, is due not to total absence of kindliness, but rather to the presence of the competing tendencies of the hunting instinct, which is as much stronger in men than in women as the maternal instinct is stronger in women than in men.

RESPONSES TO THE PRESENCE, APPROVAL AND SCORN OF MEN

Gregariousness.—Man responds to the absence of human beings by discomfort, and to their presence by a positive satisfaction. Kidd's statement about Kafir children holds true of man in general. In his games and work, too, "there is much that looks like sheer animal love for gregarious fellowship."

The rich satisfaction of the presence of even a single companion consists not only in allowing various desirable activities which need a fellowman as their stimulus, but also in the mere fact that he is there. Being one of a crowd adds new instinctive exhilarations, irrespective of any particular benefits the situation may be expected to produce. McDougall and James have both emphasized the part this tendency plays in our recreations. The former says:

"In civilized communities we may see evidence of the operation of this instinct on every hand. For all but a few exceptional, and generally highly cultivated, persons the one essential condition of recreation is the being one of a crowd. The normal daily recreation of the population of our towns is to go out in the evening and to walk up and down the streets in which the throng is densest—the Strand, Oxford Street, or the

Old Kent Road; and the smallest occasion—a foreign prince driving to a railway station or a Lord Mayor's Show—will line the streets for hours with many thousands whose interest in the prince or the show alone would hardly lead them to take a dozen steps out of their way. On their few short holidays the working classes rush together from town and country alike to those resorts in which they are assured of the presence of a large mass of their fellows. It is the same instinct working on a slightly higher plane that brings tens of thousands to the cricket and football grounds on half-holidays." ['08, p. 86]

A similar argument could be made in the case of our religious worship, the organization of schools, the preference of young women for factory labor over domestic service, and almost any other human activity.

Responses of Attention to Human Beings.—Man has a special original interest in the behavior of other men. Doubtless this, in infancy, is largely due to the mere variety in movement which human beings have in common with dogs, mechanical toys, the leaves of trees and the like. But it is hardly wholly due thereto. The human face is too early singled out from other objects and too constantly a controller of attention. Chamberlain hardly exaggerates when he says that "the face of its elders is the child's chart and compass in the first voyages of life." ['oo, p. 189.] Evidence is found in the difference between the sexes in respect to it. If measurements are taken of the strength of the interest in the intellectual and moral traits of people compared to the strength of the interest in the mechanical operations of things, women differ notably from men. It seems necessary, therefore, to admit that the specific form and features and characteristic behavior of man, as in smiling, crying, or jabbering, attract attention to him and what he does.

Attention-getting.—There seems to be, though one cannot

be sure, a real, though easily counteracted, tendency to respond to the presence of an inoffensive human being by approaching, gesticulating, calling, and general restless annoyance until he notices one. A man entering a room where another stands absorbed will often, in spite of the conventions of cityfied habits, feel a measurable irritation, walk past him, ring for a waiter, or the like, though he would not have felt and done so, had the room been empty. Children seem to act in this way irrespective both of any acquired intention to win approval, and of the more aggressive behavior which we call self-assertiveness or display.

Responses to Approving and to Scornful Behavior.—To the situation, 'intimate approval, as by smiles, pats, admission to companionship and the like, from one to whom he has the inner response of submissiveness,' and to the situation, 'humble approval, as by admiring glances, from anybody,' man responds originally by great satisfaction. The withdrawal of approving intercourse by masters and looks of scorn and derision from anyone originally provoke a discomfort that may strengthen to utter wretchedness.

The reader will understand that the approval and disapproval which are thus satisfying and annoying to the natural man are far from identical, in either case, with the behavior which proceeds from cultivated moral approbation and condemnation. The sickly frown of a Sunday-school teacher at her scholar's mischief may be prepotently an attention to him rather than the others, may contain a semi-envious recognition of him as a force to be reckoned with, and may even reveal a lurking admiration for his deviltry. It then will be instinctively accepted as approval.

Darwin long ago noted the extraordinarily ill-proportioned misery that comes from committing some blunder in society whereat people involuntarily 'look down' on one for an instant. Except for him, little attention has been paid to the originality of the hunger of man for the externals of admiration and the intolerability of objective scorn and derision.   Yet these forces of approval and disapproval in appropriate form from those above and those below us in mastery-status, are and have been potent social controls.   For example the 'discipline' of a humane home or school today relies almost entirely upon such approval from above, and finds it even more effective than severe sensuous pains and deprivations.   The elaborate para- phernalia and rites of fashion in clothes exist chiefly by virtue of their value as means of securing diffuse notice and approval. The primitive sex display is now a minor cause: women ob- viously dress for other women's eyes.   Much the same is true of subservience to fashions in furniture, food, manners, morals and religion.   The institution of tipping, which began per- haps in kindliness and was fostered by economic self-interest, is now well-nigh impregnable because no man is brave enough to withstand the scorn of a line of lackeys whom he heartily despises, or of a few onlookers whom he will never see again.

Best of all illustrations of the potent craving for objective approval, perhaps, is offered by Veblen's brilliant analysis of the economic activities of the leisure class.   These he finds to be essentially vicarious consumption and conspicuous waste, or the maintenance of a useless retinue and public prodigality in order to show that you have more than you can use, and so to fix upon you the admiring glances of those who can afford to waste less or nothing at all.

Responses by Approving and Scornful Behavior.—To mani- fest approving and disapproving behavior is as original a tendency as to be satisfied and annoyed by them. Smiles, respectful stares and encouraging shouts occur, I think, as instinctive responses to relief from hunger, rescue from fear, gorgeous display, instinctive acts of strength and daring, victory, and other impressive instinctive behavior that is harmless to the onlooker. Similarly, frowns, hoots and sneers seem bound as original responses to the observation of empty-handedness, deformity, physical meanness, pusillanimity, and defect. As in the case of all original tendencies, such behavior is early complicated, and in the end much distorted, by training; but the resulting total cannot be explained by nurture alone.

MASTERING AND SUBMISSIVE BEHAVIOR

There is, I believe, an original tendency to respond to 'the presence of a human being who notices one, but without approving or submissive behavior' by holding the head up and a little forward, staring at him or not looking at him at all, or alternating staring and ignoring, doing whatever one is doing somewhat more rapidly and energetically and making displays of activity, and by satisfaction if the person looks on without interference or scorn. There is a further tendency to go up to such an unprotesting human being, increasing the erection and projection of the head, looking him in the eye, and perhaps nudging or shoving him. There is also an original tendency to feel satisfaction at the appearance and continuance of submissive behavior on the part of the human beings one meets. These tendencies we may call the instinct of *attempt at mastery*. Such behavior is much commoner in the male than in the female. In her the forward thrust of the head, the approach, displays of strength, nudging and shoving are also commonly replaced by facial expressions and other less gross movements.

If the human being who answers these tendencies assumes a submissive behavior, in essence a lowering of head and

3

shoulders, wavering glance, absence of all preparations for attack, general weakening of muscle tonus, and hesitancy in movement, the movements of attempt at mastery become modified into attempts at the more obvious swagger, strut and glare of triumph. The submissive attitude may also provoke the master to protect the submissive one. If the human being protests by thrusting *his* head up and out, glaring back, and not giving way to advance, the aggressor either becomes submissive or there is more or less of a conflict of looks, gestures, yells, or actual attacks, until, as was described under the fighting instinct, the submission of one or the exhaustion of both.

There is an original tendency to respond to the situation, 'the presence of a human being larger than oneself, of angry or mastering aspect,' and to blows and restraint, by submissive behavior. When weak from wounds, sickness or fatigue, the tendency is stronger. The man who is bigger, who can outyell and outstare us, who can hit us without our hitting him, and who can keep us from moving, does originally extort a crestfallen, abashed physique and mind. Women in general are thus by original nature submissive to men in general. Submissive behavior is apparently not annoying when assumed as the instinctive response to its natural stimulus. Indeed, it is perhaps a common satisfier.

Every human being thus tends by original nature to arrive at a status of mastery or submission toward every other human being, and even under the more intelligent customs of civilized life somewhat of the tendency persists in many men.

The original behavior in mastery and submission, and in approving, disapproving, being approved and being scorned, derided and neglected, becomes very much complicated by differences in the sex of the person who is the situation, and in the sex and maturity of the person who is responding, by an increase in the number of persons who are the situation, and by the presence in the situation of elements provocative of curiosity, fear, anger, repugnance, the hunting instinct, kindliness, sexual attraction and coy behavior. My account of attempt at mastery, for instance, would be only partly true of any cases save those where the situation and the response were the behaviors of two males of about the same degree of physical maturity. Mastery and submission are fit illustrations of the universal fact that the many unit tendencies to respond to characteristic situations combine in elaborately complex totals. This fact makes the original social tendencies of man seem, at first sight, like a hopelessly unpredictable muddle of domineering, subservience, notice, disregard, sex pursuit, aversion, showing off, shyness, fear, confidence, cruelty and kindness. It also makes such unit-tendencies as I have described under approval, scorn, mastery and submission seem abstract and schematic, as indeed, they are.

Space is lacking in this book, and knowledge in its author, to trace in the bewildering complexes of human intercourse, the combined effect of the unit-tendencies which I have outlined. We may be confident, however, that, did we know enough, we should find that whether a person will in a given case be shy, or indulge in display, or alternate between the two —whether he will domineer or plead in courtship—whether he will respond toward a given child by approval, domineering, bullying, protection, hunting or fondling—could in every case be prophesied from knowledge of the situation and of him.

OTHER SOCIAL INSTINCTS

Rivalry.—No one can doubt that the facts vaguely referred to by Emulation or Rivalry have some basis in man's inborn organization; but, as with maternal affection, pugnacity or the hunting instinct, it is necessary to define the tendencies and separate out those elements of them which are original from those into which they grow in the course of man's social training.

The two essential facts in rivalry are: the increased vigor in man's activity when other men are engaged in the same activity and the satisfyingness of superiority to them. It may be that in the course of life any sort of fellow-working or playing becomes a stimulus, and any sort of superiority a satisfier. But original nature has no such desire for abstract superiority, and its responses to fellow-working and playing are limited to the work and play which one's fellows instinctively pursue. Original emulation or rivalry is, in the first place, a group of tendencies to respond more vigorously in trying to get some one's attention upon perceiving a fellow creature's attempts to get it, in chasing some animal upon perceiving a fellow creature chasing it, in pulling toward one's self a thing when a fellow creature is pulling it toward himself, in running toward an object toward which he runs, and the like. In the second place, it is the responses of annoyance at being deprived of some one's attention by another, of satisfaction at getting some one's attention in spite of another, of annoyance at being outdone in the chase, the seizure or the struggle, of satisfaction in getting the prey, retaining the toy or being on top in spite of competitors, and the like.

It is upon such special stimulations and satisfactions rather than upon a diffuse imitativeness and craving for superiority that education at the start has to rely. As Dr. Ordahl, who has given the best single account of the facts of animal and human rivalry, says: "That it has become an instinctive response to all situations involving a possible chance of surpassing another, we have, I think, much evidence to show improbable. It is an instinctive response only when the situation involves the natural tendencies of the animal." ['08, p. 506.]

Envious and Jealous Behavior.—It is an original tendency of man to be annoyed by the perception of another* receiving certain attention and treatment which his own behavior would otherwise get for himself. Young children are thus intolerant of the fondling of others by their mother; lovers, of the attentiveness of their mates to others; mothers, of the affection and notice given by their children to others. There seems, however, to be no uniform behavior characteristic of these jealous discomforts. Attacks on the competing object, seizure and holding of the person whose attitude toward one is being made inadequate, general raging, sulking, pining, grief and other activities are manifested. The original basis of envy seems to be simply discomfort at seeing others approved, and at being outdone by them.

Ownership.—By the instinct of ownership may be meant either original tendencies to resist the abstraction from one's person or immediate neighborhood of an object which one is using or has recently (within a few minutes) acquired, or original tendencies to be satisfied by having on one's person or within the range of one's senses many objects with which no one interferes. The former have already been listed under the instinct of possession; the latter are more doubtful. The very common enjoyment of owning, that is, having complete power over, things rather than merely using them subject to possibilities of interference or despoiliation, no matter how remote, is the outgrowth of training coöperating with one or both of these tendencies.

*The 'other' may be a thing or an event as well as a person.

Kindliness.—The situation, 'a living thing displaying hungry, frightened or pained behavior by wailing, clinging, holding out its arms and the like,' provokes attention and discomfort and may, if attendant circumstances do not shunt behavior over to the hunting, avoiding or triumphing responses, provoke acts of relief.

Another aspect of original kindliness is the positive satisfyingness of witnessing behavior characteristic of welfare in our fellows. Even the mean and brutal man naturally likes, apart from periods of rage and hunting, to see people happy. The happy behavior of others is pleasant, as flowers, sunshine and food are. It provokes, if competing responses are not too strong, kindly behavior in the shape of welcome, smiles, laughter, and the sharing of food. This kindly behavior is not necessarily confined to human beings; the child may offer a part of his cooky to a toy, or caress a flower. As Cooley says, "it flows out upon all the pleasantness the child finds about him." ['02, p. 47.] In an ordinary environment, however, people are its main stimuli and recipients.

Teasing, Tormenting and Bullying.—Teasing, tormenting and bullying are the most notable inborn exceptions to childish kindliness. They are due, I judge, to the competing tendencies to manipulation and curiosity, hunting, scorn and mastery. Manipulation and curiosity easily develop into teasing. A child tends to do all sorts of things to people as well as to things, and is restless at the quiescence of a person as he is at that of any object. If the person who is pulled, poked, hit, called to, run after or jumped upon plays back, the natural course of development is toward what is called play. If the person reacts by energetic and victorious angry behavior, the child abandons its manipulation and pleased interest in what the person will do in favor of fighting, flight or submissive appeal. If the person neither plays back nor punishes, but behaves in a vexed, sullen, frightened or insufficiently punitive angry way, the child will, according to its total make-up and the temporary set of its mind, abandon, continue or increase his curious manipulation of the person, and the observer will call his behavior teasing or tormenting. Teasing those who are unable or unwilling to revenge themselves then inevitably becomes a habit in the case of children of mean and brutal natures.

When the hunting responses are called forth by a human being, they (alone or in combination with attempted mastery) produce a special form of play typically characterized, as Burk has shown, by "pursuing, throwing down, holding down, putting knee on vanquished victim, pinching, pulling hair, pulling ears, striking, shaking, throwing missiles, dancing about conquered victim, laughing, clapping hands, . . . smiling, a triumphant air." ['97, p. 228.] In the course of training, threats may to any extent replace the actual treatment of the person as prey or slave. Many degrees of intermixture of the responses provided to an animal to be caught, torn to pieces and eaten, and of those provided to an antagonist before and after he gives instinctive tokens of submission, are found. Obviously such cruelty and bullying can occur only when the one who arouses the hunting and mastering responses is unwilling or unable to protect himself. Such a one also probably specially arouses them.

The history of slave-driving, hazing, persecution, and the almost universal inequitable use of delegated powers by governors, generals, popes, school-masters and all those in authority, warrants the conviction that the hunting response does not originally distinguish man from other animals at all surely, and that submissive behavior does not as uniformly bring release from aggression in man as it does in the mammals in general.

Motherly behavior and the other instinctive forms of kindliness are very inadequate protections against the inborn impulses to cruelty.   In children of mean and brutal nature, bullying is therefore almost sure to occur unless it is deliberately stamped out by education.

IMITATION

Imitation is a word of too many different meanings to be used without qualifications.   It may mean a tendency to make movements similar to those made in the animal's presence, or a tendency to produce a result similar to a result produced in the animal's presence, or a tendency to use the behavior of other animals in any way as a model or guide influencing one's behavior toward some degree of likeness thereto.   The behavior of other animals may be regarded as working immediately, making the animal do the like in the same way that a loud noise makes him jump; or by arousing an idea of the movement; or by arousing an idea of the result produced; or by arousing an idea that has by habit led to the movement; or by arousing ideas of various sorts that indirectly make his behavior more like the behavior of the other animal than it would otherwise have been. Indeed, imitation is used by Tarde and other sociological writers, to mean little more than the repetition, for any reason, of ideas and acts and feelings like those which other men have or have had.

It is better, therefore, instead of asking vaguely whether imitation of other men is an original tendency in man, to put separately the following questions:—

A1.   Do the sense-presentations (chiefly through sight) of all movements as made by another produce in man, apart from all training, *identical* movements?

A2.   *Similar* movements?

A3. *Tendencies to make similar* movements?

A4. If some, but not all movements, have this power, which are they?

B1. Do the sense-presentations of all positions of the body taken by another, all sounds made, all facial expressions assumed and other *results* of movement upon the mover's body, produce in man, apart from all training, movements resulting in *identical* positions, sounds and looks?

B2. *Similar* ones?

B3. *Tendencies to make* movements resulting in identical or similar ones?

B4. If some but not all positions, sounds, looks, and the like have this power, which are they?

GENERAL IMITATIVENESS

In spite of the frequency of statements that the child makes every gesture that he sees and every sound that he hears, no one who has tried to teach infants to talk, or five-year-olds to write and sing, will for a moment believe that behavior witnessed produces identical behavior by any original potency. Writers who have seemed to say so cannot, if possessed of any sense for fact, have meant what they said. Questions A1 and B1 can be dismissed each with a flat NO. At the most a general tendency to imitate can only be as in A2 and B2 a tendency to make movements, or get results, that are *somewhat like* whatever ones are witnessed.

I can find no evidence that any such tendency is original in man. As will be stated later, certain particular sorts of behavior do originally provoke in the spectator behavior that resembles them, but, so far as I can see, behavior in general does not. Consider the difficulty of getting an infant to even approximately 'wave a bye-bye,' 'pat-a-cake,' 'blow a kiss,' or 'spit it out;' and the extreme difficulty of getting him to blow his nose, clear his throat, or gargle. Sit before him and perform time after time a score of such novel but simple acts as putting your right hand on your head and your left on your right shoulder. He does not in nine cases out of ten do anything more like the act you perform than like any other one of the twenty.

Of course, after he has performed many acts as sequents to many situations, the latter including often the perception or idea of the act, you may frequently, by performing an act, get him to perform it also. But his act is then a result of learning, not of instinct; and your behavior provokes it in the same way that a verbal suggestion might. The course of human education is such that among the situations to which acts are bound as sequents, ideas of the acts are frequent. A human being's behavior thus often provokes similar behavior in another by provoking an idea to which it is, by past learning, a sequent. Such influence of one person upon another illustrates, however, the laws of habit, and nothing more.

Cooley, who watched especially for evidence of general instinctive imitativeness in his children, found none that could not be explained better as the result of general activity or of learning. He notes sagaciously that, in one of the most plausible appearances of imitation, the behavior of another person probably acted simply as the first step in a habit, since a verbal request produced the behavior in question even more surely. "M. had a trick of raising her hands above her head, which she would perform, when in the mood for it, either imitatively, when someone else did it, or in response to the words 'How big is M?', but she responded more readily in the second or non-imitative way than in the other." ['02, edition of 1910, p. 27.]

I believe the same absence of evidence of any general original production of similar behavior by behavior witnessed holds good for sounds as well. To the hypothesis that seeing the movements of another's mouth-parts or hearing a series of sounds in and of itself produces similar movements or sounds, I find the following objections:—

First of all, no one can believe that *all* of a child's speech is acquired by direct imitation. On many occasions the process is undoubtedly one of the production of many sounds, irrespective of the model given, and the selection of the best one by parental reward. Any student who will try to get a child who is just beginning to speak, to say *cat, dog* and *mouse* and will record the sounds actually made by the child in the three cases, will find them very much alike. There will in fact be little that even *looks* like direct imitation until the child has 'learned' at least forty or fifty words.

The second difficulty lies in the fact that different children, in even the clearest cases of the imitation of one sound, vary from it in so many directions. A list of all the sounds made in response to one sound heard is more suggestive of random babble as modified by various habits of duplicating sounds, than of a direct potency of the model. Ten children of the same age may, in response to 'Christmas,' say, kiss, kissus, krismus, mus, kim, kimus, kiruss, i-us and even totally unlike vocables such as hi-yi or ya-ya.

The third difficulty is that in those features of word-sounds which are hard to acquire, such as the 'th' sound, direct imitation is inadequate. The teacher has recourse to trial and chance success, the spoken word serving as a model to guide satisfaction and discomfort. In general no sound not included in the instinctive babble of children seems to be acquired by merely hearing and seeing it made.

A fourth difficulty is that by the doctrine of direct imitation it should not be very much more than two or three times as hard to repeat a two- or three-syllable series as to repeat a single syllable. It is, in fact, enormously harder. This is, of course, just what is to be expected if learning a sound means the selection from random babbling plus previous habits. If, for instance, a child makes thirty monosyllabic sounds like pa, ga, ta, ma, pi, gi, li, mi, etc., there is, by chance, one chance in thirty that in response to a word or phrase he will make that one-syllable sound of his repertory which is most like it, but there is only one chance in nine hundred that he will make that *two-syllable* combination of his repertory which is most like it.

Perhaps the advocates of imitation as an original mental function would admit that witnessed behavior does not originally produce its like in any such uniform, mechanical way as a shock produces winking, or pain a cry. They would perhaps claim only a tendency or potentiality or disposition toward the production of similar movements or results. They would, that is, insist that questions (A3) and (B3) on page 41 are the really important questions.

This doctrine that there is an original general potency of witnessed behavior to evoke its like, but only in the shape of a tendency to make like behavior appear a little oftener than it would by the laws of exercise and effect alone, is one that can at present be neither demonstrated nor refuted. It does not much matter, for if by original general imitativeness is meant only a dubious possibility that witnessed behavior will produce behavior that is occasionally somewhat more like it than would otherwise be expected, it is of little practical consequence. For even such a remnant of general original imitativeness, however, I cannot find adequate evidence; and it has many fundamental difficulties.

I judge, therefore, that the original attentiveness of man to the acts, movements, positions, sounds and facial expressions of other men and the original satisfyingness of the approval so often got by doing what other men do, which have been described in this Chapter, are really the tendencies or predispositions or potentialities that do the work in question.

THE IMITATION OF PARTICULAR FORMS OF BEHAVIOR

There being no general original imitativeness, are there perhaps certain particular movements, positions, sounds and facial expressions the perception of which does produce their like?

McDougall's answer is that, first, the responses involved in the principal instincts which he lists (i.e., flight—fear, repulsion—disgust, curiosity—wonder, pugnacity—anger, self-abasement—subjection, self-assertion—elation, parental instinct —tender emotion) when made by one man, serve each as a situation that originally provokes the same response in a spectator.

There is something peculiarly attractive and plausible in this doctrine that "the instinctive behavior of one animal directly excites similar behavior on the part of his fellows," but it is doubtful whether nature has worked to so simple a wholesale result. The similarity of the behavior is not sure in any case, and seems contrary to fact in the case of the tendencies of pugnacity—anger and parental instinct—tender emotion.

The spectators of an infuriated man, or of two men raging at each other, are not thereby provoked to similar acts and feelings. They manifest rather 'curiosity-wonder,' forming a ring to stare, the world over. So with other mammals. When Professor McDougall wrote that "anger provokes anger" he probably had in mind the fact that angry behavior of A toward B provokes angry behavior of B toward A.   But that is irrelevant to his purpose, since he surely does not wish to contend that A's fleeing from B makes B flee from A, that A's shrinking from B makes B shrink from A, that A's self-abasement before B makes B abase himself before A.

The instinctive behavior of the mother in holding, cuddling and fondling does not excite similar behavior on the part of her fellow men and women.   They need not be moved thereby to cuddle it, her, one another, their own babies, or anything else. The chief response in them may be approval, envy or mild amusement, as often as tender emotion of the same sort as her behavior expresses.   The sight of a child *not* being tenderly treated is in fact probably more likely to arouse tender emotion in spectators than the sight of one on whom it is lavished.   It is indeed the unloved rather than the loved or the loving who move the motherly spirit in the spectator.

No one common rule for the original effect of the perception of instinctive behavior in another man can be given.   His behavior in attention, cautious approach, the avoiding reactions and the hunting instinct, produces something much like itself. His behavior in anger, combat for mastery, courtship and parental affection produces in the spectator something as a rule quite unlike itself.   The effect of his behavior in attempted mastery and submission is dubious, varying greatly with its concomitants and being little known in any case.   Seeing a man in the attitude of submission may make the spectator more submissive or more aggressive.   Whether the perception of instinctive behavior originally produces like behavior is a question to be studied separately in the case of each instinct.

The question is often very difficult.   Under present conditions children would usually learn by training to run from

whatever others ran from, to look at whatever others looked
at, and the like, even if there were no original tendencies to do
so. Moreover the object or event, the perception of which
causes A to respond by a certain instinctive behavior which
then spreads to B, is likely to be perceived by B also, so that
whether his behavior is a response to A's behavior or to the
object itself is often in doubt. For example, A's fear at a
snake may arouse B's fear indirectly by merely calling B's
attention to the snake. Finally A's response may, upon his
perception of B, be modified to include certain behavior which
acts as a special signal to provoke approach, fear, or whatever
the response may be, in B. Thus the danger-signal might be
given by A when frightened in company, though not when
frightened alone; and B might respond, not to A's general
fright, but to the danger signal.

The most probable cases for the production, by behavior
witnessed, of similar behavior in the witness, are *smiling when
smiled at, laughing when others laugh, yelling when others
yell, looking at what others observe, listening when others
listen, running with or after people who are running in the
same direction, running from the focus whence others scatter,
jabbering when others jabber and becoming silent as they become silent, crouching when others crouch, chasing, attacking
and rending what others hunt,* and *seizing whatever object
another seizes.*

In my opinion these probabilities are all, or nearly all, real,
and are the chief, or even the only components of "the imitative
tendency which shows itself in large masses of men, and produces panics, and orgies, and frenzies of violence, and which
only the rarest individuals can actively withstand."

In the second division of his account of what particular

acts originally provoke similar acts in the spectator, McDougall says:—

"For the sake of completeness a fifth kind of imitation may be mentioned. It is the imitation by very young children of movements that are not expressive of feeling or emotion; it is manifested at an age when the child cannot be credited with ideas of movement or with deliberate self-conscious imitation. A few instances of this sort have been reported by reliable observers; e.g., Preyer stated that his child imitated the protrusion of his lips when in the fourth month of life. These cases have been regarded, by those who have not themselves witnessed similar actions, as chance coincidences, because it is impossible to bring them under any recognized type of imitation. I have, however, carefully verified the occurrence of this sort of imitation in two of my own children; one of them on several occasions during his fourth month repeatedly put out his tongue when the person whose face he was watching made this movement. For the explanation of any such simple imitation of a particular movement at this early age, we have to assume the existence of a very simple perceptual disposition having this specific motor tendency, and since we cannot suppose such a disposition to have been acquired at this age, we are compelled to suppose it to be innately organized. Such an innate disposition would be an extremely simple rudimentary instinct. It may be that every child inherits a considerable number of such rudimentary instincts, and that they play a considerable part in facilitating the acquisition of new movements, especially perhaps of speech movements." ['08, p. 106]

There may be such odds and ends of tendencies to duplicate particular acts. If so, no one knows what the acts are. So far, the list begins and ends unimpressively with sticking out the tongue!

On the whole, the imitative tendencies which pervade human life and which are among the most powerful forces with and against which education and social reform work, are, for the most part, not original tendencies to respond to behavior seen by duplicating it in the same mechanical way that one responds to light by contracting the pupil, but must be explained as the results of the arousal, by the behavior of other men, of either special instinctive responses or ideas and impulses which have formed, in the course of experience, connections with that sort of behavior. Man has a few specialized original tendencies whose responses are for him to do what the man forming the situation does. His other tendencies to imitate are habits learned nowise differently from other habits.

CHAPTER IV

ORIGINAL SATISFIERS AND ANNOYERS

THE ORIGINAL NATURE OF WANTS, INTERESTS AND MOTIVES

Reason finds the aim of human life the improvement and satisfaction of wants. By reducing those to which the nature of things and men denies satisfaction, or by increasing those which can be fulfilled without injuring the fate of others, man makes his wants better. By changing the environment into a nature more hospitable to the activities he craves, he satisfies them. The sciences and arts arose by the impetus of wants, and continue in their service. They are the ultimate source of all values.

The original basis of the wants which so truly do and should rule the world is the original satisfyingness of some states of affairs and annoyingness of others. Out of such original satisfiers and annoyers grow all desires and aversions; and in such are found the first guides of learning.

By a satisfying state of affairs is meant roughly one which the animal does nothing to avoid, often doing such things as attain and preserve it. By an annoying state of affairs is meant roughly one which the animal avoids or changes.

Samples of original satisfiers or instinctive likes are:— *To be with other human beings rather than alone, To be with familiar human beings rather than with strange ones, To move when refreshed, To rest when tired, To be "not altogether unenclosed" when resting and at night.*

Samples of original annoyers or instinctive aversions are: *—Bitter substances in the mouth, Being checked in locomotion*

*by an obstacle, Being hungry, Being looked at with scorn by
other men, The sight and smell of "excrementitious and putrid
things, blood, pus, entrails."*

To satisfy is not the same as to give sensory pleasure and
to annoy is not the same as to give pain. The latter confusion
is specially misleading, for pain is only one of many annoyers,
and does not inevitably annoy. Being gently held when one
wants to fight, tho not painful, is exceedingly annoying. A
mother may welcome the pain she suffers for her child. With
pleasure the case is somewhat different. If by it is meant
simply the felt tolerability and welcomeness of a state of affairs,
pleasure is a close symptom—almost a synonym—of satisfyingness. But the pleasurableness of certain sensations as commonly described in psychological treatises is a very partial
symptom. Thus a sweet taste may be annoying and a bitter
taste welcomed.

A long list could be made of such states of affairs as feeding when hungry, rest when weary, being cuddled when sleepy,
running after an animal that arouses hunting behavior, getting
nearer to it in the course of the running, jumping upon it when
near, seizing it after the jump, subduing it after seizing it,
holding a baby after giving birth to one, having it smile when
held, cooing to it when it smiles. Such a list, however, can be
replaced by one law which any of its items would exemplify,—
that *when any original behavior-series is started and operates
successfully, its activities are satisfying and the situations
which they produce are satisfying.* The absence of food when
hungry, being held so that one cannot chase the passing rabbit, being out-distanced by it, clutching the air instead of the
prey at which one leaps, having the offered toy withdrawn as
one reaches for it, immovability in the obstacle one pushes, are
samples from a similar long list of original annoyers, all of the

class described by the law that *when any original behavior-series. is started, any failure of it to operate successfully is annoying.* For these laws to be adequate to guide theory and practice, however, the word 'successfully' must be defined objectively.

Successful operation cannot be defined adequately in terms of gross behavior without returning in a larger or shorter circle to satisfyingness itself. To say that successful means the 'normal' action and 'normal' consequences of instinctive behavior leaves us with 'normal' to define, and in the end it will be defined back again as the successful or satisfying. To say that 'successful' means what furthers the life-processes of the animal leaves on our hands as exceptions such cases as the sacrifice of the mother's own life-processes to those of the child on the one hand, and such cases as rest rather than motion when freezing and intemperance of all sorts, on the other.

To replace the life-processes of the individual by the perpetuation of the species cuts out some of these exceptions, but adds others. Victory is satisfying, though gained by accident or numbers; bullying is satisfying, though due to qualities that weaken the species.

To say that successful means 'unimpeded' or 'unthwarted' or 'uninterfered with' tells fairly well what *movements* will be satisfying, since for a movement to be impeded is for it to fail as a movement. But to say that to fail to clutch the prey, clutching the air instead, is to be impeded or thwarted or interfered with is simply to say that an annoying situation is produced. It is true that mere freedom to complete the motions to which original nature impels in a given situation is satisfying, but the majority of original satisfiers involves also the production by the movement of some one effect rather than another. To run when nature so moves is satisfying, but to get from this place, or to that place, or nearer that animal, or ahead of this man, is commonly the larger satisfier in instinctive responses of flight and pursuit.

THE PRINCIPLE OF READINESS

Successful operation can in fact be satisfactorily defined, and what will originally satisfy and annoy can be safely predicted, only as a characteristic of the internal behavior of the neurones. By original nature a certain situation starts a behavior-series: this involves not only actual conduction along certain neurones and across certain synapses, but also *the readiness of others to conduct.* The sight of the prey makes the animal run after it, and also puts the conductions and connections involved in jumping upon it when near into a state of excitability or readiness to be made. Even the neurone-connections involved in the response of 'clutching' to the situation of 'jumping and reaching it' and those involved in triumphing over it and rending it or taking it to one's lair are in a different condition when a chase is started than they otherwise are. The activities of the neurones which cause behavior are by original nature often arranged in long series involving all degrees of *preparedness* for connection-making on the part of some as well as *actual* connection-making on the part of others. When a child sees an attractive object at a distance, his neurones may be said to prophetically prepare for the whole series of fixating it with the eyes, running toward it, seeing it within reach, grasping, feeling it in his hand, and curiously manipulating it.

The fact is that it is the neurones, not the body as a whole, whose life processes are primarily concerned in the 'successful' operation of a behavior-series. By 'normal' or 'successful' operation we mean the externally observable signs of the action of neurones that are ready to act. And by the failure, or thwarting, of an original tendency we mean the observable signs of failure to conduct and connect in neurones which are ready to so act. Such satisfying states of affairs as those listed at the beginning of this chapter are states of affairs which stimulate, or at least permit, the action of neural connections and neural conductions that are in readiness to act; and the annoying states of affairs listed prevent such from acting.

The essential satisfyingness in these cases is then the conduction along neurones and across synapses that are ready for conduction and the essential annoyingness in these cases is the absence of such conduction.

Now this law holds good not only in the case of such definite behavior-series as feeding, hunting, fighting or sex-indulgence, but throughout behavior. Call the neurone, neurones, synapse, synapses, part of a neurone, part of a synapse, parts of neurones or parts of synapses—whatever makes up the path which is ready for conduction—*a conduction unit.* Then *for a conduction unit ready to conduct to do so is satisfying,* and *for it not to do so is annoying.*

Along with this concept of readiness to conduct, the opposite fact of *unreadiness* or *refractoriness* must be considered. If, as I believe, any conduction unit may be in a condition of repugnance to conduction in the sense that its own activities at the time make it less excitable by stimuli to conduction than is the case with the average condition of the average conduction unit, and if the law of readiness is true, we should expect as a law of *unreadiness* that *for a conduction unit unready to con· duct to be forced to conduct would be annoying.**

*It is probably also the case that for a conduction unit that is *unready* for conduction *not to conduct* is *satisfying;* but evidence is so slight upon

This seems to be the case. Unreadiness to conduct, if such a thing existed, would be expected, as a result of long exercise of conduction across a fatiguable synapse and as a result of weakening of the conduction unit by disease. For, in either case, the common response of protoplasm would be to protect itself against less remunerative action in favor of feeding and rest. Little is known of conduction units, their exhaustion or their diseases, but that little seems to show that conduction along an exhausted or diseased conduction unit is annoying. In neurasthenia and in so-called psychasthenia, activities of the nervous system which in health are satisfying or indifferent become annoying. When, on the other hand, the nervous system is in fine fettle from health and abundant sleep, activities which on the average are slightly distasteful, are welcomed.

I believe that the original tendencies of man to be satisfied and to be annoyed—to welcome and reject—are described by these three laws of readiness and unreadiness:—(1) that *when a conduction unit is ready to conduct, conduction by it is satisfying, nothing being done to alter its action,* (2) that *for a conduction unit ready to conduct not to conduct is annoying, and provokes whatever responses nature provides in connection with that particular annoying lack;* (3) that *when a conduction unit unready for conduction is forced to conduct, conduction by it is annoying.*

Ordinarily, then, any situation not only produces full action in certain conduction units, but also predisposes other units further on in the chain toward or against conduction. Thus this complementary hypothesis that it will not be discussed here. It is a question whether the positive satisfyingness of rest for a function after its exercise, of peace after worry, of safety after fear, and the like is due to relief from conduction for unready conduction-units or to the actual conduction of ready units concerned in sensing bodily languor, gentle speech, familiar faces and the like.

the mechanism of even so simple a behavior-series as fixating a bright light, chasing a rabbit, or seizing and eating a berry is extremely complex. Such a complexity of excitants, checks and releases, as well as straightforward connections, is, however, exactly what human behavior requires and what the physiology of the neurones suggests. We have, therefore, the problem of deciding what original tendencies are found or put in readiness and unreadiness, by any given situation, as well as what bonds are aroused to immediate and total action by it.

The detailed solution of this problem for each important situation I shall not attempt. In listing the readinesses and unreadinesses which different situations produce or call into play, psychology can at present make little advance beyond what any shrewd observer can see for himself once he understands the general principles. If each behavior-series is thought of as an army sending scouts ahead, or as a train whose arrival at any one station means the sending of signals on before whereby this switch is opened, that one closed, and the other left dependent on the size or speed or color of the train, —if the sight of a small object in indirect vision is realized as a cause of remote readinesses of the neurones connected with the fovea, the neurones concerned in reaching and grasping, even possibly of the neurones concerned in tasting,—enough has been accomplished for our purpose. To discover the exact nature of such readinesses is one of the notable tasks of the sciences of human behavior.

THE EXPLANATION OF 'MULTIPLE RESPONSE' OR 'VARIED REACTION'

One further general fact with respect to original annoyers and satisfiers requires mention. The details of very many of the forms of original behavior which have been and will be listed in this inventory involve *varied response* to an annoying state of affairs until a certain satisfying condition is attained. That is, the situation provokes, not one fixed response, but any one of several responses, the failure on the part of the one first made to produce a satisfying state of affairs being (in connection with the rest of the situation) the stimulus to one of the other responses, so that the animal does many things and does them over and over again until some one of them, or some external event, puts an end to the annoying state of affairs or brings the requisite satisfaction. Thus, in responding to an attractive object seen, a variety of reaching movements may be made until the contact with the object ends the series. The contact then sets off a variety of grasping movements until the satisfying clutch of the object ends the series. The clasping of the object may then in turn set off a variety of retractions and flexions until the presence of the object in the mouth quiets these new cravings. Similarly, the situation 'being held' when the neurones concerned in running about are ready to act, provokes a variety of wrigglings, stiffenings, pushings and the like. The failure of any one of these to relieve the annoying confinement leads (in connection with the rest of the original situation) to a more energetic or different movement, the series being terminated when some one of the varied reactions ends the annoyance by securing escape. The process is easily observable in the behavior of the lower animals. A kitten which is utterly devoid of any acquired habits of response to the situation 'being confined alone in a small cage, when hungry, with food outside,' will respond to that situation quite instinctively as follows. "It tries to squeeze through any openings; it claws and bites at the bars or wire; it thrusts its paws out through any opening and claws at everything it reaches; it continues its efforts when it strikes anything loose and shaky; it may claw at things within the box. It does not pay very much attention to the food outside, but seems simply to strive instinctively to escape from confinement. The vigor with which it struggles is extraordinary. For eight or ten minutes it will claw and bite and squeeze incessantly."

The importance of the original tendencies whereby the annoyingness of a certain state of affairs causes a series of varied movements until the required satisfier is produced* is very great, not only because of their number and frequent action, but also because of their very easy modification into special habits by the selection of the 'successful' response and its association with the situation. Variation is the first requisite for progress in the behavior of an individual as it is in the development of the race.

*Or until the animal is distracted from the situation, as by fatigue, sleep, or new sensory appeals.

CHAPTER V

TENDENCIES TO MINOR BODILY MOVEMENTS AND CEREBRAL CONNECTIONS

VOCALIZATION, VISUAL EXPLORATION AND MANIPULATION

A little child, apart from training, makes all sorts of movements of the vocal cords and mouth-parts resulting in cooings, babblings, yellings, squealings and squawkings of great variety. He moves his eyes so as to bring different parts of any object which attracts visual attentiveness upon the fovea. He pulls, pokes, turns, picks up, drops, shoves, rolls, scratches, waves, and otherwise manipulates an object that permits it. This behavior is characterized, at least to superficial observation, by aimlessness, ubiquity, and indiscriminateness. The movements seem to do nothing for the animal, to be made to any one situation (of a certain class) as well as to another, and to be made hit-or-miss in any order. Vocal play seems to occur with no ulterior consequence. Any stimulus from without or within, which does not connect with some antagonistic vocal activity, seems to evoke it. One sound or another, one sequence of sounds or another, seems to occur indifferently. So, also, the manipulation of objects under consideration seems quite without an ulterior end such as the 'reach-grasp-put in mouth' responses display. It seems to be a response to *any* object that permits it; and turning, poking, scratching seem to occur as fortuitous emergences from a set of indifferent responses. A general tendency to aimless exercise of the neurones controlling the movements of the eyes, vocal apparatus and free forelimbs seems thus a just description of the tendency.

For a rough and elementary description it *is* just. But a more critical consideration of the behavior will show that it is conformable to the general type of a connection of a definite response with a definite situation, perpetuated in inheritance by its utility.

All original tendencies are aimless in the sense that foresight of the consequences does not effect the response. The animal does not originally run from a tiger because he intends to get away. He runs because of the tiger and because running in that situation is a satisfier to his neurones. He equally fingers the block because it is what it is and because fingering it satisfies him. As to the aim seen *ab extra,* the end as gained rather than as foreseen, no instincts have surer utility than the apparently objectless voice-, eye-, and finger-play. For the end of voice-play is language; the end of eye- and finger-play is knowledge. In the long run, the apparently random voice-play is more useful to the species than the specific calls of hunger, pain, fright, protection and wooing; and the puttering with eyes and fingers is more useful than the movements of flight, pursuit, attack, capture and eating. What might appear to be perverse luxuries in the business of keeping one's self and one's offspring alive, turn out to be, in connection with certain other tendencies, means of exterminating all enemies, securing food in regular abundance, and remaking the environment to suit man's almost indefinite multiplication.

The definiteness of the situations and responses would be revealed if observation could include what goes on in the nervous system as well as in more external behavior. The apparent identity of the response to different things (as when a child prattles alike to his mother, his doll, and the sky), and the apparent indiscriminateness of the selection from poking, pulling, scratching, and so on in response to apparently the same thing, would then be seen to be illusions. The inner action of nutrition, fatigue and growth plays here a larger part in deciding which of the many possible movements shall be made, than it does in the case of flight or fighting, and so justifies the rough usage of the term 'multiple response to the same situation.' The situation, too, may be, in addition to the proper inner conditions in the neurones, so general as 'anything that contrasts with the rest of the visual field' or 'anything touching the palm of the hand' or even simply 'being alive, awake and with one's vocal apparatus not otherwise engaged.'

Vocalization, visual exploration and manipulation are then to be described as general tendencies to random exercise of the neurones concerned in making many sounds, many eye movements and many manual experiments only if we mean by general and random this particular generality and randomness. When Spencer and others speak of 'excess' movements or the 'overflow of nerve energy' into 'all sorts of' movements or the 'chance' action of the muscles of speech, facial expression, gesture and manual play, they are not describing the facts of early motor play accurately. These movements are in excess of those needed for eating, fighting and the like, but they are as grounded in fundamental tendencies of the organism as the latter. It is not that the nerve energy of man (and in some measure of the monkeys) *over*-flows as that of fishes and many mammals does not, but that it flows into some hundreds of channels productive of movements of the vocal cords, mouthparts, facial muscles, eyes and hands, as it does not in a fish or mammal. The actions are 'chance' ones only in the sense that observation of the external situation alone can not predict them nearly so well as it can the actions of eating, flight or attack. They do not even *seem* to be *perfectly* random. We can at least predict that an infant will say 'ah goo' at an earlier age than he will say 'ĭ dä,' that he will pat an object far oftener than he will place his little finger on it, and many other facts of the same sort. We can predict with very great surety that a child will not roll his eyes independently at a toy or grasp it with his thumb and ring-finger. The randomness is, in any case, limited to the choice from among certain responses which, as a total group, are thoroughly defined.

Lest this somewhat subtle discussion of the more exact description of these tendencies distract attention from the sheer external behavior, I repeat that vocalization means, roughly, the responding by many different sounds in many different sequences to many different external situations, and that from it develop, under training, speech, song and other vocal arts. Visual exploration means, roughly, responding by many eye movements so as to bring various parts of an object upon the spot of clearest vision, and from it develops much in our perceptions of 'things,' our habits of purposive examination, reading and the like. Manipulation means, roughly, responding by many different arm, hand and finger movements to many different objects, and gives the possibility of the habits of using tools, writing, drawing, and the bulk of modern skilled occupations.

OTHER POSSIBLE SPECIALIZATIONS

Constructiveness.—In the ordinary descriptions of original tendencies by the consequences to which they lead, 'destructiveness' and 'constructiveness' occupy prominent places. This apparent contradiction is due simply to the impropriety of describing a tendency by its consequences instead of by the actual situation and response. Original nature knows nothing of destroying or creating—of changing an object into a status less or more profitable to the welfare of the world in general.

Its tendency is simply to manipulate objects in the fashion that has just been described. With this go the satisfactions of doing something rather than nothing, of getting a more varied and novel series of impressions, and of having acts produce perceptible changes, which are taken account of under the proper instinctive interests. Waving of arms and legs, kicking and rolling, grimacing, prattling, dropping toys, blowing whistles, tearing books, digging holes in the sand, and building with blocks are all of the same pattern. No one would think it proper to speak of instincts of constructing and destroying the air in the sense of making words and making senseless jabber. One word, vocalization, is wisely used to describe the tendency to make babbling movements. So one word, manipulation, may replace constructiveness and destructiveness to signify the tendency to make certain hand, arm and finger movements.

Adornment and Art.—Kirkpatrick and others think that there is an original specific tendency to adorn one's body. But it seems more probable that painting, tattooing, decoration with shells, flowers, clothes, feathers and the like are all learned responses selected by their value in connection with gaining notice, approval, mastery, and success in courtship.

The originality of a specific tendency to make beautiful objects may also be doubted. Constructiveness of all sorts seems to be the result of experience acting on general manipulative play. Habits of making admired, rather than unnoticed or disliked, objects would easily be selected for survival.

Curiosity.—Curiosity is a term which we use vaguely for tendencies whose result is to give knowledge. Many of these exist in man as gifts of nature. Attention to novel objects and human behavior, cautious approach, following with the eyes, reaching, grasping, putting in the mouth, tasting, visual exploration, and manipulation thus make up a large part of 'curiosity.' Such of these as need description have been already described.

The element not hitherto listed may best be named the love of sensory life for its own sake. Merely to have sensations is, other things being equal, satisfying to man. Mental emptiness is one of his great annoyers. We may justly picture the brain of man as containing many neurones, in connection with the sensory neurones, which crave stimulation—are in "readiness to conduct"—though no immediate gratification of any more practical want follows their action. Man wants sense impressions for sensation's sake. Novel experiences are to him their own sufficient reward. It is because they satisfy this want as well as because of their intrinsic satisfyingness, that visual exploration and manipulation are the almost incessant occupations of our waking infancy.

The Instinct of Multiform Mental Activity.—The hypothesis that man's brain contains many neurones in 'readiness to act' besides those whose action is concerned in the behavior-series of the specific instincts must, I think, be carried further. There are not only neurones ready to be set in action by direct stimuli from the sense-organs, but also neurones ready to be set in action by more remote or secondary connections. For example, a baby likes not only to see a pile of blocks tumble or a wheel go around, but also to find the blocks tumbling *when he hits them,* or the wheel revolving *when he pushes* a spring. Satisfactions of the second sort are, indeed, if anything the more potent. Merely hearing the toot of a horn is a feeble joy compared to blowing it. Now 'tumbling when I hit them,' 'whirling when I push,' and 'tooting when I blow' are samples of *secondary* connections, a step removed from mere sensations. They represent the action of the neurones concerned in the child's manipulations, those concerned in his sensations and *those concerned in connecting the latter with the former.* They possess the satisfyingness of manipulation, of the love of sensory life *per se,* and something more, which, for lack of a better name, I shall call the *satisfyingness of mental control.* To do something and have something happen as the consequence is, other things being equal, instinctively satisfying, whatever be done and whatever be the consequent happening.*

Now mental control, or doing something and having something happen, is satisfying in *very many concrete forms.* Not only making movements and thereby getting sensations, but also making an ideal plan and thereby getting a conclusion, making an imaginary person and thereby getting further imaginations of how he would act, and countless other 'gettings from doings,' are satisfying. They are originally satisfying since, as soon as training gives the ability to make the plan or image and get the result, nature gives satisfyingness to the connection.†

Mental activity is then, other things being equal, satisfying almost or quite in general. The neurones concerned in the special instincts are not the only ones in readiness to act. Neurones are roused to action in the course of learning which also were ready to act and whose action therefore is satisfying. It is as instinctive or 'natural' for certain men to enjoy the un-

*This is, I judge, the fact which Groos and others have in mind, or should have in mind, when they speak of man's instinct of 'pleasure at being a cause,' or of 'experimentation.' A typical illustration of the earlier appearances of such behavior is the following from Shinn ['99, p. 10]: "In the twentieth month she would often cover her eyes with her hands and take them away; hide her face in a cushion, or on her own arms, often saying, 'Dark,' then look up,—'Light now.' "

† The *'other things being equal'* is of course implied throughout. Making a connection that has to be made against strong cravings to rest or to do something else may be very annoying.

5

forced exercise of thought and skill as to enjoy food, sleep, companionship, approval or conquest.

The Instinct of Multiform Physical Activity.—A similar line of observation and reasoning justifies the conclusion that, other things being equal, many unforced movements besides those specifically made in response to food to be got, foes to be subdued and the like, are originally satisfying. It is as instinctive for the baby to curl its toes, wave its arms and wriggle its head as to suckle. The boy instinctively enjoys a gymnasium as well as chasing cats. The grasping, chasing, wrestling and pulling in response to the real situation of the hunt doubtless have a richer zest than the club-swinging or fancy tumbling done, as it were, in a biological vacuum, but what satisfaction these latter do give may be instinctive. After long rest almost any unforced movement is more satisfying to the child than further inaction would be.

PLAY

No doubt much of the behavior called play represents original bonds between certain situations and certain responses. Play, in any one of the common meanings of the word, is more original, less a product of training, than the occupations which are distinguished as work. But, as has repeatedly been the case with other tendencies, the vague assumption of a tendency to manifest, apart from training, more or less of the behavior called play, needs specification. The majority of the disputes about the service of play in education hark back to vagueness in defining what play is to be taken to mean; and in deciding which elements in it are original and which are learned. It is therefore well to remind oneself first of all of what the original tendencies to play are *not*.

There is no original tendency to act uselessly rather than

usefully, or to make-believe rather than to accept matters of fact. Nor is there a full set of tendencies to mock in a sportive way all the separate behavior-series of feeding, hunting, seeking shelter, running away, and so on which have been listed in this and the previous chapters. Man has not two original natures—one matter of fact, the other playful,—from one to the other of which he shifts by inner magic.

The majority of the original tendencies from which human play develops are not peculiar to play, but originate serious activities as well. Such are manipulation, facial expression, vocalization, multiform mental activity and multiform physical activity. The same original tendency, manipulation, is the root of making mud-pies and apple-pies. Vocalization produces matter-of-fact, utilitarian speech and playful screams or songs. To explain the greater part of original play, no additions whatever to the account of original nature so far given are needed.

Another fraction of original play is accounted for by the fact that original tendencies, which I have so far described for convenience as if they manifested themselves in distinct unitary situation-response series, do not in life come thus neatly separated. Any situation in life may be enormously complicated, so that a mixture from responses of, say; curiosity, hunting, kindliness, and manipulation may be its result. A two-year-old child may be to a six-year-old child, at one and the same time, a novelty, a small object passing him, a fellow-man, and a stimulus to secondary connections, and so may be stared at, run after, patted and felt of. So the six-year-old may not hunt and subdue, nor feed and protect, but, as we say, 'play with' the baby. Any situation in life may be only a fragment—in the artificial life of civilization, a mutilation—of any of the total situations to which original nature is previously adapted. Consequently, it may produce only a fragment of the response which the total situation would have produced. A dig in the ribs, unpreceded by threatening approach and unaccompanied by projected head, angry face, growling and snarls, *must* call forth a different response from that which it would call forth if with these accompaniments.

In a similar way the 'mutilation' of the conditions within the organism may give to a tendency an appearance of being playful beyond its deserts. If infants from a year to three years of age lived in such a community as a human settlement seems likely to have been twenty-five thousand years ago, their restless examination of small objects would perhaps seem as utilitarian as their father's hunting.

There are left, as possible instincts of play proper, not already listed, the special tendencies to hunt for hunting's sake in ways notably different from the 'real' hunt; to fight for fighting's sake in ways notably different from the 'real' fight; to fondle and pet in ways notably different from the 'real' mothering. It may be, that is, that in these cases nature provides preparation for food-getting, for the struggle for females and for motherhood by connecting special play-responses in early life to situations like, though not identical with, those to be met in earnest. Whether the chasing, fleeing, catching, wrestling, jumping upon domestic animals and other children, fisticuffs, hair-pulling, and the like, and the holding, fondling and petting babies, dolls, pets and toys, by the young, require such special instincts or are explainable as the 'real' instincts, modified by complication or distortion of the situations and by training, I shall not try to decide. In any case, in playful hunting, fighting, mothering, fleeing, home-making and the like, training early permeates and overlays man's original nature.

CHAPTER VI

THE CAPACITY TO LEARN

Our inventory so far has not included the original tendencies of the original tendencies themselves—the original tendencies not *to* this or that particular sensitivity, bond or power of response, but *of* sensitivities, connections and responses, in general. Thus, it is a fact of original nature that being impressed by this, that and the other situation and making this, that and the other connection occupies time, may produce the inner life which a man has as his consciousness, and may leave an effect upon the man's nature long after the situation and response of that time are ended. It is a fact of original nature that certain states of affairs are satisfying to a man's neurones—are such as they do nothing to avoid, whereas other states of affairs are annoying to the neurones—stimulate them to do something until the annoying state of affairs gives way to a satisfying one which they do nothing to avoid. That is, reflexes, instincts and capacities (1) always take place in time, (2) sometimes produce or modify the inner conscious life of the animal whose they are, and (3) sometimes change the organism more or less permanently. The neurones which are concerned in them have roughly the original tendency (4) to do nothing different when their life processes are being facilitated and to make whatever changes are in their repertory when their life processes are disturbed.

The first and second of these general tendencies everyone properly takes for granted. No more need be said of them.

The third fact noted above refers to the capacity for permanent modifiability or 'learning,' which is, from the point of view of man's welfare, the most important fact in nature.

THE LAWS OF LEARNING

The Law of Use.—To the situation, 'a modifiable connection being made by him between a situation S and a response R,' man responds originally, other things being equal, by an increase in the strength of that connection.   By the strength of a connection is meant roughly the probability that it will be made when the situation recurs.   Greater probability that a connection will be made means a greater probability for the same time, or an equal probability but for a longer time.* Thus, strengthening the connection between 'being asked how many six and seven are' and 'saying "thirteen," ' may mean that the probability of that response during the next six days is eight out of ten instead of seven out of ten, or that the probability is seven out of ten for sixty days instead of for forty.

The Law of Disuse.—To the situation, 'a modifiable connection not being made by him between a situation S and a response R, during a length of time T,' man responds originally, other things being equal, by a decrease in the strength of that connection.

The tendencies of use and disuse may be listed together under one name as the *Law of Exercise.*

As corollaries of the law of use we have the facts that the degree of strengthening of a connection will depend upon the vigor and duration as well as the frequency of its making.   To think '6+7=13' attentively and for ten seconds will thus in-

---

*Certain additions and qualifications are necessary to make this definition adequate, but it will serve provisionally.

crease ihe strength of its bond more than to think of it lightly and for only half a second.

The Law of Effect.—To the situation, 'a modifiable connection being made by him between an S and an R and being accompanied or followed by a satisfying state of affairs' man responds, other things being equal, by an increase in the strength of that connection. To a connection similar, save that an *annoying* state of affairs goes with or follows it, man responds, other things being equal, by a decrease in the strength of the connection.

As a corollary to the law of effect we have the fact that the strengthening effect of satisfyingness varies with its intimacy with the bond in question as well as with the degree of satisfyingness. Such intimacy, or closeness of connection between the satisfying state of affairs and the bond it affects, may be due to close temporal sequence or to attentiveness to the situation and response. Other things being equal, the same degree of satisfyingness will act more strongly on a bond made two seconds previously than on one made two minutes previously,—more strongly on a bond between a situation and a response attended to closely than on a bond equally remote in time in an unnoticed series.

These tendencies for connections to grow strong by exercise and satisfying consequences and to grow weak by disuse and annoying consequences should, if importance were the measure of the space to be allotted to topics, preëmpt at least half of this inventory. As the features of man's original equipment whereby all the rest of that equipment is modified for use in a complex civilized world, they are of universal importance in education. They are the effective original forces in what has variously been called nurture, training, learning by experience, or intelligence.

Since, however, they are so clear and straightforward, they need no comment at this point* save this reminder of their importance, a statement of which connections are modifiable, and a defense of them against certain wrong accounts of the original tendencies to strengthen and weaken bonds in behavior.

LIMITATIONS TO MODIFIABILITY

Which connections are modifiable is not known with absolute surety and precision. At one extreme are connections, such as that between 'being supported by only the air' and 'falling toward the centre of the earth,' which are utterly unmodifiable. At the other extreme are connections, such as that between the situation just mentioned and 'screaming,' which are obviously modifiable. One will always tend to fall but he may learn not to tend to scream.

The doubtful cases are the connections found in reflexes like the contraction of the pupil to brighter light, or sneezing at certain irritations of the mucous membrane of the nose, and in the still more purely physiological behavior of circulation, digestion, metabolism and the like.   It is chiefly in hygiene and medicine that doubt arises whether a certain change can or cannot be regulated by use, disuse, satisfyingness and discomfort.

THE SUPPOSED FORMATION OF CONNECTIONS BY 'FACULTIES'

There are three current opinions concerning the original capacities of man to learn, that is, to strengthen and weaken

---

*Since these original tendencies for use and satisfying consequences to strengthen connections, and for disuse and annoyingness to weaken them, are the efficient forces in learning, they will be discussed again in the second division of this treatise from the point of view of an inquiry into man's acquired tendencies or the results of learning.

bonds in behavior, which seem contrary to fact. First is the opinion that attention, memory, reasoning, choice and the like are mystical powers given to man as his birthright which weight the dice in favor of thinking or doing one thing rather than another, however the laws of instinct, exercise and effect make the throw. This opinion is vanishing from the world of expert thought and no more need be said about it than that it is false and would be useless to human welfare if true.

THE SUPPOSED FORMATION OF CONNECTIONS BY THE PERCEPTION OF THEIR ACTION IN ANOTHER

The second opinion is that for a man to perceive an S-R* sequence in another man's behavior in and of itself predisposes him to respond to that S by that R—that imitation exists as a force whereby the perception of R, in connection with S, in another man's behavior creates a bond between R and S in the perceiving individual. Of this I can find no evidence.

It is, of course, the case that imitation of a certain sort is potent in man's learning. First, certain behavior of other men, as has been shown, stirs the percipient to the same behavior. Smiling at a smile, following a leader, and being pleased at another's pleasure are, like most instincts, educative in their limited sphere. In the second place, the behavior of other men again and again provides models which decide, in whole or in part, the satisfyingness of one's own responses, and so are accessories in the action of the law of effect. But this is not the imitation required by the opinion in question. The enunciation or gesture of another man, acting as a model, forms one's habits of speech or manners in just the same way that the physical properties of trees form one's habits of climbing.

* 'S' here and later stands for 'Situation' ; 'R' stands for 'Response'.

In the third place, the behavior of other men may, as a child's intellect develops, suggest to him all sorts of ideas; these ideas may lead to acts by the laws of exercise and effect; these acts may often be like those which gave the suggestion. Thus seeing someone taking a drink of water may suggest awareness of my own thirst, or the fact that I shall not again have an opportunity to get water during the afternoon, or the mere thought of getting a drink. Any one of these thoughts has strong connections by previous habit with the response of getting a drink. The behavior of others is a very important provider of situations to which habit has bound responses like the behavior seen. But the binding force is habit —that is, the laws of exercise and effect—not imitation in the sense required by the theory in question.

For the sheer direct potency of an S-R connection witnessed to reproduce itself in the witness, the evidence alleged is that from infant life referred to on pages 41-48 (which we found, shrank to the pitiable mystery of one or two babies sticking out their tongues) and that from men in mobs who are supposed to display this sheer direct modifiability by imitation because they act *against* habit and their own essential desires. It is beyond the scope of this book to explain mob-psychology, but a recital of the details in such cases would, I think, show that fleeing, attacking, pouncing on and rending, and other wholes or fragments of instinctive coöperative activities, were all that happened supposedly as a consequence of imitation. Such would happen by reason of specific original bonds with the specific situations, irrespective of any general imitative tendency, if acquired restraints were dissipated by excitement, temporary monomania or the suggestions of a magnetic leader.

There is then no more evidence for thoroughgoing imitation as a general capacity for learning than we found for it as a general instinctive response to the behavior of other men. The two senses would indeed be the same, and the facts noted here and in Chapter III could as well have been combined in one contra-argument.

THE SUPPOSED FORMATION OF CONNECTIONS BY THE POWER OF AN IDEA TO PRODUCE THE ACT WHICH IT REPRESENTS

Next, and even more orthodox, is the theory of ideo-motor action, that the idea of an act or of the result of an act, or of some part of such result, tends, in and of itself, to produce or connect with that act. Accordingly an act may be bound to any situation by connecting with that situation some conscious representation of that act.

The classic statement of the power to bind acts to situations by so linking ideas of them is given by James in the often quoted dictum:—

"We may then lay it down for certain that *every representation of a movement awakens in some degree the actual movement which is its object; and awakens it in a maximum degree whenever it is not kept from so doing by an antagonistic representation present simultaneously to the mind.*" ['93, vol. 2, p. 526.]

McDougall, in listing ideo-motor action as a 'general or non-specific innate tendency,' describes it thus:

"In the special case in which the object to which we direct our attention by a volitional effort is a bodily movement, the movement follows immediately upon the idea in virtue of that mysterious connection between them of which we know almost nothing beyond the fact that it obtains" ['08, p. 242]; and elsewhere " . . . the visual presentation of the movement of another is apt to evoke the representation of a similar movement of one's own body, which, like all motor representations, tends to realize itself immediately in movement." ['08, p. 105]

Against this orthodox opinion, I contend that the idea of a movement (or of any response whatever) is, in and of itself, unable to produce it. I contend that an idea does not tend to provoke the act which it *is an idea of,* but only that which it *connects with as a result of the laws of instinct, exercise and effect.*

In particular I contend that any idea, image, sensation, percept, or any other mental state whatever, has, apart from use, disuse, satisfaction and discomfort, no stronger tendency to call up a movement like itself or meant by it than to call up any other movement. Two intelligible meanings can be attached to 'the representation of a certain movement by an idea,' or to 'an idea having a certain movement as its object,' or to 'an idea being of a certain movement,' and the like. The first is that the idea is like the movement in the same way that the mental image of a red inch square *is like* such a square. The second is that the idea *means* the movement in the same way that the image of the words 'red inch square' means such a square. I hold that in neither meaning does an idea tend to produce what it represents or has as its object, or is an idea of —that, in and of itself, an idea tends to do so no more when what it represents is a movement of one's own body than when what it represents is a red-inch-square.

The upholders of the orthodox view have not stated what 'the mysterious connection' is. They may mean by 'represent,' 'have as object' and 'be of' simply 'tend to produce,' 'lead to,' 'evoke as response.' In that case the doctrine of the 'impulsive power of ideas' is a mere tautology, stating that an idea produces what it does produce, evokes as a response what it does evoke. Just this may indeed have been James' meaning. For he was interested primarily in the negative fact that no special *ad hoc* consciousness of 'willing' was a necessity. It was indifferent to his main purpose *how* an idea was able to lead to action.

They may mean by 'to represent' or 'to have as object' simply 'to have been connected with in accordance with the laws of exercise and effect.' In that case, the doctrine of the 'impulsive power of ideas' is precisely, as I assert, one small feature of the general law that any situation tends to produce the response that original nature and these laws of learning have bound to it. So Angell states, in discussing this matter, that "the appropriate muscular activity never follows an idea unless one's previous experience has in some fashion or other established a nexus of the habit type." ['04, p. 356 f.]

In general, however, as the use of the doctrine of ideomotor action in applications to education, medicine and ethics shows, its adherents do assume an intrinsic tendency of an idea to produce the movement which it is like, or which it means, or both. This appears in a recent statement of the doctrine made, with awareness of the contrary view, by Washburn. She says: "A movement idea is the revival, through central excitation, of the sensations, visual, tactile, kinesthetic, originally produced by the performance of the movement itself. And when such an idea is attended to, when, in popular language, we think hard enough of how the movement would "feel" and look if it were performed, then, so close is the connection between sensory and motor processes, the movement is instituted afresh. This is the familiar doctrine expounded by James in Chapter XXVI of his "Psychology." ['08, p. 280.]

Professor Calkins still more explicitly states that in voluntary action we arouse a certain response by getting in mind an idea that is *like* the response. An 'outer' volition being a volition to act in a certain way and an 'inner' volition being a volition to think in a certain way, "The volition is the image of an action or of a result of action which is normally *similar* and antecedent to this same action or result. My volition to sign a letter is either an image of my hand moving the pen or an image of my signature written, and my volition to purchase something is an image of myself in the act of handing out money or an image of my completed purchase—golf stick or Barbedienne bronze." ['01, p. 299.] Inner volitions "do not so closely resemble their results. The volitional image of an act may be, in detail, like the act as performed;" but the volitional image of a thought is followed by only á "partially similar" thought. ['01, p. 303.]

Whatever be the precise opinions of these particular authors, there is a general belief that the likeness of an act to an idea creates an efficient bond between them. Since this belief, or something to the same effect, is at the bottom of widespread practices in medicine, moral education, school management, business and politics, it and the denial of it which I have made, must be examined.

First of all, if James' 'representation of a movement' and McDougall's 'idea' are taken in their ordinary meanings, cases can be found where such cannot awaken the actual movements which they are representations of ideas of. A little child may have made a certain movement a thousand times and may be entirely willing and eager to make it, but, no matter how vividly the movement is described to him, he cannot make it as a result of the ideas of it evoked by such a description and his own best efforts if, hitherto, he has made the movement only in response to sensory stimuli. The idea has to be connected with the movement or with the sensory stimuli to which the movement is the response by exercise or effect before it has an iota of efficiency in awakening the movement.

An idea of an act, not bound to that idea by use and effect

certainly *need* not be immediately followed by that act. If all the readers of this page summon the most lively and accurate ideas that they can of sneezing, vomiting and hiccuping, one after another, not once in a hundred times will the actual movements be made. Either the reader cannot get a representation of those movements of the sort the theory has in mind, or the theory fails. But if the representation of the movement needed by the theory is such as not one in a hundred well-intentioned students of psychology can get, the theory becomes *a priori* very dubious. Why should men in general have the capacity to provoke an act by an idea of it, but only such an idea as not one man in a hundred can summon?

In the second place, in at least the majority of connections where the idea of an act does produce the actual movement, the connection can be proved to have been built up by the laws of exercise and effect. When one has the idea of going to bed and goes, or of writing the word 'cat' and writes it, the explanation is found in the previous training that has put the idea of going to bed with being sleepy and other situations to which going to bed was the original or acquired response, or has put the act of going to bed with the idea of doing so. Let the reader now, as he sits in his chair, summon unopposed the idea of standing up. He may do it, for the idea of standing up has gone with many direct sensory situations which have, by exercise and effect, led to rising from a chair. It has, indeed, itself been bound as situation to that response. But let him summon the idea of diving off a post and he will not make the corresponding movements,* but, if he does anything, will stand up. Then of course he may make the diving movements. What 'follows immediately upon the idea'

---

*That is, such portions of them as could be made from a sitting position.

of a movement is the act that *has followed* it or some element of it often or with resulting satisfaction, not the act that *is like* the idea.

In the third place, it is certain that, apart from exercise and effect, such ideas of movements as one commonly gets do not as a rule produce the movements, and that such movements as one makes do not often come from ideas of them. Let the reader think of the following movements one after another :—reaching for an apple on his knee, grasping it, putting it in his mouth, biting it, chewing the pieces, swallowing the chewings; getting out of bed, walking to his bath, turning the faucet, climbing into the tub, splashing himself, getting out, shivering, taking towels from the rack, rubbing himself; taking a book, opening at page 1, moving the eyes as in reading; and so on through a thousand movements of daily life. Consider also the thousand or more different voluntary movements last made by you. How few were responses to ideas of them and how many were responses to sensory situations or ideas totally different from them but with which they had been connected by habit! In the illustrations given by James in the very section in which he announces the doctrine of ideo-motor action, all but one show the movement led up to by a sensorial situation or an idea that is not of the movement at all. That one shows the person *making the movement in order to get the idea of it!*

Since these illustrations are typical of the evidence that has been used to support the doctrine that 'we think the act and it is done,' they may profitably be examined one by one. The first two are as follows: "Whilst talking I become conscious of a pin on the floor, or of some dust on my sleeve. Without interrupting the conversation, I brush away the dust or pick up the pin. . . . the mere perception of the object and the fleeting notion of the act seem of themselves to bring the latter about" ['93, vol. 2, p. 522]. Now what would be the probable response to the 'mere perception' of the dust on the sleeve supposing there had been no 'notion of the act'? Surely to brush it away. And with what would 'the notion of the act' have been bound by the laws of exercise and effect alone? Surely with the response of brushing the dust away. So also with picking up the pin. By the laws of exercise and effect the sensorial situation without the idea is adequate to produce the response; and the idea itself needs no potency from its likeness to the act.

"Similarly I sit at table after dinner and find myself from time to time taking nuts and raisins out of the dish and eating them . . . the perception of the fruit and the fleeting notion that I may eat it seem fatally to bring the act about." [ibid., p. 522 f.] It seems clear that for the behavior in question no other force than the perception of the fruit and the laws of exercise and effect is needed. The notion 'that I may eat it' is here not only one to which the act might well be bound by exercise and effect, but is apparently nowise like the acts to which it leads. The notion seems to be a rather vague one, 'all right to eat it,' occurring once, while the act is a very complex one of reaching, grasping, carrying to the mouth, etc., and is repeated over and over again.

The fourth illustration is getting out of bed :—. . . "the idea flashes across me, 'Hollo! I must lie here no longer'—an idea which at that lucky instant awakens no contradicting or paralyzing suggestions, and consequently produces immediately its appropriate motor effects." [ibid., p. 524.] Here the idea is patently not a representation of the movement at all. The 'Hollo' and 'I must' show clearly that it is in words,* not in

---

*If by any sophistry it could be twisted into a representation of leg and trunk movements, it would be only the representation of lying still plus the idea of negation.

6

images of leg, trunk and arm movements. Its motor effects are appropriate, not in the sense of being in the least *like* it or *represented by* it, but in the sense of being the effects which that idea, when uncontested, had, by exercise and effect, come to produce in that man. The 'Hollo! I must' is a lineal descendant of the sensory admonitions from others received during life and connected each with its sequent response by use, satisfaction, and the discomforting punishment attached to opposite courses.

These four cases are all such as a believer in the entire sufficiency of the laws of exercise and effect might properly choose as illustrations of their action. Moreover, in three the sensorial situation is adequate, and in the fourth the idea nowise represents or is like the movements.

The fifth case is: "Try to feel as if you were crooking your finger, whilst keeping it straight. In a minute it will fairly tingle with the imaginary change of position; yet it will not sensibly move because *its not really moving* is also a part of what you have in mind. Drop *this* idea, think of the movement purely and simply, with all brakes off; and, presto! it takes place with no effort at all." [*ibid.*, p. 527.] Now the essential fact here is that when one is told to try to feel as if he were crooking his finger, he tends, in the case of many subjects, to respond by taking an obvious way to get that feeling— namely, by actually crooking his finger. He responds to the request, regardless of any ideas beyond his understanding of the words, by a strong readiness to crook his finger. Being forbidden, he restrains the impulse. The 'tingling' is not from the *imaginary change* of the finger's position but from the *real restraint from changing* its position. The tingling occurs with individuals who cannot imagine the finger's movement. Far from showing that the imagined movement is adequate, in and of itself, to cause the movement, such cases show that it is unsafe to infer that the image comes first in cases where deliberately evoked images of movements are accompanied by the movements or parts thereof.

It appears then that the great majority of movements are not produced by ideas of them and that the majority of ideas of movements do not produce the movements which they represent. When an idea does produce the movement which it is an idea of, that movement gives evidence of having been bound to that idea by exercise or effect. The connection whereby the idea of a movement could, in and of itself, produce that movement would indeed be mysterious if it existed, but it does not exist.

CHAPTER VII

THE ANATOMY AND PHYSIOLOGY OF ORIGINAL TENDENCIES

Intellect, character and skill have their physiological basis in the structure and activities of the neurones and accessory organs which compose the nervous system. The original nature of man in these respects depends on the original structure and activities of the neurones.

The neurones are essentially threads of specialized protoplasm each connecting one part of the body with another. Like other elements of the body, they eat, excrete, grow and die; but their special functions in the animal's life are *sensitivity, conductivity,* and *modifiability.* Sensitivity means the capacity to be excited to action at one end by one or many agencies. Conductivity means the capacity to transmit the action thus excited, or some consequence of it, to the other end of the neurone. Modifiability means the capacity to change in accordance with use shortly to be described.

They are arranged in an elaborate system of *receptors,* easily accessible to important influences within and without the body, *effectors* in intimate connection with organs for action, and *connectors* which lead from the receptors to the effectors. Each neurone of this total system has its special connections with the outside world, with the other organs of the body, or with other neurones.

THE STRUCTURE OF THE NEURONES

Figures 4 and 5 show typical neurones, varying widely in shape, but maintaining the common element of a thread-like

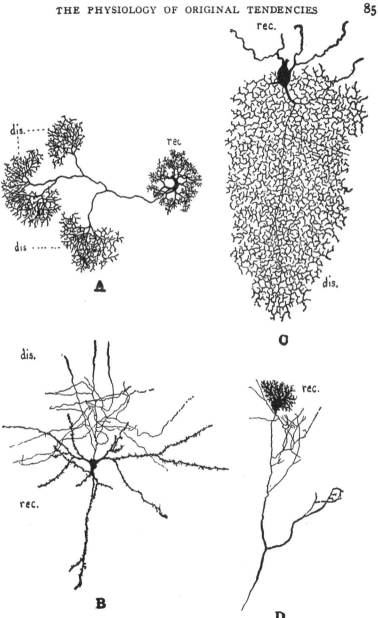

FIG. 4. A, B, C, and D. Four neurones. The discharging end of D is not fully shown, being far beyond the limits of the drawing.
A is after Kölliker ['02, p. 834], after Marenghi.
B is after Kölliker ['96, p. 654].
C is after Van Gehuchten ['oo, vol. 2, p 175].
D is after Kölliker ['96, p. 349].

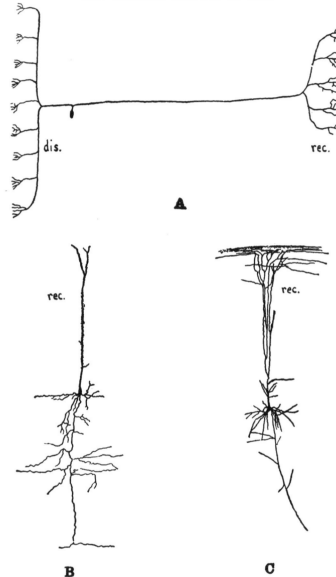

dis.

rec.

A

rec.

rec.

B   **C**

FIG. 5. A, B, and C. Three neurones. The discharging ends of B and C are
not shown, being far beyond the limits of the drawing.
B is after Barker ['01, p. 70]   C is after Kölliker ['96, p. 46]

body suitable to put one part of the animal in touch with other parts—to conduct stimuli from one part of the body to another —to let what happens to one part influence what is done by another part. For convenience I have marked the receiving end in certain cases *r*, and the discharging or transmitting end *dis*. It should be noted that in the drawings the diameter ot the neurones is necessarily enormously exaggerated in comparison with their length. A neurone may be two feet long, but so small in diameter that a hundred side by side would make a line no wider than one of the lines in the drawings.

Figures 6 and 7 show representative structures where the receiving ends of the neurones are in connection with events outside or inside the body.

Figures 8 and 9 show representative structures where the discharging ends of neurones are in connection with muscles.

Figures 10, 11 and 12 show representative synapses or places of connection between the discharging end of one neurone and the receiving end of another neurone.

THE ARRANGEMENT OF THE NEURONES

Figures 13, 14 and 15 show, more or less schematically, certain cases of the arrangement of neurones in series to form conduction-lines or conduction-chains. The whole nervous system is a combination of millions of such conduction-chains. The neurones concerned in the behavior of a single man probably exceed in number by a thousand-fold all the telephone lines* in the world, and a description of the details of their arrangement, if such were known, would be an almost endless task.

Four general features of the original arrangement of man's

*Counting as a "line" every wire length which acts as a unit.

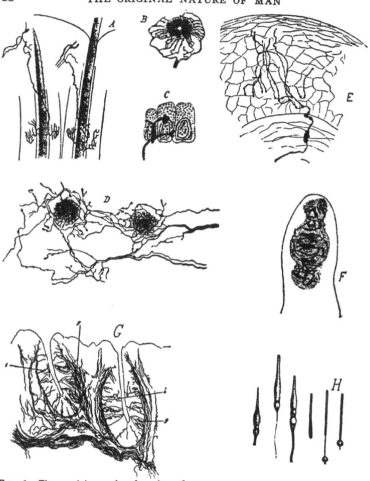

FIG 6. The receiving ends of various first sensory neurones, or receptors.
A. Receiving ends around the base of hairs (in the mouse).
B. Cross section of the tissue shown in A.
C. Neurone endings in epithelial cells
D. Endings around pigment cells.
E. An ending in the lining of the oesophagus.
F. An ending in a tactile corpuscle
G   Endings in the *papilla foliata;* g, taste-buds with *intra-* and *circum-*gemmule neurone-endings; *i, inter-*gemmule neurone endings.
H. Endings of the rods and cones in the retina of man
A, B, C, and D are after Edinger ['96, p. 42], C being after Bethe and D being after Eberth and Bunge   E is after Barker [o1, p. 362], after Retzius. F is after Barker ['o1, p 386], after Smirnow.   G and H are after Kölliker ['o2, p. 28 and p 820]

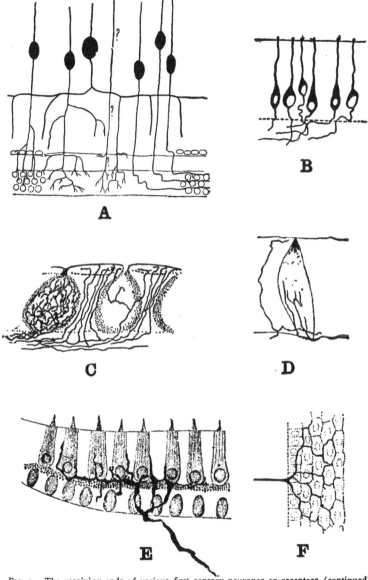

FIG. 7.   The receiving ends of various first sensory neurones or receptors (continued).
A   Ends of neurones in the *Lamina spiralis* and organ of Corti.   The ending
marked ? may be a discharging end
B.   Ends of the first olfactory neurones in the nose.
C and D.   Taste-buds and the receiving ends of gustatory neurones.
E   A receiving end of a neurone in the *macula acustica sacculi.*
F   A sensory neurone ending in the skin.
A is after Kölliker ['02, p 952]   B is after Van Gehuchten ['00, vol. 1, p.
244].   C is after Barker ['01, p. 527], after v. Lenhossék.   D is after Kölliker
['02, p. 29].   E is after Barker ['01, p. 502], after v. Lenhossék.   F is
after Van Gehuchten ['00, vol 2, p 372]

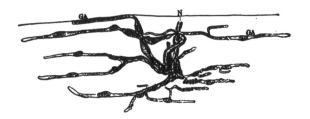

FIG. 8.

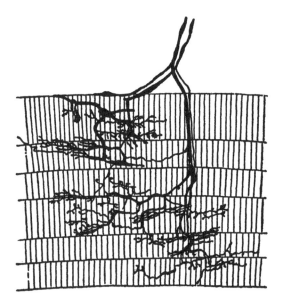

FIG. 9.

FIG. 8. The discharging end of a motor neurone on the gastrocnemius muscle of the frog. After Barker, after Schiefferdecker, after W. Kühne.

FIG. 9. The discharging ends of neurones in striped muscles of the white rat. After Van Gehuchten ['oo, vol. 1, p. 205].

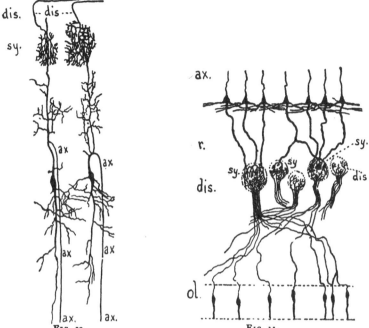

FIG. 10.

FIG. 11.

FIG. 10. The discharging ends of two neurones of the optic nerve (dis.) in synapse (sy) with portions of the receiving ends of two neurones of the optic lobe. These two neurones are shown in part only in the figure. Their axones (ax.) continue far beyond the limits of the drawing After Van Gehuchten ['oo, vol. 2, p. 250].

FIG 11. The olfactory receptors, or first sensory olfactory neurones (ol), their discharging ends (dis), in synapse (sy) with the receiving ends (r.) of seven of the second sensory olfactory neurones The axones of the latter (ax.) continue far beyond the limits of the drawing After Van Gehuchten ['oo, vol. 2, p. 287]

neurones may be specially noted.   First, the system as a whole is on the plan of a system of conduction-units running from parts of the body where events important to the life of the animal are 'sensed' or allowed to impress him, to parts of the body by which he 'reacts to' or adapts himself to, or changes his behavior as result of, these events, *via* a very complex switchboard or set of relay stations permitting a very great variety of combinations, redirections, shuntings and retard-

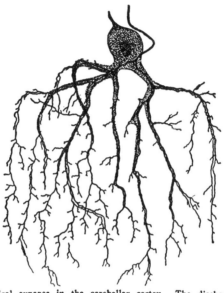

Fɪɢ. 12. A typical synapse in the cerebellar cortex. The discharging end-branch of a neurone intertwined with and applied closely to the surface of the receiving end of a Purkinje neurone. The former is shown in full black; the latter in stipple. The full detail of the latter is not shown. After Johnston ['06, p. 241].

ations of the conducted currents. Second, in particular, there are arrangements whereby several neurones may discharge into one neurone as shown schematically in Figure 16, and in a real case in Fɪɢ. 17, so that there can be a convergence of stimuli separately initiated toward a common final path. Third, there are arrangements whereby one neurone may discharge into several neurones as shown schematically in Figure 18, and in a real case in Fig. 19, so that there may be a distribution or diffusion or varied transmission of one initial stimulus to many final paths.

Fourth, the connecting, or associative, or 'switchboard,' neurones form, especially in man, an apparatus for redirection of stimuli which is almost infinitely complex and which is

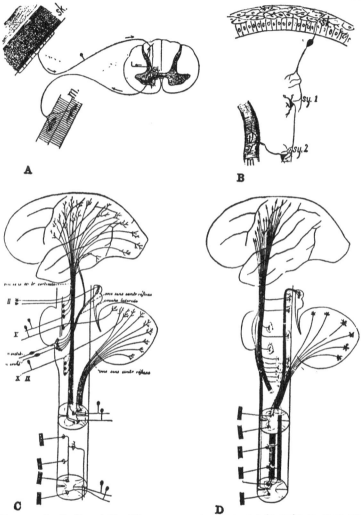

FIG. 13. A, B, C, and D. The arrangement of neurones in series to form conduction lines or continuous chains. A shows two neurones forming a chain
from the skin (sk.) to the muscle (m.) via the synapse (sy.) in the spinal
cord. B shows three neurones forming a chain from the skin (sk.) to the
muscle (m.) via the synapses sy. 1 and sy. 2   C shows at the bottom chains
such as are shown in A and B except that the skin and receiving part of the
first neurone are not shown. C shows, in the upper three-fourths of the diagram,
parts of other chains, leading from the first or second sensory neurones to
the cortex. D shows parts of chains leading from the cortex to the muscles.
A is from Van Gehuchten ['oo, vol. 1, p. 517]. B is after Edinger ['96, p.
31]. C and D are after Van Gehuchten ['oo, vol. 2, p. 513 and p. 512].

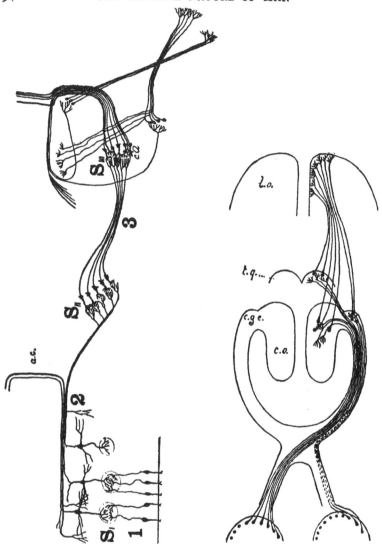

FIG. 14. Shows the chain of neurones conducting stimuli from the olfactory sense organ to the Cornu Ammonis, (c a.) and thence in various directions to make further connections. The neurones marked 1, 2 and 3 designate in order the first three links of this chain, the synapse between the first and the second sets of neurones, the second and the third and so on being marked S1, S11, and S111 The neurones of group 2 shown cut off at a. c. are neurones which conduct across to the other hemisphere of the brain After Van Gehuchten ['oo, vol 2, p. 294].

FIG. 15. Shows part of the chain of neurones which, beginning in the rods and cones of the retina, continue to the occipital lobe of the brain The last two links in the chain are shown here—the neurones which form the sensory part of the optic nerve receiving stimuli in the retina and discharging across synapses in the corpora quadrigemina, external geniculate bodies and optic layer to neurones which conduct thence to the occipital lobe. After Van Gehuchten ['oo, vol. 2, p. 253].

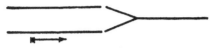

FIG. 16.   Schema of Convergence.

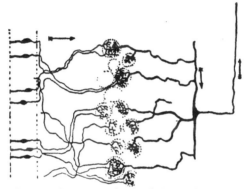

FIG. 17.   Convergence in the Olfactory Receptors.

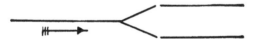

FIG. 18.   Schema of Distribution.

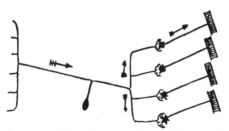

FIG. 19.   Distribution in a Spinal Reflex Path.

extraordinarily apt for varied transmission, so that the same stimulus may, according to minor coöperating conditions, be conducted to many different final paths, and so that many different stimuli may, according to some common feature, be conducted to the same final path. The varieties of connections which appear in the case of the instincts of multiform mental and physical activity, curiosity, manipulation, visual exploration and vocalization, and in the millions of habits which develop from these instincts, have a fit mechanism in this very sensitive, very complex and very modifiable switchboard arrangement of man's neurones.

An original bond between a situation and a response in human behavior has as its physiological basis an original ease of conduction of the physiological action aroused in certain neurones toward a certain final path rather than toward any other. The original arrangement of the neurones whereby the discharging end of a given neurone A, is near to the receiving ends of B, C, D, etc., and remote from the receiving ends of X, Y, Z, etc., is the main determinant of what responses of sensation and movement the given situation will provoke. Original connections in behavior depend in large part upon the original location of neurones in the brain—the original distances between the discharging ends of the neurones severally and the receiving ends of all others.

They may depend upon other facts also. The synapses between the discharging end of A and the receiving ends of B, C, and D might conceivably be identical, so far as concerns the distances A_{dis} to B_r, A_{dis} to C_r, and A_{dis} to D_r; and yet the ease of conduction might be very different in the three cases. Just as three membranes may vary in permeability by a certain substance, or as three joints, one of copper, one of gold and one of rubber, would vary in resistance to the electric current, so the three synapses—A→B, A→C and A→D—may vary in resistance to the stimuli conducted by A, otherwise than by differences in mere distance.   If there were such variations in the permeability of 'synapses of equal distances,' and if they were original in man, they would be a second determinant of the path that any given stimulus would take—and so of the response that any given situation would originally provoke. Proximity of neurones in space, then, there must be as a basis for connections in behavior; a nerve impulse cannot jump an inch from the discharging end of one to the receiving end of another.   Permeability of some special sort may be an additional requirement.

SENSITIVITY AND CONDUCTIVITY

About the detailed physiology of *sensitivity*—the capacity of a neurone to be aroused by certain events at its receiving end (or, much less frequently, along its course)—very little is known.   That little is not specially relevant to our purpose. The same is true of *conductivity* within a single neurone. What the action of a neurone is, whereby something happening at the receiving end makes something happen at the discharging end, is unknown; and the acceptance of one or another of the various present hypotheses would not alter any conclusion to be stated here.   Conductivity over a chain of neurones involves obviously sensitivity, discharge, and conduction across the synapses, as well as mere conductivity within the neurones taken singly.   That there is some specialized action corresponding to the discharge and conduction across the synapse seems probable, but what it is cannot be affirmed.

THE PHYSIOLOGY OF THE CAPACITY TO LEARN AND OF READINESS

The modifiability of a neurone might consist in changes in it:—(1) whereby its form was altered so that its receiving end was in different spatial relations to the stimulating agents, or so that its discharging end was in different spatial relations to the neighboring receiving ends; (2) whereby its receiving end was more or less sensitive to forces acting on it; (3) whereby it offered more or less resistance as a conductor, or otherwise changed its conducting action; (4) whereby it discharged in a different way, or (5) whereby other differences were produced.

Its modifications in the course of growth obviously include the first sort—alterations of its spatial relations,—as is shown roughly in Figures 20 and 21. So also do the modifications produced in it by certain diseases. What modifications are produced in a neurone by its own ordinary activities are matters largely for hypothesis.

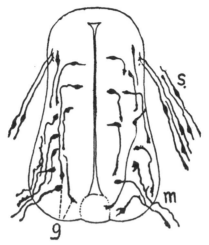

F IG 20.

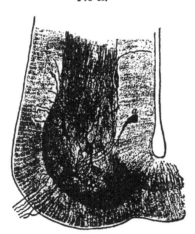

FIG. 21.

FIG. 20. Immature neurones in a section of half of the spinal cord of a chick
at the third day of incubation After Van Gehuchten ['oo, vol. 1, p 282],
after Ramón y Cajal. The neurones shown here will grow to a complexity
equal to that of those shown in Figs. 4 and 5 The ends of the five neurones
shown under s. which run toward the centre of the diagram will grow into
the spinal cord to form long axones with many collaterals each branching in
an elaborate terminal arborization in close proximity to some associative or
motor neurone; the other ends of these neurones will grow out to the surface
of the skin or elsewhere.
The four neurones at the left of m will grow out into the body to connect
with certain muscle fibres. The other neurones will also grow in such a
way that their ends assume special space relations to the ends of other sensory
or motor neurones. The two ends of neurones at g. are growing parts or
growing 'cones'
FIG. 21. Neurones in various stages of growth. A very early stage is shown at
a; a somewhat later stage at b; neurones whose receiving ends have something like their eventual complexity are shown at c. After v. Lenhossék ['95,
p. 92]

CHAPTER VIII

THE ORDER AND DATES OF APPEARANCE AND
DISAPPEARANCE OF ORIGINAL TENDENCIES

Different original tendencies appear at different dates after
the fertilization of the ovum—the beginning of a new individual life. Some are delayed only until birth; some, till long
after birth. The order of appearance and the length of the
intervals from the start of life to the appearance of each tendency are not random. Typical conditions exist for man as a
species, with, of course, very wide variations. For this typical
order and these typical intervals there must be a reason.

Original tendencies also may persist for different lengths
of time after their first appearance. The influence of the
discomfort produced by them is often the only explanation
needed for this transitoriness and its degree. But in some
cases the original tendency seems to be *inherently* transitory,
to disappear from the organism's repertory even though its
exercise produces no discomfort to the individual. For these
wanings and their dates also there must be a reason.

Two theories have been suggested to account for the order
and the dates of appearance and disappearance of original
tendencies. The first is the *Recapitulation Theory*. The
second is the *Utility Theory*.

THE RECAPITULATION THEORY

The Recapitulation Theory in its clearest form is that the
order of appearance of original tendencies in the individual
is more or less exactly that in which they have appeared in

the race—that is, in the entire ancestry of the individual,—and
that the intervals from the fertilization of the ovum to the
dates of appearance of the individual's original tendencies
bear more or less exactly the same proportions one to another
that the intervals from the beginning of life in the animal
kingdom to the dates of appearance of the same tendencies
in the race bear one to another. The order and dates of disappearance in the individual parallel in a similar manner the
corresponding facts in man's ancestry. The reason assigned
for this parallelism between an individual and his entire ancestry in the order and dates of appearance and disappearance
of original tendencies by the recapitulation theory is the supposed bionomic law. This is a law of the germ's development
whereby any change made in it is made with an additional
mechanism that sets the date of the change's effect on the individual developing from that germ later than the dates of the
effects of changes made hitherto in the germ. Suppose, for
example, that for a thousand centuries from the origin of life,
man's ancestors floated aimlessly, then for a thousand swam
by cilia, then for a thousand wriggled like snakes, then for a
thousand walked on four feet, then for a thousand both walked,
climbed and swung as do the monkeys. Let us suppose further that each new tendency was accompanied by the loss of
the old one. Then, by this extreme form of the recapitulation
theory, the human individual should, beginning at the start
of his individual life, possess these tendencies in that same
order, retain each for an equal time, and lose them one after
another (except of course the last, whose loss would depend
upon whether the individual's ancestry had lost it).

A more general illustration in graphic form will help to
fix this extreme form of the Recapitulation Theory in memory.
Suppose tendencies A, B, C, D, etc., to have appeared in man's

ancestry at the times shown by the upper ends of the lines at
the left hand of Fig. 22 and to have been lost at the times

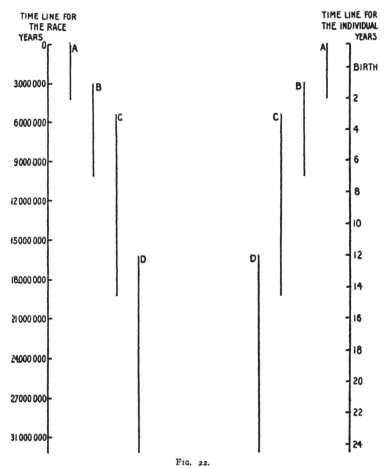

FIG. 22.

shown by the lower ends of these lines.   Then tendencies A,
B, C, D, etc., will appear in man's life and, apart from outside
influence, will disappear therefrom, as shown by the lines at
the right of Fig. 22.

This clear and extreme form of the recapitulation theory is probably held by no student of human nature; for, obviously,

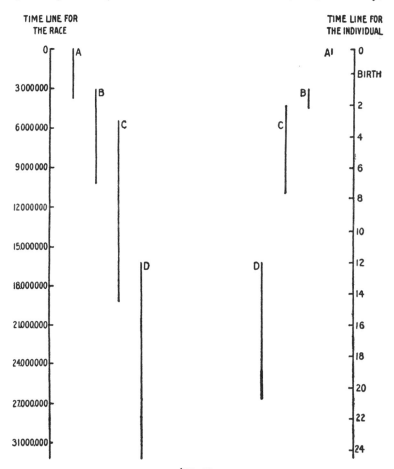

FIG. 23.

the time during which the early ancestral tendencies are possessed by the individual is, if not zero, at least a far smaller fraction of the time during which the late ancestral tendencies are possessed by him than is the case with the times in the case of the race. So the parallelism of individual and race is universally amended by supposing the early racial tendencies to be in the individual abbreviated in some rough proportion to their earliness.

Instead of Fig. 22, then, we would have something like Fig. 23, wherein A's stay in the individual is one-tenth as long a fraction of the period from conception to the adult condition, as A's stay in the individual is of the period from the protozoa to modern man; B's stay is two-tenths; C's is four-tenths and D's is seven tenths.

To make sure that the reader gets a just idea of what the recapitulation-theory means to its adherents and of how they use it in explaining human nature, I quote at some length from their most instructive statements about it. The following are samples of the more general statements:

"The course of mental development is exactly determined through the relation of ontogenesis (individual development) to phylogenesis (the development of the race). The development of the higher (purposive and rational) activities is regulated in every respect in accord with the previously developed instincts, and is primarily conditioned by them. No influence that works in opposition to this development and to the law of inheritance of racial traits in order can ever reach a suitable adaptation, but only disturbs the natural course of development, and creates abnormal misdirected endeavor." [Schneider, '82, p. 489]

"The individual, from conception to senescence, follows the order of development of the race." [Burk, F. L., '98, p. 36]

"As in the physical world, so in the psychical there is a natural order of growth. Since it is the order of nature that the new organism should pass through certain developmental stages, it behooves us to study nature's plan and seek rathei to aid than to thwart it. For nature must be right; there is no higher criterion. There is, therefore, no study of more vital importance to the educationist than this of the natural development of organisms. The parallelism of phylogeny and ontogeny enforces the argument in favor of natural development and the doctrine of katharsis or vaccination as applied to the moral growth of the child. It furnishes a double support to the view that education should be a process of orderly and gradual unfolding, without precocity and without interference, from lower to ever higher stages; that forcing is unnatural and that the mental pabulum should be suited to the stage of development reached. So long as we keep the end in view and do not cause the child to linger in any of the stages, we need not fear the discipline that each stage is calculated to give as a preparation for the next. For what Von Baer long ago said of animals is true also of the child: 'The type of each animal appears to fix itself at the very beginning in the embryo and to dominate the whole development.'

"The period of animal recapitulation is short. In this work the attempt has not been made to deal with the recapitulation of human stages of development, but reasoning from the fact that the length of time taken to recapitulate a period does not depend upon the duration of that period phylogenetically, but upon its recency, we may conclude that the recapitulation of human stages of development is much longer than that of the longest animal stage, viz., the ape stage." [Guillet, '00, pp. 427-428]

THE UTILITY THEORY

The Utility Theory explains the dates of original tendencies by the same causes as account for their existence—*variation* and *selection*. Other things being equal, the date at which a tendency appears is that one of the many varying dates at which it has appeared in our ancestry which has been most serviceable in keeping the stock alive. Thus suckling, though late in the race, is early in the individual. The sex instincts, though early in the race, are very late in the individual. Walking on all fours, though the possession of the race for perhaps millions of years, is evanescent or non-existent as a human instinct; creeping, though not a duplicate of any important form of locomotion possessed and then lost in our ancestral line, is one of the most emphatic transitory tendencies of infancy.

An advocate of the Utility Theory should not assert that the actual order is in every particular useful (that is, more useful than a chance order) ; much less that it is the most useful order for survival that there could be. An order of original tendencies has to be very injurious if the individual possessing it is to be very frequently eliminated. For a better order than whatever order exists to be selected for survival, it must first appear as a variation. That is, the theory that the order and dates of appearance and disappearance of original tendencies are due to natural selection is subject to the same interpretation as the theory of natural selection elsewhere.

I have not found instructive quotations representing the utility theory. It has been, perhaps, assumed by opponents of the recapitulation theory, but they have generally been satisfied to point out the latter's impossibilities, without advancing a constructive doctrine. As held by the writer, the utility theory of the order of appearance and dates of the original tendencies in human intellect and character is *that the same causes which account for the origin and perpetuation of a tendency account for its time relations to other tendencies. Whatever makes the tendency happen at all makes it happen at some date and place in the total order of the animal's development. Whatever makes it vary at all makes it vary in its date. Other things being equal, the date which will be perpetuated will be that one of the many varying dates at which it appears, which proves most serviceable in keeping the species alive. Similarly for its date of disappearance.* What the time relations of human original tendencies are, like what the tendencies themselves are, is thus the result of *variation by whatever influences the germplasm* and *selection by utility.*

THE GRADUAL WAXING OF DELAYED INSTINCTS AND CAPACITIES

It is a favorite dictum of superficial psychology and pedagogy that instincts lie entirely dormant and then spring into full strength within a few weeks. At a certain stage, we are told, such and such a tendency has its 'nascent period' or ripening time. Three is the age for fear, six is the age for climbing, fifteen is the age for cooperativeness, and the like. The same doctrine is applied to the supposed 'faculties' or very general capacities of the mind. Within a year or two around eight the child is said to change from a mere bundle of sensory capacities, to a child possessed of imagination; somewhere around thirteen another brief score of months brings his reasoning up from near zero to nearly full energy; a year or two somewhere in the 'teens creates altruism!

These statements are almost certainly misleading. The one instinct whose appearance seems most like a dramatic rushing upon life's stage—the sex instinct—is found upon careful study to be gradually maturing for years. The capacity for reasoning shows no signs by any tests as yet given of developing twice as much in any one year from five to twenty-five as in any other. In the cases where the differences between children of different ages may be taken roughly to measure the rate of inner growth of capacities, what data we have show nothing to justify the doctrine of sudden ripening in a serial order. Thus the results in the case of the rate of tapping (as on a telegraph key) for boys are shown in Figure 24. The dash line represents the average ability year by year from six to sixteen as determined by Bryan ['92]* and the continuous line that determined by Gilbert ['94]. Figure 25 shows the average of the two curves. These

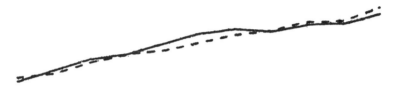

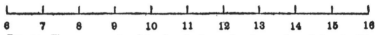

| 6 | 7 | 8 | 9 | 10 | 11 | 12 | 13 | 14 | 15 | 16 |

FIG. 24. The average rate of tapping for boys of each age from 6 to 16. The continuous line represents Gilbert's estimate; the dash line represents Bryan's estimate (for the left-wrist-movement).

curves suggest fluctuations, notably a failure of the thirteen-year-olds to surpass the twelve-year-olds, a notable superiority of the sixteen-year-olds over the fifteen-year-olds, and a greater gain from six to eleven than thereafter, but the development of the capacity is, as a whole, gradual. At least, that word would seem to most observers to fit the progress measured by Figures 24 and 25.

* For one of eight movements used by him, the 'Left Wrist.'

The few interests whose strength, period by period, have
been more or less well measured, give no evidence of any
sudden accession to power.   Thus collecting * seems to increase
in vigor gradually from before six to ten.   The capacities

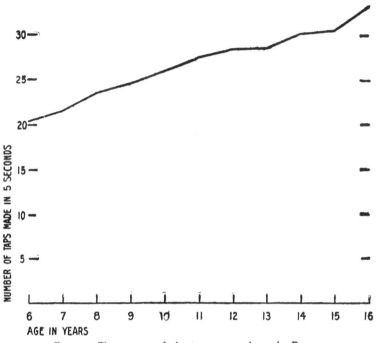

FIG. 25.   The average of the two curves shown in FIG. 24.

of sensory discrimination, memory, observation and the like
which have been measured in children at different ages, are
of course in the conditions that they are at any age because of

* According to C. F. Burk ['oo] twelve hundred boys and girls reported
to their teachers the names of the objects which they were at the time
collecting. The average number of collections reported by those of each
age from six to seventeen is given as follows:

training as well as inner growth, and the facts concerning their rates of gain cannot be used at their face value in our argument. But so far as they do go, they give no support to the theory of the sudden rise of inner tendencies. Indeed every tendency that has been subjected to anything like rigid scrutiny seems to fit the word gradual rather than the word sudden in the rate of its maturing.

In the case of the lower animals, where control of training and accurate measurement of the animal's performance is feasible, gradualness of development is found the rule for delayed instincts. Thus the author ['99] found that a dozen days or so were required from the first beginnings to the full development of fear of large moving objects in chicks, that the fighting of roosters shows its first feeble beginnings as early as the sixth day of the chick's life, that the balancing reaction (on a swinging perch) develops gradually from the sixth day on.

AVERAGE NUMBER OF ACTIVE COLLECTIONS FOR DIFFERENT AGES

Age	Av. per Boy	Av. per Girl	Av. per Child
6 years	1.2	1.9	1 4 collections
7 "	2.1	2.6	2 3 "
8 "	3.5	4.5	4 "
9 "	3.9	4 1	4 "
10 "	4.4	4.4	4.4 "
11 "	3.4	3.3	3.3 "
12 "	3	3	3 "
13 "	3.5	3.4	3.4 "
14 "	3	3	3 "
15 "	2.7	3.2	3 "
16 "	2 1	3.3	2 8 "
17 "	2	3	2 5 "

Such errors as children would make in their reports probably would act to make the rise from six to ten seem *more* sudden than it really was. Even as reported, the rise is very gradual.

THE PROBABLE FREQUENCY OF TRANSITORINESS IN ORIGINAL

TENDENCIES

James' description of the fact of transitoriness and of its
extent in man is the best introduction to the topic of this
section. He says:

"Leaving lower animals aside, and turning to human instincts, we see the law of transiency corroborated on the widest
scale by the alternation of different interests and passions as
human life goes on. With the child, life is all play and fairy-
tales and learning the external properties of 'things;' with the
youth it is bodily exercises of a more systematic sort, novels of
the real world, boon-fellowship and song, friendship and love,
nature, travel and adventure, science and philosophy; with the
man, ambition and policy, acquisitiveness, responsibility to
others, and the selfish zest of the battle of life. If a boy
grows up alone at the age of games and sports, and learns
neither to play ball, nor row, nor sail, nor ride, nor skate, nor
fish, nor shoot, probably he will be sedentary to the end of his
days; and, though the best of opportunities be afforded him for
learning these things later, it is a hundred to one but he will
pass them by and shrink back from the effort of taking those
necessary first steps the prospect of which, at an earlier age,
would have filled him with eager delight. The sexual passion
expires after a protracted reign; but it is well known that its
peculiar manifestations in a given individual depend almost
entirely on the habits he may form during the early period of
its activity. Exposure to bad company then makes him a loose
liver all his days; chastity kept at first makes the same easier
later on. In all pedagogy the great thing is to strike the iron
while hot, and to seize the wave of the pupil's interest in each
successive subject before its ebb has come, so that knowledge
may be got and a habit of skill acquired—a headway of interest,
in short, secured, on which afterward the individual may float.
There is a happy moment for fixing skill in drawing, for mak-

ing boys collectors in natural history, and presently dissectors
and botanists; then for initiating them into the harmonies of
mechanics and the wonders of physical and chemical law.
Later, introspective psychology and the metaphysical and religious mysteries take their turn; and last of all, the draw. ot
human affairs and worldly wisdom in the widest sens of the
term." ['93, vol. 2, p. 400 f.]

The particular statements of this characteristic passage form
a sagacious commentary on the loss of interests as a man grows
up and becomes engaged in new pleasures and duties, but it is
doubtful whether they do show the law of transiency to be very
widely active in human instincts. Two forces, other than the
law of transitoriness, must be considered, before attributing the
ebbs in man's activities so exclusively to it. The first is the
force of new situations—changed circumstances about man—
rather than a changed nature in him. The second is the force
of changes in his nature due to special acquisitions—learned
habits—not to mere losses of transitory instincts and capacities.

Consider, for example, the loss of zeal for 'play and fairy
tales and learning the external properties of things' by the
youth and grown man. Is not a part of the loss due to
changed circumstances? Would not a man regain a portion
of his zeal for play, if, say, all the fellow-members of his stock
exchange or club or factory began by a miracle to play? Is it
not, in part, the avoidance of the disapproval of his fellows
which makes the youth or man cast off childish things. Given
a situation such that play adds no discomforting moral or social
results, and the youth or man *does* seem to act as if the supposedly lost zest had simply been held down by lack of a con-
genial situation such as it customarily had in childhood. So
the student body of a college may all spin tops or play marbles;
hard-headed brokers may gambol in an initiation festivity; and

joyless politicians may jump up and down and dance in a ring. Are not the pleasures of travel and the stock sports of amusement-parks both evidence that the love of 'learning the external properties of things' persists in fair measure into adult years? New places, new sights, new experiences attract grown men and women also. It is even a stock item in everyday humor that the boy's craving for the circus is his father's excuse. The displays of aeroplanes of the last two years seem to be frequented by adults because of the same interest in learning the external properties of things which makes the child besiege the engine-house.

Of the difference between the child and the adult in this respect which remains after changed circumstances have been allowed for, is not a part due to the addition of habits rather than the loss of instincts? 'To design a real engine in competition with other inventors under the stimulus of the world's needs expressed in money price and personal distinction' is so much more satisfying to man's nature—even to his original nature—than 'playing cars' or 'playing build bridges,' that the serious habit eventually makes the play out of which it sprang an inferior interest. If a man gets only innocent pleasure from hearing fairy tales, and gets not only innocent pleasure but also comforts for his family from writing them, we must expect that the habit will displace the less remunerative instinct. The youth may be more interested in the *internal* properties of things revealed by mechanics, electricity, chemistry and biology, just because he has already had, and used up, the satisfactions of knowing external facts about chairs and tables, tops and balls, horses and dogs. His apparently new interests may be the same fundamental interest turned to new objects because of a change produced in him by experience. The old objects have lost their appeal because of the connections they have

8

acquired in the course of his training—not because of an inevitable decay of some original welcoming force.

The discounts for changes in the situation and acquired changes in the man, which I have suggested as necessary in the case of 'play and fairy tales and learning the external properties of things,' can be shown to be appropriate in the case of the other losses incurred by the process of maturity which James has chosen as illustrations.

If this is the case with James's temperate account, what shall we say of those who describe the inner growth of man's instincts and capacities altogether as a series of tendencies, appearing, waiting, lasting a brief space and vanishing unless then and there fixed as habits—like the ripening of fruits which soon decay unless preserved by the housewifery of habits, or like a procession of candidates which pass through an office, disappearing for good and all unless enlisted at the time and drilled by some recruiting officer of the mind. Such a sharp definition of the rise and fall of original tendencies in a serial order of stages or epochs seems to me to be a gross exaggeration, corresponding only here and there to the actual progress of inner development.

To refute such extravagant notions of the suddenness of appearance of original tendencies, their brevity of stay and their disappearance without other cause than an inherent original transitoriness of the neural bonds, it should suffice to think over the tendencies themselves, each in connection with the treatment it receives at the hands of the changes produced by circumstances in the stimulating situation and responding organism. For example, the readiness of the hunting response persists even in spite of the inadequate stimuli and absence of rewards of a modern village or town, so that, if habitual restraints are removed, men will gladly leave their work to chase an escaped cat. They will, with slight encouragement, undergo notable privations and expense to spend a few days in tracking game and possessing themselves of animal carcasses got by so near an approach as is possible to man's original naked-handed pursuit. Collecting and hoarding survive the penalties which follow childish scavenging and adult waste of time. The drawers, closets and attics of five houses out of ten bear some witness to the tendency. Whole trades maintain themselves by ministering to its continued strength.

Transitoriness is a fact; instincts do wax and wane; but the waning is far less frequent, far more gradual and far later in its onset, than the ordinary descriptions of stages, epochs, fluctuations and the like would lead one to believe. Much of human behavior can be explained by certain original tendencies which wane slowly or not at all, except in so far as the consequences of their manifestations stamp them out, or the law of disuse slowly weakens them.

CHAPTER IX

THE VALUE AND USE OF ORIGINAL TENDENCIES

At the beginning of this volume it was stated that human welfare required that some original tendencies be cherished, that some be redirected or modified, and that others be eliminated outright.

To most of my readers it will seem evident that original nature includes tendencies that are good, tendencies that can be used for good, and tendencies that had best be abolished. The fact that maternal affection, curiosity and cruelty are original tendencies would seem sufficient proof of the statement, but it has been denied by two extreme views, one that original nature is essentially wrong and untrustworthy, the other that original nature is always right. The former view, though probably as fair as the latter, is now in universal disrepute and need not detain us. The latter, by being attractive to sentimentalists, absolutist philosophers and believers in a distorted and fallacious form of the doctrine of evolution, has been of great influence upon educational theories. Since it is also championed to some extent by so eminent a student of human nature as Stanley Hall, it must be considered seriously.

THE DOCTRINE OF NATURE'S INFALLIBILITY

By the 'Nature is Right' doctrine, the actual terminus of evolution is the moral end of human action. What is going to be, is right. Our duty is to abstain from interfering with nature, supposing such interference to be possible. A child should be trained up in the way that the inner impulse of development leads him to go. The *summum bonum* for the race is to live out its own evolution with interest and freedom. No stage to which nature impels, should by human artifice be either hastened or prolonged, lest the magic order be disturbed. The ideal for humanity is to be sought in its natural outcome, in what it of itself tends to be, irrespective of training. Human effort should be to let the inner forces of development do their perfect work.

This doctrine that the unlearned tendencies of man are right is assumed in a vague way as a support for one or another proposal about educational practice more often than it is stated straightforwardly as a general principle. But the quotations that follow will serve as a composite statement and illustration of it as a general principle.

"No influence that works in opposition to this development (that of original nature) and to the law of the inheritance of racial traits in order can ever reach a suitable adaptation, but only disturbs the natural course of development, and creates abnormal, misdirected endeavor." [Schneider, '82, p. 489]

"Only here (in the original tendencies or 'natural development' of the individual and of the race) can we hope to find true norms against the tendencies to precocity in home, school, church, and civilization generally, and also to establish criteria by which to both diagnose and measure arrest and retardation in the individual and the race." [G. Stanley Hall, '04, Preface, p. viii]

Guillet says: "Since it is the order of nature that the new organism should pass through certain developmental stages, it behooves us to study nature's plan, and to seek rather to aid than to thwart it. For nature must be right; there is no higher criterion." [Guillet, '00, p. 427]

To these extraordinary renunciations of any hope of improving upon the unguided course of inner growth common sense at once opposes the facts that lying, stealing, torturing, ignorance, irrational fears, and a hundred weaknesses and vices, are original in man.

Schneider, Stanley Hall, and others who have proclaimed that 'Nature is right' and used the doctrine as a pillar of their theories of education, were not ignorant of these facts. Nor did they forget such facts temporarily in zeal for their attractive doctrine. They offer, or could offer, three explanations of these apparently wrong original tendencies in man.

First, an original tendency that is undesirable, in and of itself, may be the *prerequisite of some desirable tendency* and hence, on the whole, desirable.

"Children," writes Burk, "frequently persist in following some strange, useless or even savage interests quite foreign to our civilization . . . these strange and useless experiences nevertheless may be essential as a platform out of which a higher coördination, useful for modern life, may be reached. The intermediate stage or level may be useless or even inimical to our civilization, but yet as a link in evolution, be none the less essential." [Burk, F. L., '98, p. 24]

In Stanley Hall's words, "Many an impulse seeks expression, which seems strong for a time, but which will never be heard of later. Its function is to stimulate the next higher power that can only thus be provoked to development, in order to direct, repress or supersede it. . . . Nearly every latency must be developed, or else some higher power, that later tempers and coördinates it, lacks normal stimulus to develop." ['04, vol. 2, pp. 90-91] Thus the miscellaneous and apparently futile finger movements of babies may be a necessary fore-runner of reaching, grasping, holding, and the like.

Second, An original tendency, undesirable in and of itself, may on the whole be desirable because it is the *necessary corre-late or result of some desirable tendency.*

The tendency to righteous anger may involve a tendency to mere raging. Love may be unable to exist in full measure without jealousy of the irrational, cruel and mean sort. In Stanley Hall's opinion, "An able-bodied young man, who can not fight physically, can hardly have a high and true sense of honor, and is generally a milk-sop, a lady-boy, or a sneak." ['04, vol. 1, p. 217]

Third, a tendency undesirable in and of itself would, on the whole, be desirable, if *by its presence in early life, man is pro-tected from the same tendency later.*

If being a thief at five and a bully at ten kept one from being a thief and a bully from twenty-five to seventy, these original tendencies would of course be desirable as lesser evils. That original tendencies do sometimes thus preventively inocu-late and immunize has been asserted by Stanley Hall and many of his followers.

The extent to which this doctrine of immunization by early wrong-doing is carried is well illustrated in the following recommendations of selfishness, greed, lying and cheating by Kline and France :—

"Do we believe that the child recapitulates the history of the race? If so we may not be surprised to find the passion for property-getting a natural one, nor that the child lies, cheats and steals to acquire it or that selfishness rules the child's actions. Selfishness is the cornerstone of the struggle for existence, deception is at its very foundation, while the acquir-ing of property has been the most dominant factor in the his-tory of men and nations. These passions of the child are but the pent up forces of the greed of thousands of years. They must find expression and exercise, if not in childhood, later. Who knows but what our misers are not those children grown up whom fond mothers and fathers forced into giving away their playthings, into the doing of unselfish acts, in acting out a generosity which was neither felt nor understood. Not to let these activities have their play in childhood is to run a great risk. It does no good to make the child perform moral acts when it does not appreciate what right and wrong mean, and to punish a child for not performing acts which his very nature compels him to do, is doing that child positive injury.

During the period of adolescence, generosity and altruism spring up naturally. Then why try to force the budding plant into blossom? Instruct them by all means, teach them the right; but if this fails, do not punish, but let the child be selfish, let him lie and cheat, until these forces spend themselves. Do not these experiences of the child give to man in later life a moral virility?"   ['99, p. 455]

DEFECTS IN MAN'S ORIGINAL NATURE

These three subsidiary hypotheses (that an intrinsically undesirable tendency may be the prerequisite of some desirable tendency, or its necessary correlate, or the means of immunization from a similar but worse tendency later) do not, however, supply all the shortcomings of the 'Nature is Right' doctrine. The first and second of them, while very probably true of certain tendencies, do not provide greed, insane rage, cruelty, and many others, with any adequate excuse. The experience of families, schools and states, has not found that interference with these instincts withers the hopes of any noble traits. Nor does present knowledge of the relations of mental traits lead us to expect that these instincts are necessarily bound to any compensating advantages. The great majority of the original tendencies which can be defended by the hope that they are bound as cause or effect or correlative to some valuable quality of mind are either such as no wise judge would consider wrong —for example, general activity of body and of mind; or such as produce the good quality *only by being interfered with, re-directed, modified* in situation, response, or both.

The third hypothesis, that rage, teasing, bullying, envy, neglect of absolute values, and the like, will, if denied exercise, inhibited or redirected when they appear as man's original nature decrees, be all the more potent and mischievous in the long run, is then necessary if nature's infallibility is to be saved. It was in fact invented to save it.

Very strong evidence should be required before believing that the exercise of any function thus weakens it. For such mental immunization is directly contrary to one of the most nearly universal laws of mental life, the law of exercise. Still stronger evidence should be required before believing that the exercise of any function to which an original impulse leads weakens it. For the exercise of an *original* tendency is almost always satisfying, other things being equal. Hence mental immunization by an early attack is here directly contrary to the law of effect.

There can, indeed, be no doubt that the laws of habit are the rule, that ordinarily the exercise of any tendency with satisfying or indifferent results strengthens the tendency, and that an original tendency will persist unless it is transitory by nature, is prevented from functioning, or is checked or redirected by other forces. If immunization by early indulgence occurs at all, it occurs as an exception for which adequate special reasons must be given.

No one has given adequate special reasons, or indeed reasons of any kind worth mentioning. In fact, Stanley Hall himself often abandons the doctrine and returns to the orthodox theory that education must redirect original tendencies. For example, he writes that we shall "utilize most of the energy now wasted in crime by devising more wholesome and natural expressions for the instincts that motivate it" ['04, vol. 1, p. 342]. Anger's "culture requires proper selection of objects and great transformation, but never extermination." ['04, vol. 1, p. 355] "The popular idea, that youth must have its fling, implies the need of greatly and sometimes suddenly widened liberty, which nevertheless needs careful supervision and wise direction." ['04, vol. 2, pp. 89-90] Hall even says flatly that "the spontaneous expressions of this best age and condition of life (youth in college), with no other occupation than their own development, have shown reversions as often as progress." ['04, vol. 2, p. 399]

Finally it must be said that under the pressure of obvious facts even the most ardent advocates of nature's infallibility always somewhere give the doctrine up. So Stanley Hall writes:—

. . . "now another remove from nature seems to be made necessary by the manifold knowledges and skills of our highly complex civilization . . . the child must be subjected to special disciplines and be apprenticed to the higher qualities of adulthood, for he is not only a product of nature, but a candidate for a highly developed humanity. To many, if not most, of the influences here there can be at first but little inner response. . . . The wisest requirements seem to the child more or less alien, arbitrary, heteronomous, artificial, falsetto." ['04, Preface, p. xii]

Guillet, who asserts that 'Nature must be right,' later unconsciously recants fully. "These instincts, then, which every child has . . . must be turned into worthy grooves. Not suppression, but a generous control." ['00, p. 445]

The imperfections and misleadings of original nature are in fact many and momentous. The common good requires that each child learn countless new lessons and unlearn a large fraction of his natural birthright. The main reason for this is that original equipment is archaic, adapting the human animal for the life that might be led by a family group of wild men in the woods, amongst the brute forces of land, water, wind, rain, plants, animals, and other groups of wild men. The life to which original nature adapts man is probably far more like the life of the wolf or ape, than like the life that now is, as a result of human art, habit and reasoning, perpetuating themselves in language, tools, buildings, books and customs.

It is a useful, if trite, exercise to consider this enormous gap between the fate of man left to what the human germ plasm has learned and the opportunity to which the learning of men themselves calls each new generation. How easily we revert to a nearly simian brutality when the records and restraints of civilization fail is the best proof and illustration of the unfitness of original nature to rule the behavior of man.

Other illustrations in abundance can be found of the archaic unreason of original nature, or, more scientifically, of the thoroughgoing transformation which life undergoes in proportion as human reason works back upon the conditions of things and the wants of men. By the germs' decree we fear, not the carriers of malaria and yellow fever, but thunder and the dark; we pity, not the gifted youth debarred from education, but the beggar's bloody sore; we are less excited by a great injustice than by a little blood; we suffer more from such scorn as untipped waiters, cabmen, and barbers show, than from our own idleness, ignorance and folly.

It is also true that even to a brute's life in the woods human instincts are not perfectly adapted, or without gross errors. To exist, a species needs to behave so as to exist, but not so as to exist well. A species can, and most species do, make many blunders in life. 'Good' means in evolution only 'good enough to keep the species from elimination,' and 'best' means only the surest aids to survival that have happened to happen.

The original tendencies of man have not been right, are not right, and probably never will be right. By them alone few of the best wants in human life would have been felt, and fewer still satisfied. Nor would the crude, conflicting, perilous wants which original nature so largely represents and serves, have had much more fulfilment. Original nature has achieved what goodness the world knows as a state achieves order, by killing, confining or reforming some of its elements. It progresses, not by *laissez faire,* but by changing the environment in which it operates and by renewedly changing itself in each generation. Man is now as civilized, rational and humane as he is because man in the past has changed things into shapes more satisfying, and changed parts of his own nature into traits more satisfying, to man as a whole. Man is thus eternally altering himself to suit himself. His nature is not right in his own eyes. Only one thing in it, indeed, is unreservedly good, the power to make it better. This power, the power of learning or modification in favor of the satisfying, the capacity represented by the law of effect, is the essential principle of reason and right in the world.

PART II

The Psychology of Learning

CHAPTER X

THE LAWS OF LEARNING IN ANIMALS

The intellect, character and skill possessed by any man are the product of certain original tendencies and the training which they have received. His eventual nature is the development of his original nature in the environment which it has had. Human nature in general is the result of the original nature of man, the laws of learning, and the forces of nature amongst which man lives and learns.

SAMPLES OF ANIMAL LEARNING

The complexities of human learning will in the end be best understood if at first we avoid them, examining rather the behavior of the lower animals as they learn to meet certain situations in changed, and more remunerative, ways.

Let a number of chicks, say six to twelve days old, be kept in a yard (YY of Figure 26) adjoining which is a pen or maze (A B C D E of Figure 26). A chick is taken from the group and put in alone at A. It is confronted by a situation which is, in essence, *Confining walls and the absence of the other chicks, food and familiar surroundings.* It reacts to the situation by running around, making loud sounds, and jumping at the walls. When it jumps at the walls, it has the discomforts of thwarted effort, and when it runs to B, or C, or D, it has a continuation of the situation just described; when it runs to E, it gets out and has the satisfaction of being with the other chicks, of eating, and of being in its usual habitat. If it is repeatedly put in again at A,

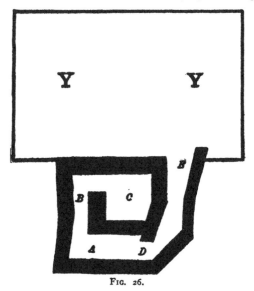

FIG. 26.

one finds that it jumps and runs to B or C less and less often, until finally its only act is to run to D, E, and out. It has formed an association, or connection, or bond, between the situation due to its removal to A and the response of going to E. In common language, it has learned to go to E when put at A—has learned the way out. The decrease in the useless running and jumping and standing still finds a representative in the decreasing amount of time taken by the chick to escape. The two chicks that formed this par-

ticular association, for example, averaged three and a half
minutes (one about three and the other about four) for their
first five trials, but came finally to escape invariably within
five or six seconds.

The following schemes represent the animal's behavior
(1) during an early trial and (2) after the association has
been fully formed—after it has learned the way out perfectly.

(1)

BEHAVIOR IN AN EARLY TRIAL.

SITUATION.	RESPONSES.	RESULTING STATES OF AFFAIRS.
As described above, in the text	To chirp, etc.	Annoying continuation of the situation and thwarting of the inner tendencies.
	To jump at various places.	
	To run to B.	" " "
	" " " C.	" " "
	" " " D.	" " "
	" " " E.	Satisfying company, food and surroundings.

(2)

BEHAVIOR IN A TRIAL AFTER LEARNING.

SITUATION.	RESPONSES.	RESULTING STATES OF AFFAIRS.
Same as in (1).	To run to E.	Satisfying as above.

A graphic representation of the progress from an early
trial to a trial after the association has been fully formed is
given in the following figures, in which the dotted lines represent the path taken by a turtle in his fifth (Fig. 27) and
fiftieth (Fig. 28) experiences in learning the way from the
point A to his nest. The straight lines represent walls of
boards. Besides the useless movements, there were, in the
fifth trial, useless stoppings. The time taken to reach the

nest in the fifth trial was seven minutes; in the fiftieth, thirty-five seconds. The figures represent typical early and late trials, chosen from a number of experiments on different

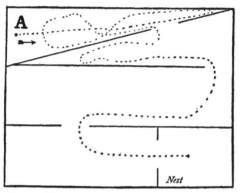

FIG. 27. The path taken by a turtle in finding his way from A to his nest, in his 5th trial.

individuals in different situations, by Dr. R. M. Yerkes, to whom I am indebted for permission to use these figures.

Let us next examine a somewhat more ambitious performance than the mere discovery of the proper path by a chick

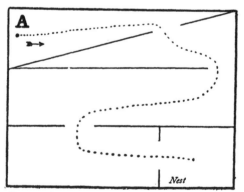

FIG. 28. The path taken by a turtle in finding his way from A to his nest, in his 50th trial.

or turtle. If we take a box twenty by fifteen by twelve
inches, replace its cover and front side by bars an inch apart,
and make in this front side a door arranged so as to fall
open when a wooden button inside is turned from a vertical
to a horizontal position, we shall have means to observe such.
A kitten, three to six months old, if put in this box when
hungry, a bit of fish being left outside, reacts as follows:
It tries to squeeze through between the bars, claws at the
bars and at loose things in and out of the box, stretches its
paws out between the bars, and bites at its confining walls.
Some one of all these promiscuous clawings, squeezings, and
bitings turns round the wooden button, and the kitten gains
freedom and food. By repeating the experience again and
again, the animal gradually comes to omit all the useless
clawings, and the like, and to manifest only the particular
impulse (e. g., to claw hard at the top of the button with
the paw, or to push against one side of it with the nose)
which has resulted successfully. It turns the button around
without delay whenever put in the box. It has formed an
association between the situation, *confinement in a box of a
certain appearance,* and the response of *clawing at a certain
part of that box in a certain definite way.* Popularly speaking,
it has learned to open a door by turning a button. To the
uninitiated observer the behavior of the six kittens that thus
freed themselves from such a box would seem wonderful and
quite unlike their ordinary accomplishments of finding their
way to their food or beds, but the reader will realize that the
activity is of just the same sort as that displayed by the chick
in the pen. A certain situation arouses, by virtue of accident
or, more often, instinctive equipment, certain responses. One
of these happens to be an act appropriate to secure freedom.
It is stamped in in connection with that situation. Here the act

9

is clawing at a certain spot instead of running to E, and is selected from a far greater number of useless acts.

In the examples so far given there is a certain congruity between the 'set' associated with the situation and the learning. The act which lets the cat out is hit upon by the cat while, as we say, trying to get out, and is, so to speak, a likely means of release. But there need be no such congruity between the 'set' and the learning. If we confine a cat, opening the door and letting it out to get food only when it scratches itself, we shall, after enough trials, find the cat scratching itself the moment it is put into the box. Yet in the first trials it did not scratch itself in order to get out, or indeed until after it had given up the unavailing clawings and squeezings, and stopped to rest. The association is formed with such an 'unlikely' or 'incongruous' response as that of scratching, or licking, or (in the case of chicks) pecking at the wing to dress it, as truly as with a response which original nature or previous habit has put in connection with the set of the organism toward release, food, and company.

The examples chosen so far show the animal forming a single association, but such may be combined into series. For instance, a chick learns to get out of a pen by climbing up an inclined plane. A second pen is then so arranged that the chick can, say by walking up a slat and through a hole in the wall, get from it into pen No. 1. After a number of trials the chick will, when put in pen No. 2, go at once to pen No. 1, and thence out. A third pen is then so arranged that the chick, by forming another association, can get from it to pen No. 2, and so on. In such a series of associations the response of one brings the animal into the *situation* of the next, thus arousing its response, and so on to the end. Three chicks thus learned to go through a sort of long labyrinth without mistakes, the 'learning' representing twenty-three associations.

The learning of the chick, turtle and kitten in the cases quoted is characterized negatively by the absence of inferential, ratiocinative thinking; and indeed by the absence of effective use of 'ideas' of any sort. Were the reader confined in a maze or cage, or left at some distance from home, his responses to these situations would almost certainly include many ideas, judgments, or thoughts about the situation; and his acts would probably in large measure be led up to or 'mediated' by such sequences of ideas as are commonly called reasoning. Between the annoying situation and the response which relieves the annoyance there might for the reader well intervene an hour of inner consideration, thought, planning and the like. But there is no evidence that any ideas about the maze, the cage, the food, or anything else, were present to determine the acts of the chicks or kittens in question. Their responses were made directly to the situation as sensed, not *via* ideas suggested by it. The three cases of learning quoted are adequately accounted for as the strengthening and weakening of bonds between a situation present to sense and responses in the nervous system which issue then and there in movement. The lower animals do occasionally show signs of ideas and of their influence on behavior, but the great bulk of their learning has been found explainable by such direct binding of acts to situations, unmediated by ideas.

CHARACTERISTICS OF ANIMAL LEARNING

These cases, and the hundreds of which they are typical, show the laws of readiness, exercise, and effect, uncomplicated by any pseudo-aid from imitation, ideo-motor action, or superior faculties of inference. There are certain states of affairs which the animal welcomes and does nothing to avoid—its satisfiers. There are others which it is intolerant of and rejects, doing one thing or another until relieved from them. Of the bonds which the animal's behavior makes between a situation and responses those grow stronger which are accompanied by satisfying states of affairs, while those accompanied by annoyance weaken and disappear. Exercise strengthens and disuse weakens bonds. Such is the sum and substance of the bulk of animal learning.

These cases exemplify also five characteristics of learning which are secondary in scope and importance only to the laws of readiness, exercise, and effect.

The first is the fact of *multiple response to the same external situation.* The animal reacts to being confined in the pen in several ways, and so has the possibility of selecting for future connection with that situation one or another of these ways. Its own inner state changes when jumping at the wall at B produces a drop back into the pen, so that it then is less likely to jump again—more likely to chirp and run. Running to C and being still confronted with the confining walls may arouse an inner state which impels it to turn and run back. So one after another of the responses which, by original nature or previous learning, are produced by the confining walls *plus* the failure of the useless chirpings, jumpings and runnings, are made.

This principle of *Multiple Response* or *Varied Reaction* will be found to pervade at least nine-tenths of animal and human learning. As ordinarily interpreted, it is not universal, since, even if only one response is made, the animal may change its behavior—that is, learn—either by strengthening the connection so as to make that response more surely, more quickly and after a longer interval of disuse; or by weakening the connection so as to be more likely to do nothing at all in that situation, inactivity being a variety of response which is always a possible alternative. If we interpret variety of reaction so as to include the cases where an animal either makes one active response or is inactive—that is, either alters what it was doing when the situation began to act, or does not alter what it was doing—the principle of varied response is universal in learning.

The second of the five subsidiary principles is what we may call the law of the learner's *Set* or *Attitude* or *Adjustment* or *Determination*. The learning cannot be described adequately in a simple equation involving the pen and a chick taken abstractly. The chick, according to his age, hunger, vitality, sleepiness and the like, may be in one or another attitude toward the external situation. A sleepier and less hungry chick will, as a rule, be 'set' less toward escape-movements when confined; its neurones involved in roaming, perceiving companions and feeding will be less ready to act; it will not, in popular language, 'try so hard to' get out or 'care so much about' being out. As Woodworth says in commenting upon similar cases of animal learning:

"In the first place we must assume in the animal an adjustment or determination of the psycho-physical mechanism toward a certain end. The animal desires, as we like to say, to get out and to reach the food. Whatever be his consciousness, his behavior shows that he is, as an organism, set in that direction. This adjustment persists till the motor reaction is consummated; it is the driving force in the unremitting efforts of the animal to attain the desired end. His reactions are, therefore, the joint result of the adjustment and of stimuli from various features of the cage. Each single reaction tends to become associated with the adjustment." [Ladd and Woodworth, '11, p. 551.]

The principle that in any external situation, the responses made are the product of the 'set' or 'attitude' of the animal, that the satisfyingness or annoyingness produced by a response is conditioned by that attitude, and that the 'successful' response is by the law of effect connected with that attitude as well as with the external situation *per se*—is general. Any process of learning is conditioned by the mind's 'set' at the time.

Animal learning shows also the fact, which becomes of tremendous moment in human learning, that one or another element of the situation may be prepotent in determining the response. For example, the cats with which I experimented, would, after a time, be determined by my behavior more than by other features of the general situations of which that behavior was a part; so that they could then learn, as they could not have done earlier, to form habits of response to signals which I gave. Similarly, a cat that has learned to get out of a dozen boxes—in each case by pulling some loop, turning some bar, depressing a platform, or the like—will, in a new box, be, as we say, 'more attentive to' small objects on the sides of the box than it was before. The connections made may then be, not absolutely with the gross situation as a total, but predominantly with some element or elements of it. Thus, it makes little or no difference whether the box from which a cat has learned to escape by turning a button, is faced North, South, East or West; and not much difference if it is painted ten per cent blacker or enlarged by a fifth. The cat will operate the mechanism substantially as well as it did before. It is, of course, the case that the animals do not, as a thoughtful man might do, connect the response with perfect strictness just to the one essential element of the situation. They can be much more easily confused by variations in the element's concomitants; and in certain cases many of the irrelevant concomitants have to be supplied to enable them to give the right response. Nevertheless they clearly make connections with certain parts or elements or features of gross total situations. Even in the lower animals, that is, we find that the action of a situation is more or less separable into the action of the elements that compose it— that even they illustrate the general *Law of Partial Activity** —that a part or element or aspect of a situation may be prepotent in causing response, and may have responses bound more or less exclusively to it regardless of some or all of its accompaniments.

If a cat which has never been confined in a box or cage of any sort is put into a box like that described a few pages back, it responds chiefly by trying to squeeze through the openings, clawing at the bars and at loose objects within the box, reaching out between the bars, and pulling at anything then within its grasp. In short, it responds to this artificial situation as it would by original nature to confinement, as in a thicket. If a cat which has learned to escape from a number of such boxes by manipulating various mechanical contrivances, is confined in a new box, it responds to it by a mixture of the responses originally bound to confining obstacles and of those which it has learned to make to boxes like the new one.

In both cases it illustrates the *Law of Assimilation* or *Analogy* that to any situations, which have no special original or acquired response of their own, the response made will be that which by original or acquired nature is connected with some situation which they resemble. For S_2 to resemble S_1 means for it to arouse more or less of the sensory neurones which S_1 would arouse, and in more or less the same fashion.

* Or, better, the law of *piecemeal activity*, or *activity by parts*.

The last important principle which stands out clearly in the learning of the lower animals is that which I shall call *Associative Shifting*. The ordinary animal 'tricks' in response to verbal signals are convenient illustrations. One, for example, holds up before a cat a bit of fish, saying, "Stand up." The cat, if hungry enough, and not of fixed contrary habit, will stand up in response to the fish. The response, however, contracts bonds also with the total situation, and hence to the human being in that position giving that signal as well as to the fish. After enough trials, by proper arrangement, the fish can be omitted, the other elements of the situation serving to evoke the response. Association may later be further shifted to the oral signal alone. With certain limitations due to the necessity of getting an element of a situation attended to, a response to the total situation A B C D E may thus be shifted to B C D E to C D E, to D E, to E. Moreover, by adding to the situation new elements F, G, H, etc., we may, subject to similar limitations, get *any response of which a learner is capable* associated with *any situation to which he is sensitive*. Thus, what was at the start utterly without power to evoke a certain response may come to do so to perfection. Indeed, the situation may be one which at the start would have aroused an exactly opposite response. So a monkey can be taught to go to the top of his cage whenever you hold a piece of banana at the bottom of it.

These simple, semi-mechanical phenomena—multiple response, the coöperation of the animal's set or attitude with the external situation, the predominant activity of parts or elements of a situation, the response to new situations as to the situations most like them, and the shifting of a response from one situation to another by gradually changing a sit-nation without disturbing the response to it—which animal learning discloses, are the fundamentals of human learning also. They are, of course, much complicated in the more advanced stages of human learning, such as the acquisition of skill with the violin, or of knowledge of the calculus, or of inventiveness in engineering. But it is impossible to understand the subtler and more planful learning of cultivated men without clear ideas of the forces which make learning possible in its first form of directly connecting some gross bodily response with a situation immediately present to the senses. Moreover, no matter how subtle, complicated and advanced a form of learning one has to explain, these simple facts— the selection of connections by use and satisfaction and their elimination by disuse and annoyance, multiple reaction, the mind's set as a condition, piecemeal activity of a situation, with prepotency of certain elements in determining the response, response by analogy, and shifting of bonds—will, as a matter of fact, still be the main, and perhaps the only, facts needed to explain it.

CHAPTER XI

ASSOCIATIVE LEARNING IN MAN

VARIETIES OF LEARNING

We may roughly distinguish in human learning (1) connection-forming of the common animal type, as when a ten-months-old baby learns to beat a drum, (2) connection-forming involving ideas, as when a two-year-old learns to think of his mother upon hearing the word, or to say candy when he thinks of the thing, (3) analysis or abstraction, as when the student of music learns to respond to an overtone in a given sound, and (4) selective thinking or reasoning, as when the school pupil learns the meaning of a Latin sentence by using his knowledge of the rules of syntax and meanings of the word-roots.

Connection-forming of the common animal type occurs frequently in the acquisitions of early infancy, in 'picking up' swimming or skating undirected, in increasing the distance and precision of one's hits in golf or baseball by the mere try, try again method, and in similar unthinking improvement of penmanship, acting, literary style, tact in intercourse, and indeed almost every sort of ability. Such direct selection of responses to fit a situation, irrespective of ideas of either, appears in experimental studies of human learning.

Thus, a person absorbed in reading the copy, holding it in mind and getting it typewritten as fast as he can, will modify his responses to various elements in the situations met so as to write more efficiently, without thinking of the element in question, or of how he has responded to it, or of the change he is actually making in the response. Book indeed says: "The special introspective notes of our learners . . . revealed . . . that *all* new adaptations or short cuts in method were unconsciously made, i.e., fallen into by the learners quite unintentionally . . . The learners suddenly noticed that they were doing certain parts of the work in a new and better way, then purposely adopted it in the future." ['08, pp. 92 and 95]. Similarly a person whose general aim is to solve a mechanical puzzle may hit upon the solution, or some part of it, in the course of random fumbling, may hit upon it sooner in the next trial, and so progress in the learning—all with little help from ideas about the puzzle or his own movements. Ruger, who studied the process of learning in the case of such puzzles, quotes ['10, p. 21 ff.] samples of such approach to learning of the animal type, such as; "I have no idea in the world how I did it. I remember moving the loop of the heart around the end of the bar, and the two pieces suddenly came apart." He says, in a general account of this matter:

"The behavior of human subjects in the puzzle tests . . . showed many of the features usually accredited to the behavior of animals in contrast with that of human beings. The times for repeated successes in a number of cases remained high and fluctuating, the time for later trials in a given series being often greater than that for the first success. Acts which made no change in the situation whatever were at times repeated indefinitely and without modification. In successive trials of a series, after an essential step toward a solution had been performed correctly, it was reversed and done over several times with irrelevant movements interspersed before the subject passed on to the next step . . . In practically all of the cases random manipulation played some part and, in many cases, a very considerable part in the gaining of success." [*ibid.*, p. 9.]

If the reader will trace, fairly rapidly, the outline of, say, a six-pointed star, looking only at the reflection of it and his hand given by a mirror, he will get a useful illustration of the animal-like learning by the gradual elimination of wrong responses. As Starch has shown ['10], one may make, again and again, responses which thought could have told us were wrong. As he says ['10, p. 21], "Apparently the only way to reach the line is to keep on trying till one succeeds."

Learning is indeed theoretically, and perhaps in fact, possible without any other factors than a situation, an animal whose inner conditions it can change, the retention of certain of these conditions in the animal because they favor, and the abandonment of certain others of them because they disturb, the life-processes of the neurones concerned at the time. The bare fact of selective association of response to situation is all that is needed for certain cases of learning.

Other cases follow the same simple associative plan, save that *ideas* are terms in the associated series. The familiar mental arithmetic drills of childhood, wherein we were made to "Take 6, add 5, subtract 2, divide by 3, multiply by 5, add 9, divide by 6, and give the answer," differ from the long maze through which the chicks were put, essentially in that the situations, after the first 'Take 6,' and the responses, until final announcement of the answer, include ideas as components.

The formation of connections involving ideas accounts for a major fraction of 'knowledge' in the popular sense of the term. Words heard and seen, with their meanings, events with their dates, things with their properties and values, numerical problems, such as $9 + 3$ or $36 \div 4$, with their answers, persons with their characteristics, places with their adjuncts, and the like, make up the long list of situation-response bonds where one term, at least, is the inner condition in a man which we call an idea or judgment or the like. Man learns also to isolate and respond to elements which for the lower animals remain inextricably imbedded in gross total situations. The furniture, conversation.or behavior which to a dog are an undefined impression (such as the reader would have from looking at an unfamiliar landscape upside down or hearing a babel of Chinese speeches, or being submerged ten feet under water for the first time, or being half awakened in an unfamiliar room by an earthquake), become to man intelligible aggregates of separate 'things,' 'words,' or 'acts,' further defined and constituted by color, number, size, shape, loudness, and the many elements which man analyzes out of the gross total situations of life for individual response.

Of this analytic learning and also of the longer or shorter inferential and selective series, fuller account will be given later. The simpler connection-forming, without or with ideas as features of the situation or the response, is obviously the primary fact and will be considered first.

THE LAWS OF HABIT

This sort of learning, more or less well named connection-forming, habit-formation, associative memory and association, is an obvious consequence of the laws of readiness, exercise, and effect described in Chapters IV and VI of the previous discussion. By it things are put together and kept together in behavior which have gone together, often enough or with enough resulting satisfaction, and are put apart and kept apart which have been separated long enough, or whose connection has produced enough annoyance. The laws of connection forming or association or habit furnish education with two obvious general rules :—(1) Put together what should go together and keep apart what should not go together. (2) Reward desirable connections and make undesirable connections produce discomfort. Or, in combined form: Exercise and reward desirable connections; prevent or punish undesirable connections. These psychological laws and educational rules for the learning process are among the elementary principles taught to beginners. They may seem so obvious as not to need statement even to beginners, much less here. But an examination of the literature of educational theory and practice and of the text-books, courses of study, and classroom exercises of schools will prove that they are neglected or misunderstood and that a thoroughgoing practical use of them is almost never made.

Educational theorists neglect them when they explain learning in terms of general faculties, such as attention, interest, memory, or judgment, instead of multitudes of connections; or appeal to vague forces such as *learning, development, adaptation,* or *adjustment* instead of the defined action of the laws of exercise and effect; or assume that the mere presence of ideas of good acts will produce those acts.

School practice neglects them when it fancies that knowledge of the addition combinations in higher decades (that is, $17 + 9$, $23 + 5$, $38 + 4$, etc.) will come by magic after $7 + 9$, $3 + 5$, $8 + 4$, etc., are once known; or that the difficulty which pupils find in learning 'division by a fraction' will be prevented or cured by explanation of *why* one should 'invert and multiply' or 'multiply by the reciprocal;' or when it gives elaborate drills in declining *bonus-a-um, boni-ae-i, bono-ae-o, etc.,* or in conjugating *amo, amas, amat, amamus, amatis, amant, amabam, amabas, amabat,* etc. ; or when it uses additional lessons and retention in school as stock punishments, or grants favors to those who make the most trouble until they are granted.

The laws of readiness, exercise, and effect, operating in human associative learning, show the same subsidiary laws —multiple response, guidance by a total attitude or set of the organism, prepotency of elements, response to new situations in accord with already existing bonds, and the shifting of bonds by progressive changes in a situation—which animal learning reveals. But under the conditions provided by the different original nature which man learns with, and the different environment that he learns in, these laws work in special ways and produce special effects. Since, moreover, their general importance justifies treatment beyond the bare descriptions of them given in the previous chapter, each of them will be reviewed here.

Multiple-Response or Varied Reaction.—In the course of family and community and school life, and under the influence of self-directed education, the 'right' response is often provided from the beginning and throughout. Thus, one may not have to learn the way to the breakfast table as one path chosen from many taken, but may be led from the beginning in the way he shall go; one may be so predisposed beforehand that 9×7 always leads to 63. There are nevertheless very many cases where multiple response is the first step in learning. Try as we will to secure the right response at the start and throughout, it cannot always be done. In the pronunciation of a foreign language, in force and coherence in English composition, or in skill at billiards or tennis, the right responses cannot be guaranteed beforehand. Further, where circumstances can with enough care be so arranged that the selection is simply between the right response and doing nothing at all, the labor often outweighs the gain; so that the learner is wisely left to make responses of varying degrees of merit, from which the better are selected by their intrinsic satisfyingness or the social rewards that they bring. Further, we are often careless, or ignorant of means of predisposing the learner beforehand to the right act or thought as a sole response, so that, for example, many a pupil learns that $\frac{1}{4} \div \frac{1}{8} = 2$ only by finding that 2 rather than $\frac{1}{2}$, $\frac{1}{32}$ or 32 is approved by his teacher.

Attitudes, Dispositions, Pre-adjustments or 'Sets.'—It is a general law of behavior that the response to any external situation is dependent upon the condition of the man, as well as upon the nature of the situation; and that, if certain conditions in the man are rated as part of the situation, the response to it depends upon the remaining conditions in the man. Consequently it is a general law of learning that the change made in a man by the action of any agent depends upon the condition of the man when the agent is acting. The condition of the man may be considered under the two heads of the more permanent or fixed and the more temporary or shifting, attitudes or 'sets.'

The facts are obvious, though they have been somewhat neglected by psychologists in the interest of the supposed control of behavior by too simple mechanisms of elementary association on the one hand, and too mystical powers of consciousness on the other. The situation 'a certain printed word' has different effects upon learning, according as the child in question is bent upon reading or upon spelling; the figures $\frac{247}{126}$ obviously determine learning differently according as the pupil is predisposed to copy, to add, to subtract, or to multiply; the same hand provokes one response at cribbage and another at whist.

Carefully observed evidence of the so patent fact of the determination of response by the 'set' of the individual has been reported in connection with the experimental study of the thought-processes by Marbe, Watt, Ach, Messer, Bühler, and others. Naturally enough such experimental study finds that the course of thought is much, more closely determined by the attitude established by the instructions given or problem set, perhaps an hour previous, than by the particular sensations and images that form the bulk of the consciousness of the moment. Anybody may easily secure similar evidence for himself by observing the differences in the responses which a man makes to some one situation after different previous instructions, or in the course of different total tasks.

Still more obvious are the effects upon response of those more permanent attitudes or sets in a man which distinguish him as Englishman or Frenchman, poet or painter, father of a family or celibate, lover or neglecter of music, eager for praise or self-sustained, and the like. The response to any situation is guided by these enduring adjustments of the man as well as by the particular bonds which the situation itself has acquired in his life.

Only a little less obvious should be the fact that the attitude or set of the person decides not only what he will do and think, but also what he will be satisfied and annoyed by. Hunger not only puts certain actual connections in operation: it also makes certain conduction units more ready to conduct. This conditioning of the action of the law of readiness by the man's dispositions appears throughout behavior, though not so directly as its conditioning of gross external responses. The child 'set' on subtracting is less satisfied by thinking of '13' on seeing the $\frac{7}{6}$ than he would have been had he been 'adjusted' to adding. The same state of affairs may be

10

welcomed or rejected, and so have opposite effects on learning, according as one is 'set' toward learning to shoot to kill or to shoot to maim only; or according as one is competing to throw a ball to the utmost distance or is competing to 'throw a player out at the plate.' The player of high ambitions at golf is annoyed by and gradually eliminates shots that the more modestly adjusted man would cherish. A slight alteration of the rules of a game may dispose players to feel wretchedly at a response which their attitude of the year before would have made them welcome. The radical actor who first decided to play Shylock as a tragic rather than a comic character, thereby predisposed himself not only to new facial expressions and gestures, but also to new satisfactions at tears, hushed anxiety and awe in his audience. When, in experiments in association with words, the task being to give a synonym for each, one thinks of a word's opposite, there is often an even impressive distaste and chagrin.

The practical importance of attitudes or sets in both functions—of helping to determine what a man will think or do, and what he will be satisfied or annoyed by—should be obvious also. The child or man must be put in condition to use the situation, and a large part of the theory of education considers precisely this problem of getting him permanently disposed to respond to the subject-matter of instruction by zeal, open-mindedness, scientific method and the like, and temporarily disposed to extract the most value from the particular situations of a given lesson. The Herbartian 'step' of preparation, McMurry's insistence on a definite aim for the pupil, Dewey's doctrines that pupils should feel appropriate needs and take the problem-solving attitude, and Bagley's demand that ideals of general method and procedure should be present as controlling forces in school drills, are notable illustrations.

The Partial or Piecemeal Activity of a Situation.—One of the commonest ways in which conditions within the man determine variations in his responses to one same external situation is by letting one or another element of the situation be prepotent in effect. Such partial or piecemeal activity on the part of a situation is, in human learning, the rule. Only rarely does man form connections, as the lower animals so often do, with a situation as a gross total—unanalyzed, undefined, and, as it were, without relief. He does so occasionally, as when a baby, to show off his little trick, requires the same room, the same persons present, the same tone of voice and the like. Save in early infancy and amongst the feeble-minded, however, any situation will most probably act unevenly. Some of its elements will produce only the response of neglect; others will be bound to only a mild awareness of them; others will connect with some energetic response of thought, feeling or action, and become positive determiners of the man's future.

The elements which can thus shake off the rest of a situation and push themselves to the front may be in man far subtler and less conspicuously separate to sense than is the case in animals. Perhaps a majority of man's intellectual habits are bonds leading from objects which a dog or cat would never isolate from the total fields of vision or hearing in which they appear. Very many of his intellectual habits lead from words and word-series, from qualities of shape, number, color, intent, use and the like, and from relations of space, time, likeness, causation, subordination and the like—elements and relations which would move the lower animals only as the component sounds and relations of a symphony might move a six-year-old destitute of musical capacity and training.

Such prepotent determination of the response by some element or aspect or feature of a gross total situation is both an aid to, and a result of, analytic thinking; it is a main factor in man's success with novel situations; the progress of knowledge is far less a matter of acquaintance with more and more gross situations in the world than it is a matter of insight into the constitution and relations of long familiar ones.

Man's habits of response to the subtler hidden elements, especially the relations which are imbedded or held in solution in gross situations, lead to consequences so different from habits of response to gross total situations or easily abstracted elements of them, that the essential continuity from the latter to the former has been neglected or even denied. Selective thinking, the management of abstractions and responsiveness to relations are thus contrasted too sharply with memory, habit, and association by contiguity. As has been suggested, and as I shall try to prove later, the former also are matters of habit, due to the laws of readiness, exercise and effect, acting under the conditions of human capacity and training, the bonds being in the main with elements or aspects of facts and with symbols therefor.

Assimilation or Response by Analogy.—The laws of instinct, exercise, and effect account for man's responses to new as well as to previously experienced situations. To any new situation man responds as he would to some situation like it, or like some element of it. In default of any bonds with it itself, bonds that he has acquired with situations resembling it, act.

To one accustomed to the older restricted view of habits, as a set of hard and fast bonds each between one of a number of events happening to a man and some response peculiar to that event, it may seem especially perverse to treat the connections formed with new experiences under the same principle as is used to explain those very often repeated, very sure, and very invariable bonds, which alone he prefers to call habits. The same matter-of-fact point of view, however, which finds the laws of exercise and effect acting always, though with this or that conditioning set or attitude in the man, and with this or that element only of the total external situation influential, finds them acting also whether the situation has been experienced often, rarely, or never.

If any learned response is made to the situation—if anything is done over and above what man's original nature provides—it is due to the action of use, disuse, satisfaction and discomfort. There is no arbitrary *hocus pocus* whereby man's nature acts in an unpredictable spasm when he is confronted with a new situation. His habits do not then retire to some convenient distance while some new and mysterious entities direct his behavior. On the contrary, nowhere are the bonds acquired with old situations more surely revealed in action than when a new situation appears. The child in the presence of a new object, the savage with a new implement, manufacturers making steam coaches or motor cars, the school boy beginning algebra, the foreigner pronouncing English— in all such cases old acquisitions are, together with original tendencies, the obvious determiners of response, exemplifying the law stated above.

Were the situation so utterly new as to be in no respect like anything responded to before, and also so foreign to man's equipment as neither to arouse an original tendency to response nor to be like anything else that could do so, response by analogy would fail. For all response would fail. Man's nature would simply be forever blind and deaf to the situation in question. With such novel experiences as concern human learning, however, man's responses follow the law that a new situation, *abcdefghij*, is responded to as *abcdelmnop* (or *abcdeqrstu*, or *fghiabyd*, or the like) which has an original or learned response fitted to it, would be.

The law of response by analogy is left somewhat vague by the vagueness of the word 'like.' 'For situation A to *be like* situation B' must be taken to mean, in this case, 'for A to arouse in part the same action in the man's neurones as B would.' This may or may not be such a likeness as would lead the man to affirm likeness in the course of a logical or scientific consideration of A and B. For example, diamonds and coal-dust are much alike to the scientific consideration of a chemist, but it is unlikely that a person who had never seen a diamond would call it coal-dust as a result of the law of analogy. Science, as we know, is often a struggle to educate the neurones which compose man's brain to act similarly toward objects to which, by instinct and the ordinary training of life, they would respond quite differently, and to act diversely to objects which original nature and everyday experience assimilate.

One obvious set of habits remains to be noted, which often substitute for or alternate with, or combine with, response by analogy. Children acquire early, and we all to some extent maintain, the habits of response to certain novelties in situations by staring in a futile way, saying 'I don't know,' feeling perplexed and lost, and the like. That is, man responds to the *difference* as well as to the likeness in a situation. By original nature differences of certain sorts provoke staring, curious examination, consternation, and the like; by training, differences provoke 'I don't know,' 'What's that?' and the like. The action of any situation, as was noted in the previous volume, is the combined action of its elements. Whatever in it has been bound to certain responses acts, by the laws of habit, to produce the phenomena of assimilation or response by analogy. Its quality or feature of foreignness, bafflingness, true novelty, acts by instinct or habit to produce wonder, confessions of inability, and such questionings as have in the past brought satisfying results in similar cases. We might indeed say that these apparent exceptions to response by analogy really illustrate it, the new novelty being treated as was the old novelty like it.

Associative Shifting.—The same fact—that the response attached by instinct or habit to *abcde* may be made to *abc,* or to *abcfg*—accounts for both assimilation and association shifting. Starting with response X made to *abcde,* we may successively drop certain elements and add others, until the response is bound to *fghij,* to which perhaps it could never otherwise have become connected. Theoretically the formula of progress, from *abcde* to *abcdef* to *abcfg* to *abfgh* to *afghi* to *fghij,* might result in attaching any response whatever to any situation whatever, provided only that we arrange affairs so that at every step the response X was more satisfying in its consequences than balking or doing anything else that the person could do. And the actual extent of associative shifting verifies this theoretical expectation. It is indeed easy to shift desire from intrinsic *desiderata* to dull pieces of printed paper, to shift hatred from truly odious behavior to perfectly smooth and genial words like Progressive, Jew, or Labor Union!

Most important of all cases of this process is the shifting of satisfyingness and annoyingness. The physiological mechanisms by which these potent determiners of behavior can win attachments utterly beyond, and even opposite to, those which original nature prescribes are obscure; but the fact itself is sure. Satisfyingness and annoyingness may, under the limit-

ing condition noted above, be attached to any situation whatever. So, unhappily, man may come to be made wretched by
simple out-door sports, children's merriment, spectacles of
cheerful courage, or the daily panorama of sensory experience.
So, to his very great gain, man may come to welcome productive labor, excellence for its own sake, consistency and
verification in thought, or the symbols of welfare in men whose
faces he can never see.

CHAPTER XII

LEARNING BY ANALYSIS AND SELECTION

ANALYSIS AND SELECTION IN GENERAL

All learning is *analytic.* (1) The bond formed never leads from absolutely the entire situation or state of affairs at the moment. (2) Within any bond formed there are always minor bonds from parts of the situation to parts of the response, each of which has a certain degree of independence, so that if that part of the situation occurs in a new context, that part of the response has a certain, tendency to appear without its old accompaniments. The convenient custom of symbolizing a bond as $S_1 \rightarrow R_1$, or $S_2 \rightarrow R_2$ always requires interpretation as $(S_{1a} + S_{1b} + S_{1c} + S_{1d} \dots S_{1n}) \rightarrow (R_{1a} + R_{1b} + R_{1c} \dots R_{1n})$. Of the elements of a situation some are analyzed out to affect the animal, while others are left; of those so abstracted for efficacy on learning and future behavior, one will be picked out by one neurone group, another by another; although these neurone-groups co-act in making connection with the further response to the situation, they do not co-act indissolubly as an absolute unit, but form preferential bonds.

The bond formed never leads from absolutely the entire state of affairs outside the animal, because the original sensitivities and attentivenesses always neglect certain elements of it, and because acquired interests emphasize the welcome to these or others. This abstraction by taking or leaving, and by giving and denying special potency over further responses, will be described in more detail under Learning by Selection.

Each total situation-response bond is composed of minor bonds from parts of the situation to parts of the response, because man's equipment of sensory neurones is such a set of analytical organs as it is, and because his connecting neurones are such a mechanism as they are for converging and distributing the currents of conduction set up in these sensory neurones. The action set up in sensory neurones by the sight of a smiling mother (call it S_{1a}) plus whatever accessories the

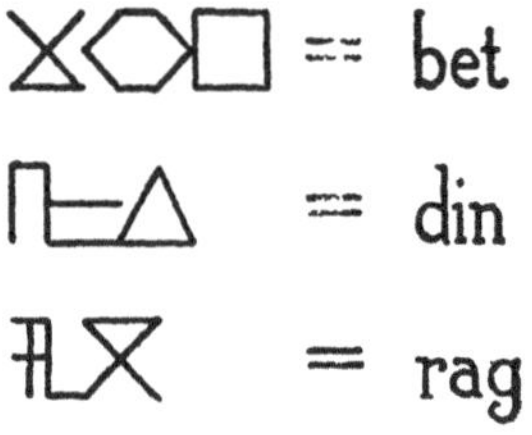

$$X\bigcirc\square \;==\; bet$$
$$\lceil\vdash\triangle \;==\; din$$
$$\dashv\!\!\downarrow X \;=\; rag$$

FIG. 29.

$$\lceil\vdash\triangle$$
$$\dashv\!\!\downarrow X$$
$$X\bigcirc\square$$
$$\dashv\!\!\downarrow X$$
$$\lceil\vdash\triangle$$
$$X\bigcirc\square$$

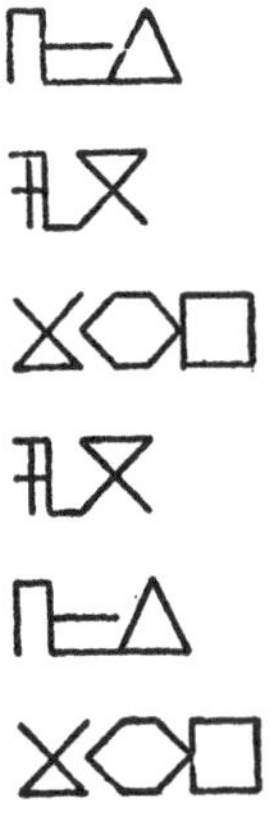

FIG. 30.

total situation contains (call these S_{1b}, S_{1c}, etc.) is as a whole bound to the baby's response, say, of saying mamma in a certain happy way; but the bond from S_{1a} to the 'in a certain happy way' part of the response is somewhat independent of other elements of the total bond. The degree of independence varies enormously. At one extreme is such great interdependence, or intimate co-action, or 'fusion,' in a total bond that the element in a new context retains almost nothing (nothing apparent to external observation) of the connecting tendency

it had acquired in the old context. Thus let the reader memorize the three-pair vocabulary of Fig. 29 so that upon seeing
anyone of the diagrams in a changed order, as in Fig. 30, he
can give the associated word. Let him do this as quickly as
possible. Let him then look at Fig. 31. It is not probable that
he will connect the letters 't r a n d i g' with it, though the
elements of which it is composed were, in order of reading,
connected, in learning the other ten pairs, with t, r, a, n, d, i, g,
respectively. At the other extreme is an independence or
separateness of component bonds within the total bond such
that the element in a new context evokes almost exactly its
old associates. Thus let a man be taught to shut his eyes and
open his right hand as a total response to the situation—*the
field of vision changing from white to red, and simultaneously
his right hand receiving a sharp prick.* Let him also be taught
to keep his eyes open and to close his right hand as a total

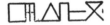

FIG 31.

response to the situation—*the field of view changing from white
to blue and his right hand receiving a cold moist bath.* These
total bonds having been made, it is very likely that if his
right hand received the same prick while the field of view
changed from white to blue, he would open his right hand
without shutting his eyes.

Consider now any part of a situation with which, as a
whole, there is, by original nature or by the action of use,
disuse, satisfaction and discomfort, some bond. When such a
part happens alone* or in a new context, it does, as was stated

* It really never happens alone, being always a part of some total state
of affairs. The *'alone'* means simply that it is a very distinct and predominant element of the total situation.

under the laws of partial activity and response by analogy, what it can. It tends to provoke the total response that was bound to it; it tends especially to provoke the minor feature of that total response which was especially bound to it. If this special preferential bond is strong, it may become the dominant feature of the response to a situation composed of the old element *plus* a new context.

In the lower animals, and in very young children, the situations act more as gross totals; and the combination of connections which we call 'the' bond between the situation and its response acts more as a unit. So, to get a dog to perform a trick, say of jumping up on a box and begging, at the appropriate verbal command, it may be necessary to have not only the words, but also the voice, intonation, sight and smell of the one person; and if he jumps up on the box he may inevitably beg. But even in the lower animals cases of decided preferential bonds of elements in situations with parts of the responses thereto may be found in abundance. In all save stupid men, the training given by modern life results in the formation of an enormous number of bonds with separate elements of situations, some of them very, very subtle elements. This training results also in the power, given the appropriate mental set, of responding alike to an element in almost complete disregard of the contexts of the gross total situations in which it appears. Indeed, the intellectual life of man seems to consist as much in discriminating, abstracting, taking apart, as in associating or connecting. His procedure in learning geometry, grammar, physics or law seems in large measure almost the opposite of his procedure in habit-formation and memory. For a first step in the description of learning, such learning by analysis does need to be distinguished from the mere associative learning, though, as wil be seen later, the same fundamental mechanism accounts for both.

All man's learning, and indeed all his behavior, is *selective*. Man does not, in any useful sense of the words, ever absorb, or re-present, or mirror, or copy, a situation uniformly. He never acts like a *tabula rasa* on which external situations write each its entire contribution, or a sensitive plate which duplicates indiscriminately whatever it is exposed to, or a galvanometer which is deflected equally by each and every item of electrical force. Even when he seems most subservient to the external situation—most compelled to take all that it offers and do all that it suggests—it appears that his sense organs have shut off important features of the situation from influencing him in any way comparable to that open to certain others, and that his original or acquired tendencies to neglect and attend have allotted only trivial power to some, and greatly magnified that of others.

All behavior is selective, but certain features of it are so emphatically so that it has been customary to contrast them sharply with the associative behavior which the last chapter described. A notable case is the acceptance of some one very subtle element of an outside event or an inner train of thought to determine further thought and action. In habit-formation, memory, and association by contiguity, the psychologist has declared, the situation determines the responses with little interference from the man, the bond leads from some one concrete thing or event as it is, and the laws of habit explain the process. In the deliberate choice of one or another feature of the present thought to determine thought's future course, on the other hand, the man directs the energy of the situation, the response which the situation itself would

be expected to provoke does not come, and new faculties
or powers of inference or reasoning have to be invoked.

Such a contrast is almost necessary for a first rough
description of learning, and the distinction of such highly
selective thinking from the concrete association of totals is
useful throughout. We shall see, however, that learning by
inference is not opposed to, or independent of, the laws of
habit, but really is their necessary result under the conditions
imposed by man's nature and training. A closer examination
of selective thinking will show that no principles beyond
the laws of readiness, exercise, and effect are needed to explain
it; that it is only an extreme case of what goes on in associative learning as described under the 'piecemeal' activity
of situations; and that attributing certain features of learning
to mysterious faculties of abstraction or reasoning gives no
real help toward understanding or controlling them.

It is true that man's behavior in meeting novel problems
goes beyond, or even against, the habits represented by bonds
leading from gross total situations and customarily abstracted
elements thereof. One of the two reasons therefor, however,
is simply that the finer, subtle, preferential bonds with subtler
and less often abstracted elements go beyond, and at times
against, the grosser and more usual ones. One set is as much
due to exercise and effect as the other. The other reason
is that in meeting novel problems the mental set or attitude
is likely to be one which rejects one after another response
as their unfitness to satisfy a certain desideratum appears.
What remains as the apparent course of thought includes
only a few of the many bonds which did operate, but which,
for the most part, were unsatisfying to the ruling attitude or
adjustment.

THE SUBTLER FORMS OF ANALYSIS

Stock cases of learning by the separation of a subtle element from the total situations in which it inheres and the acquisition of some constant element of response to it, regardless of its context, are: learning so to handle the number aspect of a collection, the shape of an object, the 'place-value' of a figure in integral numbers, the 'negativeness' of negative numbers, the pitch of sounds, or the 'amount of heat' in an object. The process involved is most easily understood by considering the significance of the means employed to facilitate it.

The first of these is having the learner respond to the total situations containing the element in question with the attitude of piecemeal examination, and with attentiveness to one element after another, especially to so near an approximation to the element in question as he can already select for attentive examination. This attentiveness to one element after another serves to emphasize whatever appropriate minor bonds from the element in question the learner already possesses. Thus, in teaching children to respond to the 'fiveness' of various collections, we show five boys or five girls or five pencils, and say, "See how many boys are standing up. Is Jack the only boy that is standing here? Are there more than two boys standing? Name the boys while I point at them and count them. (Jack) is one, and (Fred) is one more, and (Henry) is one more. Jack and Fred make (two) boys. Jack and Fred and Henry make (three) boys." (And so on with the attentive counting.) The mental set or attitude is directed toward favoring the partial and predominant activity of 'how-many-ness' as far as may be; and the useful bonds that the 'fiveness,' the 'one and one and one and one and one-ness' already have, are emphasized as far as may be.

The second of the means used to facilitate analysis is having the learner respond to many situations each containing the element in question (call it A), but with varying concomitants (call these V.C.) his response being so directed as, so far as may be, to separate each total response into an element bound to the A and an element bound to the V.C.

Thus the child is led to associate the responses—'Five boys,' 'Five girls,' 'Five pencils,' 'Five inches,' 'Five feet,' 'Five books,' 'He walked five steps,' 'I hit my desk five times,' and the like—each with its appropriate situation. The 'Five' element of the response is thus bound over and over again to the 'fiveness' element of the situation, the mental set being 'How many?,' but is bound only once to any one of the concomitants. These concomitants are also such as have preferred minor bonds of their own (the sight of a row of boys per se tends strongly to call up the 'Boys' element of the response). The other elements of the responses (boys, girls, pencils, etc.) have each only a slight connection with the 'fiveness' element of the situations. These slight connections also in large part* counteract each other, leaving the field clear for whatever uninhibited bond the 'fiveness' has.

The third means used to facilitate analysis is having the learner respond to situations which, pair by pair, present the element in a certain context and present that same context with *the opposite of the element in question,* or with something at least very unlike the element. Thus, a child who is being taught to respond to 'one fifth' is not only led to respond to 'one fifth of a cake,' 'one fifth of a pie,' 'one fifth of an apple,' 'one fifth of ten inches,' 'one fifth of an army of twenty

---

* They may, of course, also result in a fusion or an alternation of the responses, but only rarely.

soldiers,' and the like; he is also led to respond to each of these *in contrast with* 'five cakes,' 'five pies,' 'five apples,' 'five times ten inches,' 'five armies of twenty soldiers.' Similarly the 'place values' of tenths, hundredths, and the rest are taught by contrast with the tens, hundreds, and thousands.

These means utilize the laws of connection-forming to disengage a response-element from gross total responses and attach it to some situation-element. The forces of use, disuse, satisfaction and discomfort are so manoeuvred that an element which never exists by itself in nature can influence man almost as if it did so exist, bonds being formed with it that act almost or quite irrespective of the gross total situation in which it inheres. What happens can be most conveniently put in a general statement by using symbols.

Denote by a b, a g, a l, a q, a v, and a β certain situations alike in the element a and different in all else. Suppose that, by original nature or training, a child responds to these situations respectively by $r_1 r_2$, $r_1 r_7$, $r_1 r_{12}$, $r_1 r_{17}$, $r_1 r_{22}$, $r_1 r_{27}$. Suppose that man's neurones are capable of such action that r_1, r_2, r_7, r_{12}, r_{17}, r_{22} and r_{27}, can each be made singly.

Scheme A

	a	b	g	l	q	v	β
r_1	6	1	1	1	1	1	1
r_2	1	1					
r_7	1		1				
r_{12}	1			1			
r_{17}	1				1		
r_{22}	1					1	
r_{27}	1						1

If now the situations, a b, a g, a l, etc., are responded to (each once), the result by the law of exercise will be to strengthen bonds as shown in Scheme A, the situation-elements noted in the top line of the table being bound to each of the response-elements noted at the left side of the table as noted by the numbers entered in the body of the table.

The bond from a to r_1, has had six times as much exercise as the bond from a to r_2, or from a to r_7, etc. In any new gross situation, a θ, a will be more predominant in determining response than it would otherwise have been; and r_1 will be more likely to be made than r_2, r_7, r_{12}, etc., the other previous associates in the response to a situation containing a.

Suppose further that g is opposite to, or notably unlike, b; that q is opposite to or notably unlike 1; and that β is notably unlike v. Let 'opposite to' and 'unlike' have the meaning that the response elements r_2 and r_7, r_{12} and r_{17}, r_{22} and r_{27} are, in the case of each pair, *in no respect identical, and in large measure incapable of being made by the same*

Scheme B

	a	b	g(opp. of b)	1	q(opp. of 1)	v	β(opp. of v)
r_1	6	I	I	I	I	I	I
$r_{not\ 1}$							
r_2	I	I					
$r_{not\ 2}$	I		I				
r_{12}	I			I			
$r_{not\ 12}$	I				I		
r_{22}	I					I	
$r_{not\ 22}$	I						I

organism at the same time. Express this fact by replacing r_7 by r_{not2} r_{17} by r_{not12}, and r_{27} by r_{not22}. Then, if the situations, a b, a g, a l, a q, etc., are responded to each once, the result by the law of exercise will be to strengthen bonds as shown in Scheme B on the opposite page, whose plan is the same as that of Scheme A.

The bond from a to r_1 has again had six times as much exercise as the bond from a to r_2, or from a to r_7, etc. The bonds from a to r_2 and to r_{not2} tend to counterbalance each other in the sense that the tendency is for neither r_2 nor r_{not2} to occur,* the field being left free for whatever unimpeded tendency the element a possesses. Similarly for the effect of the a-r_{12} and a-r_{not12} bonds.

Denote by 'opp. of a' an element which is the opposite of, or at least very unlike, a. Let 'opposite to' and 'unlike' have as before the meaning that the original or acquired responses to 'opp. of a' have few or no elements in common with the responses to a, and in large measure cannot be made by the same organism at the same time as the response to a. Then, if the situations, a b, (opp. of a) b, a g, (opp. of a) g, a l, (opp. of a) l, etc., are responded to each once, the result by the law of exercise will be to strengthen bonds as shown in Scheme C.

The element a is thus made to connect six times with r_1 and once with each element of the counteracting pairs, r_2 and r_{not2}, r_{12} and r_{not12}, r_{22} and r_{not22}. The element opp. of a is made to connect with r_{not1} six times, and with r_2, r_{not2},

---

* They can not occur together. They may occasionally appear in alternation; or the one of them which by casual physiological happenings has an advantage may appear. But the effect of the exercise of the bonds leading from the situations, a b, a g, etc, is to make a call up neither r_2 nor r_7, neither r_{12} nor r_{17}, since another unimpeded bond and response is at hand.

Scheme C

	a	(opp. of a)	b	g(opp. of b)	l	q(opp. of l)	v	β(opp. of v)
r_1	6		1	1	1	1	1	1
$r_{not\ 1}$		6	1	1	1	1	1	1
r_2	1	1	2					
$r_{not\ 2}$	1	1		2				
r_{12}	1	1			2			
$r_{not\ 12}$	1	1				2		
r_{22}	1	1					2	
$r_{not\ 22}$	1	1						2

etc. each once. b, g, l, q, v and β are made to connect with the counteracting r_1 and $r_{not\ 1}$, each equally often. Thus, by the law of exercise, r_1 is being connected with a; the bonds from a to anything else are being counteracted; and the slight connections from b, g, l, etc. to r_1 are being counteracted. The element a becomes predominant in situations containing it; and its bond toward r_1 becomes relatively enormously strengthened and freed from competition.

These three processes occur in a similar, but more complicated, form if the situations a b, a g, etc. are replaced by a b c d e f, a g h i j k, etc., and the responses $r_1\ r_2$, $r_1\ r_7$, $r_1\ r_{12}$, etc., are replaced by $r_1\ r_2\ r_3\ r_4\ r_5\ r_6$, $r_1\ r_7\ r_8\ r_9\ r_{10}\ r_{11}$, etc.—*provided the* r_1, r_2, r_3, r_4, etc. *can be made singly.* In so far as any one of the responses is necessarily co-active with any one of the others (so that, for example, r_{13} always brings r_{26} with it and *vice versa*), the exact relations of the numbers recorded in schemes like Schemes A, B and C on pages 161 to 164 will change; but, unless r_1 has such an inevitable co-actor, the general results of schemes A, B and C will hold good. If r_1 does have such an inseparable co-actor, say r_2, then, of course, a can never acquire bonds with r_1 alone, but everywhere that r_1 or r_2 appears in the preceding schemes the other element must appear also. $r_1 r_2$ would then have to be used as a unit in analysis.

The 'a b,' 'a g,' 'a l,' . . . 'a β' situations may occur unequal numbers of times, altering the exact numerical relations of the connections formed and presented in schemes A, B and C, but the process in general remains the same.

So much for the effect of use and disuse in attaching appropriate response elements to certain subtle elements of situations. There are three main series of effects of satisfaction and discomfort. They serve, first, to emphasize, from the start, the desired bonds leading to the responses $r_1 r_2$, $r_1 r_7$, etc. to the total situations, and to weed out the undesirable ones. They also act to emphasize, in such comparisons and contrasts as have been described, every action of the bond from 'a' to r_1; and to eliminate every tendency of 'a' to connect with aught save r_1, and of aught save 'a' to connect with r_1.* Their third service is to strengthen the bonds productive of appropriate responses to 'a' wherever it occurs, whether or not any formal comparisons and contrasts take place.

The process of learning to respond to the difference of pitch of tones from whatever instrument, to the 'square-root-

---

* Of course a compound bond, say with a x y z , wherein 'a' clearly leads to r_1, and x y z, its concomitants, clearly lead to r_{61} r_{62} r_{63}, may also be confirmed by satisfaction. Suppose, for instance, that 'a' = 'sevenness,' 'x' = 'pencils,' 'y' = 'on the teacher's desk,' and 'z' = 'the general background of illumination, temperature, presence of other children and the like,' and that the response is 'seven pencils on the desk now,' then satisfyingness would strengthen the separate bond between 'a' and r_1 by strengthening the total bond of which it is a loose and largely independent part.

ness' of whatever number, to triangularity in whatever size or combination of lines, to equality of whatever pairs, or to honesty in whatever person and instance, is thus a consequence of associative learning, requiring no other forces than those of use, disuse, satisfaction, and discomfort. "What happens in such cases is that the response, by being connected with many situations alike in the presence of the element in question and different in other respects, is bound firmly to that element and loosely to each of its concomitants. Conversely any element is bound firmly to any one response that is made to all situations containing it and very, very loosely to each of those responses that are made to only a few of the situations containing it. The element of triangularity, for example, is bound firmly to the response of saying or thinking 'triangle' but only very loosely to the response of saying or thinking white, red, blue, large, small, iron, steel, wood, paper and the like. A situation thus acquires bonds not only with some response to it as a gross total, but also with responses to each of its elements that has appeared in any other gross totals. Appropriate response to an element regardless of its concomitants is a necessary consequence of the laws of exercise and effect if an animal learns to make that response to the gross total situations that contain the element and not to make it to those that do not. Such prepotent determination of the response by one or another element of the situation is no transcendental mystery, but, given the circumstances, a general rule of all learning." Such are at bottom only extreme cases of the same learning as a cat exhibits that depresses a platform in a certain box whether it faces north or south, whether the temperature is 50 or 80 degrees, whether one or two persons are in sight, whether she is exceedingly or moderately hungry, whether fish or milk is outside the box. All learning is analytic, representing the activity of elements within a total situation. In man, by virtue of certain instincts and the course of his training, very subtle elements of situations can so operate.

Learning by analysis does not often proceed in the carefully organized way represented by the most ingenious marshalling of comparing and contrasting activities. The associations with gross totals, whereby in the end an element is elevated to independent power to determine response, may come in a haphazard order over a long interval of time. Thus a gifted three-year-old boy will have the response element of 'saying or thinking *two*,' bound to the 'two-ness' element of very many situations in connection with the 'how-many' mental set, and he will have made this analysis without any formal, systematic training. An imperfect and inadequate analysis already made is indeed usually the starting point for whatever systematic abstraction the schools direct. Thus, the kindergarten exercises in analyzing out number, color, size, and shape commonly assume that 'one-ness' *versus* 'more-than-one-ness,' black and white, big and little, round and not round are, at least vaguely, active as elements responded to in some independence of their contexts. Moreover, the tests of actual trial and success in further undirected exercises usually coöperate to confirm and extend and refine what the systematic drills have given. Thus the ordinary child in school is left, by the drills on decimal notation, with only imperfect power of response to the 'place-values.' He continues to learn to respond properly to them by finding that $4 \times 40 = 160$, $4 \times 400 = 1600$, $800 - 80 = 720$, $800 - 8 = 792$, $800 - 800 = 0$, $42 \times 48 = 2116$, $24 \times 48 = 1152$, and the like, are satisfying; while $4 \times 40 = 16$, $24 \times 48 = 832$, $800 - 8 = 0$, and the like, are not. The process of analysis is the same in such casual, unsystematized formation of connections with elements as in the deliberately managed, piecemeal inspection, comparison and contrast described above.

Occasionally an element seems to pop up in a gross total situation and drag its response element out into clear relief, with little or no aid from any such extricating associations as have been described. So Ruger found in solving mechanical puzzles that sometimes a feature of the total situation, hitherto dissolved therein, would apparently suddenly crystallize out and lead to signal success. The usual fact in such cases is that the element already has its preferential minor bond in full working strength, but that this bond is kept inactive because conditions within the man keep him from the particular set of attention or questioning or preliminary action by which the element can get enough prepotency to cause its response.

There is also the possibility that the so called 'accidental' activities (that is, activities of unknown causation) of man's neurones may throw certain elements into relief and bind certain responses to them in ways unpredictable from even a complete schedule of the man's previously formed bonds. Such unearned useful bonds with elements are probably rare, and in any case cannot be profitably discussed, the hypothesis being that we do not know how they are caused.

THE HIGHER FORMS OF SELECTION

In human thought and action a situation often provokes responses which have not been bound to it by original tendencies, use or satisfaction. Such behavior, apparently in advance of, or even in opposition to, instinct and habit, appears in adaptive responses to novel data, in association by similarity, and in the determination of behavior by its aim rather than its antecedents which is commonly held to distinguish purposive thinking and action from 'mere association and habit.'

Successful responses to novel data, association by similarity and purposive behavior are, however, in only apparent opposition to the fundamental laws of associative learning. Really they are beautiful examples of it.

Man's successful responses to novel data—as when he argues that the diagonal on a right triangle of 796.278 mm. base and 137.294 mm. altitude will be 808.022 mm., or that Mary Jones, born this morning, will sometime die—are due to habits, notably the habits of response to certain elements or features, under the laws of piecemeal activity and assimilation.

Nothing, as was hinted in Chapter XI, looks less like the mysterious operations of a faculty of reasoning transcending the laws of connection-forming, than the behavior of men in response to novel situations. Let children who have hitherto confronted only such arithmetical tasks, in addition and subtraction with one- and two-place numbers and multiplication with one-place numbers, as those exemplified in the first line below, be told to do the examples shown in the second line.

Add	Add	Add	Subt.	Subt.	Multiply	Multiply	Multiply
8	37	35	8	37	8	9	6
5	24	68	5	24	5	7	3
—	—	23	—	—	—	—	—
		19					
		—					

Multiply	Multiply	Multiply
32	43	34
23	22	26
—	—	—

They will add them, or subtract the lower from the upper

number, or multiply 3 × 2 and 2 × 3, etc., getting 66, 86, and 624, or respond to the element of 'Multiply' attached to the two-place numbers by 'I can't' or 'I don't know what to do,' or the like, for the reasons stated on page 149; or, if one is a child of great ability, he may consider the 'Multiply' element and the bigness of the numbers, be reminded by these two aspects of the situation of the fact that '$\frac{9}{9}$, multiply' gave only 81, and that '$\frac{10}{10}$ multiply' gave only 100, or the like; and so may report an intelligent and justified 'I can't,' or reject the plan of 3 × 2 and 2 × 3, with 66, 86 and 624 for answers, as unsatisfactory. What the children will do will, in every case, be a product of the elements in the situation that are potent with them, the responses which these evoke, and the further associates which these responses in turn evoke. If the child were one of sufficient genius, he might infer the procedure to be followed as a result of his knowledge of the principles of decimal notation and the meaning of 'Multiply,' responding correctly to the 'place-value' element of each digit and adding his 6 tens and 9 tens, 20 twos and 3 thirties; but if he did thus invent the shorthand addition of a collection of twenty-three collections, each of 32 units, he would still do it by the operation of bonds, subtle but real.

It has long been apparent that man's *erroneous* inferences —his *unsuccessful* responses to novel situations—are due to the action of misleading connections and analogies to which he is led by the laws of habit. It is also the fact, though this is not so apparent, that his *successful* responses are due to fruitful connections and analogies to which he is led by the same laws. It is not a difference in the laws at work, but in the nature of the habits that produce the variations and select from them for the further guidance of thought. The insights of a gifted thinker seem marvellous to us because the subtle elements which are prepotent for his thought elude us; but in the same way our insights into the operations of new machines, new chemical compounds, or new electrical apparatus would seem marvellous to a savage to whom levers, screws, reducing gears, oxygen, hydrogen, electrical energy and electric potential were elements utterly concealed in the gross complexes before him. We should succeed with these novel situations as the savage could not, because we should accentuate different elements, and these elements would have bound to them different associates.

Association by similarity is, as James showed long ago, simply the tendency of an element to provoke the responses which have been bound to it. *Abcde* leads to *awxyz* because *a* has been bound to *wxyz* by original nature, exercise or effect.

Purposive behavior is the most important case of the influence of the attitude or set or adjustment of an organism in determining (1) which bonds shall act, and (2) which results shall satisfy.

James early described the former fact, showing that the mechanism of habit can give the directedness or purposefulness in thought's products, provided that mechanism includes something paralleling the problem, the aim, or need, in question.

The second fact, that the set or attitude of the man help to determine which bonds shall satisfy, and which shall annoy, has commonly been somewhat obscured by vague assertions that the selection and retention is of what is 'in point,' or is 'the right one,' or is 'appropriate,' or the like. It is thus asserted, or at least hinted, that 'the will,' 'the voluntary attention,' 'the consciousness of the problem' and other such entities are endowed with magic power to decide what is the 'right' or 'useful' bond and to kill off the others.

The facts are that in purposive thinking and action, as everywhere else, bonds are selected and retained by the satisfyingness, and are killed off by the discomfort, which they produce; and that the potency of the man's set or attitude to make this satisfy and that annoy—to put certain conduction-units in readiness to act and others in unreadiness—is in every way as important as its potency to set certain conduction-units in actual operation. Whatever else it be, purposive thought or action is a series of varied reactions or 'multiple response.' Point by point in the series, that response is selected for survival and predominant determination of future response which relieves annoyances or satisfies cravings which rule the thinker. In intellectual matters, and in the activities of man that are only indirectly connected with the common instinctive wants, these annoyances and satisfactions and their effect on learning may be, and indeed usually have been, over-looked because they lack intensity of effect and uniformity of attachment. But they should not be. The power that moves the man of science to solve problems correctly is the same as moves him to eat, sleep, rest, and play. The efficient thinker is not only more fertile in ideas and more often productive of the 'right' ideas than the incompetent is; he also is more satisfied by them when he gets them, and more rebellious against the futile and misleading ones. "We trust to the laws of cerebral nature to present us spontaneously with the appropriate idea," and also *to prefer that idea to others.*

CHAPTER XIII

MENTAL FUNCTIONS

Learning is connecting, and man is the great learner primarily because he forms so many connections. The processes described in the last two chapters, operating in a man of average capacity to learn, and under the conditions of modern civilized life, soon change the man into a wonderfully elaborate and intricate system of connections. There are millions of them. They include connections with subtle abstract elements or aspects or constituents of things and events, as well as with the concrete things and events themselves.

Any one thing or element has many different bonds, each in accordance with one of many 'sets' or attitudes, which co-act with it to determine response. Besides the connections leading to actual conduction in neurones, there are those which lead to greater or less readiness to conduct, and so determine what shall satisfy or annoy in any given case.

The bonds productive of observable motor responses—such as speech, gesture, or locomotion, are soon outnumbered by those productive, directly and at the time, of only the inner, concealed responses in the neurones themselves to which what we call sensations, intellectual attention, images, ideas, judgments, and the like, are due. The bonds productive of motor responses also include a far richer equipment than we are accustomed to list. Man's life is chock-full of evanescent, partly made, and slurred movements. These appear in so-called 'inner' speech, the tensions of eyes and throat in so-called intellectual attention, and the like.

The bonds lead not only from external situations—facts outside the man—to responses in him, and from situations in him to acts by which he changes outside nature, but also from one condition or fact or event in him to another and so on in long series. Of the connections to be studied in man's learning an enormous majority begin and end with some state of affairs within the man's own brain—are bonds between one mental fact and another.

The laws whereby these connections are made are significant for education and all other branches of human engineering. Warning is connecting; and teaching is the arrangement of situations which will lead to desirable bonds and make them satisfying. A volume could well be written showing in detail just what bonds certain exercises in arithmetic, spelling, German, philosophy, and the like, certain customs and laws, certain moral and religious teachings, and certain occupations and amusements, tend to form in men of given original natures; or how certain desired bonds could economically be formed. Such would be one useful portion of an Applied Psychology of Learning or Science of Education.*

The psychology of learning might also properly take as its task the explanation of how, starting from any exactly defined original nature, the bonds have been formed which cause the man in question to make such and such movements, attend to this rather than that feature of an object, have such and such ideas in response to a given problem, be satisfied with some of them and reject others, enjoy this picture,

---

* The more elementary and general applications of the laws of learning will be found set forth in such books as Bagley's *Educative Process;* Colvin's *Learning Process;* and the author's *Principles of Teaching.*

abstract numerical relations from a certain state of affairs, and so on through all the acquisitions which his life of learning comprises. Psychology might seek to list the bonds and elements of bonds which account for his habits, associations of ideas, abstractions, inferences, tastes and the rest, might measure the strength of each, discover their relations of facilitation and inhibition, trace their origins, and prophesy their future intrinsic careers and their effects in determining what new bonds or modifications of old bonds any given situation will form. As a geologist uses the laws of physics and chemistry to explain the modifications of the earth's surface, so a psychologist might use the laws of readiness, exercise, and effect to explain the modifications in a man's nature—in his knowledge, interests, habits, skill, and powers of thought or appreciation. This task is, however, one for the future.

The process of learning is one of simple making and keeping connections and readinesses to conduct, but the result is a mixture of organized and unorganized tendencies that, even in an average three-year-old child, baffles description and prophecy. No one has ever even listed the tendencies to respond of any one human creature above that age and of average capacity to learn, nor even begun to trace the history of their acquisition.

What psychology has done is to consider certain vaguely defined groups of tendencies, describing them roughly and observing how they change in certain important respects, notably in their efficiency in producing some desired result in living. The terms, *intellect, character, skill,* and *temperament,* thus more or less well separate off four great groups of connections in a man. Within the sphere of intellect, the terms, *information, habits, powers, interests* and *ideals,* go a step further in delimiting certain groups of connections.

The terms, *ability to add, ability to read, interest in music, courage,* and *business honesty,* are samples of compound tendencies or groups of connections much narrower than those listed above, and cutting across them in many ways. It is such compound tendencies, or groups of connections, or hierarchies of bonds that will be the subject matter of this and the five following chapters.

THE ORGANIZATION OF CONNECTIONS

There are very many points of view from which the total multitude of man's original and acquired bonds may be grouped into 'traits' or 'abilities' or 'functions' or 'compounds of tendencies.' The one most often taken regards human behavior as a means to attain ends, and so expresses the results of learning as 'knowledge of medicine,' 'ability to add,' 'ability to typewrite,' 'skill in drawing,' and the like. But all sorts of facts may be used to cut up the one gross fact of a man's nature, or to bundle together the millions of situation-response bonds which his nature really is. Thus, by relation to objects of importance, we get such traits or functions as a man's knowledge of plants, his politics, or his interests in sports, or his love of the water; by relation to certain elementary features of the world, we get such traits as color-vision, or discrimination of pitch; by relation to the organization already found in man's original nature, we get such groupings as the sexual life, feeding habits, protective responses, and the like. We may even be swayed by the existence of convenient means of measuring behavior, and consequently group man's tendencies into his ability to mark a's, rate of tapping, memory of numbers, accuracy in matching weights, and the like.

Let us then use the term Mental Function for any group

of connections, or for any feature of any group of connections or indeed for any segment or feature of behavior, which any competent student has chosen or may in the future choose to study, as a part of the total which we call a man's intellect, character, skill, and temperament. By so catholic a definition we shall have a convenient term to mean any learnable thing in man, the psychology of whose learning anybody has investigated. We can thus report the psychology of learning in so 'little' a function as *tending to say "jeb nok wif les kig sun" when, in a given total set, "zek pel tus" has been said;* or in so 'large' a function as *ability to read the vernacular,* or even *total knowledge—its quantity, quality, and serviceableness.* To utilize what has been thought and done about the dynamics of human learning, just such a range of report must be made.

In studying mental functions one might begin at the real beginning—man's original nature—and trace each formation of each bond, getting eventually the entire history of each function in terms of original tendencies and environmental circumstances coöperating under the laws of exercise, effect, and readiness. Such a thoroughgoing genetic method would be admirable in intention, but its execution is impossible in our present state of ignorance.

One might insist on analyzing the function into the actual situation-response bonds and readinesses that compose it, so far as that could possibly be done, and studying these, its elements, before attempting to say anything else about the function—for example, about its efficiency as a whole, its improvement by practice, its temporary decrease in efficiency due to illness or excessive exercise, and the like. Such a reduction to constituent bonds and readinesses before any further experimentation is surely often the part of wisdom. It is very much needed, for example, in the case of the school functions —ability to read, ability to spell, ability to add, and the like. As a matter of fact, however, almost all of the investigations of the psychology of learning concern functions unreduced to simple—not to say simplest—constituent connections. Apart from the memorizing of unrelated facts—such as series of numbers or nonsense syllables—the functions that have been studied are for the most part such vague composite ones as adding, multiplication, telegraphy, or typewriting. The results, though probably not so widely significant as those to be expected from studies of learning that is fully analyzed into its elements, are of great importance and give the best information available upon which to base plans for improving and economizing learning in schools, trades, and professions.

CHARACTERISTICS OF MENTAL FUNCTIONS

Mental functions may be 'wide' or 'narrow.' For example, 'ability to spell' differs from 'ability to spell cat;' 'motor control' differs from 'ability to draw a circle' or 'speed in tapping;' 'memory' differs from 'ability to memorize a series of nonsense syllables'—in each case by being a wider, more inclusive, compound or group of bonds and readinesses. There is, theoretically, a variation possible from a function representing a single bond between one situation and one response, or the readiness of a single conduction unit, to a function representing millions of such bonds or readinesses. And the functions actually investigated by psychologists cover nearly as wide a range.

A mental function may involve a single set, or a series of sets, of bonds—may be *'short'* or *'long.'* It is clear that sensitiveness to pain (if in the sense of the least

amount of pressure or electrical shock at a certain spot that
will cause a sensation of pain) differs from ability to draw a
circle or ability to spell cat, in that the series of neural bonds
involved is shorter. It is commonly assumed, at least, that
in the first case the function concerns the working of only
the first sensory neurones and the further connected neurones
leading to the cortical 'centers' in question; in the second and
third cases, the function concerns such first sensory neurones
and their connected neurones as far as the cortical centers,
and thence on to the muscles involved in the drawing, writing,
or speech. In any case, between such functions as sensitiveness to pain or bitter or red and such as executive ability,
power to plan a military campaign, or ability to make a
successful prognosis for a disease, there is this difference in
the number of bonds *in the series,* in the number of connec-
tion-steps between what is taken as the starting situation-group
and what is taken as the ending response-group. The difference in the number of bonds when they are arranged, so to
speak, 'in parallel' being designated conveniently by 'wide'
and 'narrow,' this difference in the number of bonds when they
are arranged 'in series' is conveniently compassed by the terms
'long' and 'short.'

A mental function may be more or less prophetic—may
involve differing proportions of actual and of possible bonds.
The functions, 'ability to spell cat,' 'knowledge that $\sqrt{289} = 17$,'
and 'speed in tapping,' refer to the actual existence of bonds.
The function, 'ability to memorize a series of nonsense
syllables,' refers to the probability that, when certain things
happen, certain bonds will be formed. The terms—skill in
drawing, motor control, business ability, and interest in
mathematics—ordinarily imply something about both the present
existence of some bonds and the future formation, under certain

conditions, of others. Similarly, terms designating functions may refer to the already existent readiness of certain conduction-units—that is, to the already existent tendency to be satisfied by such and such states of affairs; or they may refer to the future existence of that tendency, given certain conditions; or they may refer to both.

A mental function may relate primarily to the form of what is done, or to the content in connection with which something is done. Such functions as 'ability to memorize series of nonsense syllables,' 'delicacy of discrimination,' and 'attention to small details' may be contrasted with such as 'business ability' and 'efficiency in teaching' in that the former are concerned chiefly with the form, and the latter chiefly with the content, of the man's behavior. In the former, the function is defined primarily as operating on facts in a certain way—memorizing them, or discriminating them, or attending to them. In the latter, the function is defined primarily as operating successfully on certain facts, without any close specification of what the form of operation is.

This distinction between the form of a mental function—what it does to the data—and its content—the stuff to which it does something—is not a very useful one. A statement of a function in terms of the content or experiences it works on and the form of operation it exercises on them, has to be translated into terms of actual situations and responses before it can be properly handled in thought or in experimentation. The reason for making the distinction here is that, as a matter of history, psychology began its study of dynamics by assuming 'faculties' of perception, memory, imagination, discrimination. attention and the like, which were supposed to act somewhat indifferently upon many different sorts of content. Consequently, we have, as a heritage, many descriptions of functions—such as 'keen delicacy of discrimination,' or 'slight power of voluntary attention,' or 'excellent memory'—which, if they are to mean anything useful, mean some fact about all possible bonds of a certain formal aspect—the aspect of response to a difference, or the aspect of responding to one element predominantly, or the like. These descriptions play important rôles in arguments concerning the improvement of mental functions and the effect of improving one upon the efficiency of others. The distinction made above will be convenient in dealing with them.

A mental function may consist primarily in an *attitude* or primarily in an *ability*. Some mental functions—such as 'enjoyment of good reading,' 'desire for approval,' or 'misery at being scorned'—refer primarily, or even exclusively, to the satisfyingness and annoyingness of certain states of affairs. Others—such as 'speed in tapping' or 'ability to give the opposites of certain words,' or 'knowledge of Russian'—refer primarily, or even exclusively, to the mere acts or ideas excited by certain situations. Others—such as 'interest in mathematics,' 'appreciation of music,' and 'taste in household decoration'—refer obviously to a compound of tendencies to do this or that, to think this or that, and also to welcome, cherish, or be satisfied by, this and to reject, avoid, or be annoyed by, that.

A mental function refers always to some *actually or possibly observable events in behavior,* not to any mythical entities beneath behavior. Wide or narrow in its scope, short or long in the series of operations which it comprises, recording existing powers or prophesying their existence under given conditions, emphasizing the particular situations to which the man can respond in a certain way or leaving them unspecified, telling what he will do or telling what he will be satisfied by—in every case a mental function concerns some history or prophecy of behavior, and had we knowledge enough, would be found to stand for certain bonds and readinesses in the neurones, or certain probabilities of the appearance under given conditions of certain bonds and readinesses.

THE CONCEPTS OF EFFICIENCY AND IMPROVEMENT

A man may change as a total nature by adding new mental functions to his equipment or by changing the condition of functions already possessed. What we call the same function may exist in countless different conditions. Ability to add may be of a hundred different degrees; knowledge of chemistry may mean a million different things in different men at different times, according to just what concrete facts and powers the knowledge comprises in each case.

Education is especially interested in *changes* in the condition of a mental function, and more especially in the total change in it which makes it better or worse—more or less desirable from the inquirer's point of view. We wish to know what a certain training has done to 'improve' A's ability to add, or knowledge of chemistry, or power to reason, or appreciation of music. Consequently a change in the condition of a mental function in any given man is very often described in terms of so much 'gain' or 'improvement' or 'increase in efficiency,' or as so much 'loss' or 'deterioration' or 'decrease in efficiency.'

Each of the two conditions of the function by comparing which the change is described is, in such a case, judged as to its efficiency—its success, actual or possible, in attaining some end—the quantity and quality of some product produced by it—its value from some point of view.

Just exactly what we mean when we say that John Smith writes better than he did last year, or has gained in self control, or has lost skill in billiards from lack of practice, or has improved ten per cent in memory for nonsense-syllables—is a matter of importance in every case. Scientific treatment of John Smith's learning demands that the two degrees of efficiency and the difference between them be so identified that all competent thinkers can have in mind the same facts.

The terms, efficiency, improvement, and deterioration, mean, of course, something somewhat similar in all these cases. Otherwise competent students of psychology and education would not so use them. Their meanings also obviously vary somewhat with the functions respecting which they are used—efficiency in self control, for instance, being in fact different from efficiency in memory for nonsense syllables. Both in their similarities and in their diversities, they need critical examination.

The efficiency of a mental function in a given man at a given time is, as a rule, to be defined and measured by the quantity and quality of some product produced by the man under certain defined conditions. Improvement in it then means, and is measured by, the increase in the quantity or quality of the product produced under the same external conditions, or the maintenance of equal quality and quantity under more adverse conditions.* In the experiments on learning whose results are to be studied here, the external conditions have been kept as nearly identical as the experimenter could keep them, so that improvement is shown in the quantity or quality of the product produced.

The quantity and quality of the product produced—words

*Or by some net balance of superiority to the earlier performance in quantity, quality and power to combat adverse conditions.

remembered, sums done, letters made on the typewriter, puzzles solved, lines translated, and the like—are represented by some sort of score or scores. Thus, Book measured the improvement made in learning to typewrite by the gain in the number of "strokes" made. "Each letter and mark of pronunciation, not requiring a shift of the carriage, was counted as one stroke; striking the word-spacer was counted as half a stroke; making a capital or any mark requiring the use of the 'shift key' was counted as two strokes; moving the carriage back to make a line was counted as three strokes." The improvement made by school-children in adding has been measured by the number of examples (each of ten one-place numbers) added, with a discount of half an example for each wrong answer. Improvement in spelling may be measured by the difficulty of the words that can be spelled, a person being scored 25 if he can just spell words as hard as '*he*'; 30, if he can just spell words as hard as "*will*"; 35, if he can just spell words as hard as "*for*"; 50, if he can just spell words as hard as "*they*" and "*every*"; 60, if he can just spell words as hard as "*also*" and "*penny*"; and so on.

Since our thinking about efficiency, improvement and deterioration is in terms of such scores, it is always desirable to keep in mind just what the score really means. Thus, if we use the score last mentioned and find that certain children improve in spelling in the first half of the year from 25 to 35, and, in the last half, from 35 to 50, and so state that the gain the second half-year was 15 or one and one-half times the gain during the first half-year, we should ourselves remember and inform others, that the 15 really means "from words as hard as '*for*' to words as hard as '*they*' and '*every*'" and that the 10 means "from words as hard as '*he*' to words as hard as '*for*.'" A mere gain in score by itself alone may be ambiguous or even misleading.

Consider, for example, these cases: From fifty letters written per minute to one hundred—from fifty dollars earned per month at typewriting to one hundred dollars—from fifty words written per minute to one hundred—from fifty per cent of correct judgments of the difference in length of two lines, 100.0 and 100.1 mm. long, to one hundred per cent of correct judgments.

The first gain is one that any literate and fairly intelligent adult can make, and can make in a very few hours of practice; the second is a gain that only a small percentage of stenographers ever make; the third is a gain that nobody has ever made. In all these, the 'fifty' means some positive amount of ability, but in the fourth it is a true zero.   In the fourth, the change is from 'just not any' ability, or the ability that an idiot might display (mere chance producing fifty correct judgments), to an ability which no eyes and brain can anywhere nearly approach.   Not only the numerical relations of the amounts, not only the slope of the curve, but also the actual facts of behavior denoted by the score must be considered in every case.

CHAPTER XIV

THE AMOUNT, RATE, AND LIMIT OF IMPROVEMENT

PRACTICE CURVES

The most convenient means of representing the amount of improvement made in the course of a given amount of practice is by a 'practice-curve,' or line whose height at successive points represents the scores made in successive tests. Thus, in FIG. 32, each sixtieth of an inch along the horizontal, or base-line, or abscissa, represents one minute of practice in typewriting, the vertical line at the left is a scale for the score (words written per minute), and the heights of successive portions of the practice curve itself show, for each successive practice period, the score achieved, rising from 6.3 words per minute to 24.7 words per minute. FIG. 33 shows the same fact, being identical with FIG. 32 in every respect save that the practice curve is constructed by joining the mid-points of each of the horizontal sections of the curve of FIG. 32.

In the following pages the improvement in tossing balls, in typewriting, in addition, in writing German script, in shorthand, in re-writing words using a key whereby for each letter a certain number is written, and in marking the A's on sheets of printed capitals is shown in such practice-curves. An examination of these will give a general sense of the facts. In examining them one should note the amount of time spent in

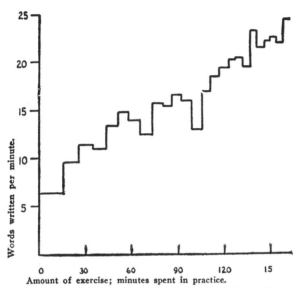

FIG. 32. Improvement in Typewriting the Same Paragraph of 100 Words. Written Once Daily. Abscissa = Time Spent in Practice: Ordinates = Amounts of Product per Unit of Time.

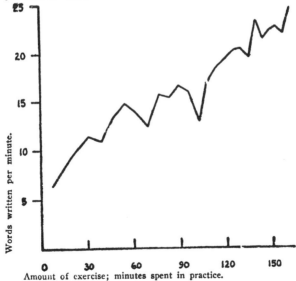

FIG. 33. Same as FIG. 32, but Using Mid-Points over Each Division of the Abscissa-Length corresponding to One Practice Daily.

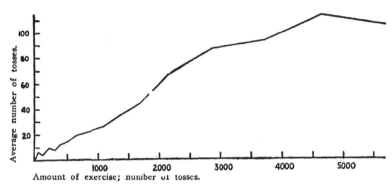

FIG. 34. Improvement in Tossing Balls: Subject F. The Average Number of Tosses without Failure in Each Successive Practice Period. (The horizontal scale is for the amount of exercise of the function, as measured by the number of tosses.)

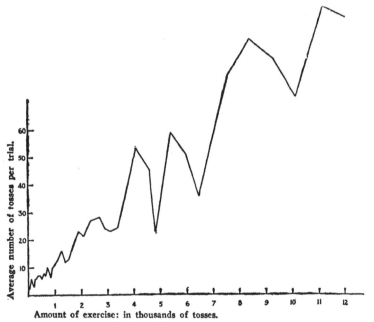

FIG. 35. Improvement in Tossing Balls. Subject A. Same Arrangement as in FIG. 34.

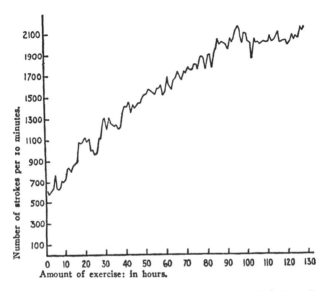

FIG. 36. Improvement in Typewriting by the Touch Method: Subject *V*, After Book, '08, Plate opposite p. 21.

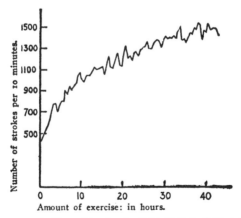

FIG. 37. Improvement in Typewriting by the Sight Method: Subject Z. After Book, '08, Plate opposite p. 21.

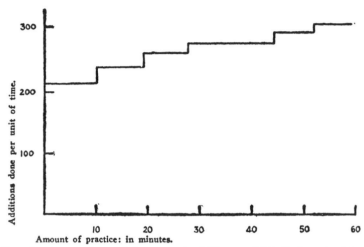

FIG. 38.   Average Curve of Improvement of Nineteen Adult Students in Column
Addition of One-Place Numbers.

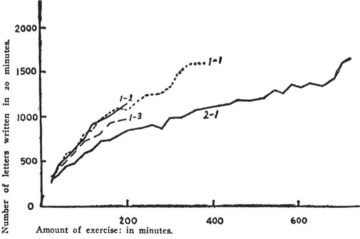

FIG. 39.   Improvement in Writing English Words in German Script.   Four Groups of
Women Students.   After Leuba and Hyde, '05, p. 362.   (The curves marked 1-1,
1-2, 1-3 and 2-1 give the improvement for the groups practicing 20 minutes once a
day, 20 minutes once in two days, 20 minutes once in three days, and 20 minutes
twice a day respectively.)

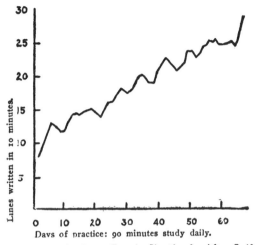

FIG. 40. Improvement in Copying a Text in Short-hand. After Swift, '03, p. 226.
A line equals   line of James *Talks to Teachers*, or about eight and a third words.

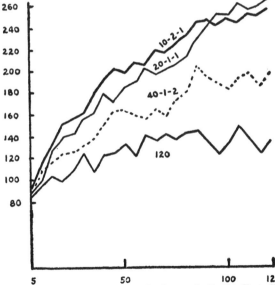

FIG. 41. Improvement in Writing Numbers for Letters in English Text: Four Groups
of College Students. After Starch, '12, p 212. (The curves marked 10-2-1,
20 1-1, 40-1-2, and 120 are for the groups practicing 10 minutes twice a day, 20
minutes once a day, 40 minutes every other day, and 120 minutes all in one period,
respectively.) The abscissa does not start at zero, but at 5 minutes.

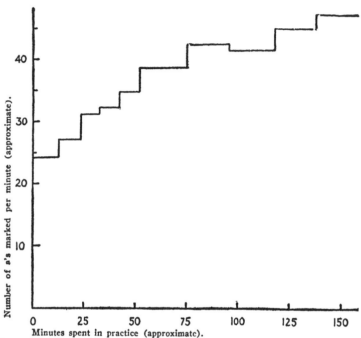

FIG. 42. Average Curve of Improvement of Nine Women Students in Marking a's in Regular Text, No Page Being Used Twice. Computed from Data Given by Whitley, '11, p. 120 ff. (The scores given by Whitley are somewhat complicated, and the curve drawn here is therefore only an approximation.)

connection with the amount of improvement made. Unless otherwise noted, this time was spent, a few minutes a day over many days. I report here also one sample of the results obtained from practice in the case of school-children under school conditions.

Kirby ['13] tested over 700 children in grade 4 before and after sixty minutes spent in practice at column addition* of

* The arrangement in the case of addition was 75 minutes practice in all, the work of the first and last fifteen minutes being compared. This comparison gives, then, the approximate effect of sixty minutes of practice.

ten one-place numbers. They changed from an average score of approximately 31 columns, 24 columns being added correctly, to a score of approximately 50 columns, 37 being added correctly. That is, they gained over fifty per cent in speed, maintaining almost exactly the same accuracy. This work was done under school conditions as an educational experiment, and it was possible for any child to spend time outside in practice with addition. It is unlikely that many children did this, however. Kirby's results have been confirmed by Hahn ['13].

Kirby also tested over 600 children in grade 3 before and after fifty minutes practice with division, * using printed blanks of mixed example such as:

$50 = $ __ 6s and __ remainder $\qquad 29 = $ __ 3s and __ remainder
$43 = $ __ 7s and __ remainder $\qquad 35 = $ __ 4s and __ remainder

The children changed from an average score of about 40 examples, with 37 correct, to a score of about 73 examples with 70 correct. They nearly doubled the amount done without any decrease in accuracy. Like the addition experiment, this is subject to possible, but probably very slight, influences from work done outside the practice periods themselves.

THE FREQUENCY AND RAPIDITY OF IMPROVEMENT UNDER
EXPERIMENTAL CONDITIONS

So far as I am aware of the facts, no mental function has ever been deliberately practiced with an eye to improv-

---

* The arrangement in the case of division was 60 minutes practice in all, the work of the first and last ten minutes being compared. This comparison gives, then, the approximate effect of fifty minutes of practice.

13

ing it, and with proper opportunity for the law of effect to operate, without some improvement as a result. There have been cases where one investigator has failed to find improvement, but where others have found it. There have been cases, of course, where certain individuals failed to improve. And there may be cases of zero improvement unreported because the investigator, finding no result from practice, said nothing about it. On the whole, however, it seems fairly safe to say that all functions that anyone is likely to ever take any theoretical or practical interest in are improvable unless the general practice of life has already put them at their limit; and that the latter case is very rare.

The rate of improvement shown in experiments with practice seems, and to some extent is, in sharp contrast to the rate shown by children in schools, workers at trades, and all of us in the learning of ordinary work and recreation. For example, let the reader get intelligent men and women to estimate the degrees of efficiency that they would expect, on grounds of general experience as workers or teachers or both, to be attained in the cases described in the following tabular arrangement (Table 1). Have the last line of each division of the table kept hidden from them. Then compare their estimates with the efficiencies actually attained in experiments on practice, shown in the last line of each division of the table. Or let the reader consider that if he should now spend seven hours, well distributed, in mental multiplication with three-place numbers, he would thereby much more than double his speed and also reduce the number of his errors; or that, by forty hours of practice, he could come to typewrite (supposing him to now have had zero practice) approximately as fast as he can now write by hand; or that, starting from zero knowledge, he could learn to copy English into German script at a rate of fifty letters per minute, in three hours or a little more.

TABLE I.

THE FACTS OF THREE TYPICAL EXPERIMENTS ARRANGED TO ALLOW
ESTIMATES OF THE AMOUNT OF IMPROVEMENT, AND COMPARISON
OF THESE WITH THE ACTUAL IMPROVEMENT

I.

Function.—Addition, of one-place numbers, each being orally announced.

Individuals.—Ten hospital nurses, 21-35 years old.

Initial Ability.—Number of one-place numbers added in five minutes; 180, 200, 225, 225, 290, 150, 220, 235, 250, 260.

Length of Practice.—2 hours, 25 minutes.

Distribution of Practice.—5 minutes daily except Sunday.

Ability after Practice.—Number of one-place numbers added in five minutes.

——, ——, ——, ——, ——, ——, ——, ——, ——, ——.
380, 430, 368, 460, 540, 280, 380, 570, 440, 540.*

II.

Function.—Addition of columns, each of ten one-place numbers, the sum of each column being written.

Individuals.—College and university students: the seven most ordinary out of nineteen individuals.

Initial Ability.—Number of one-place numbers so added in five minutes (counting the writing of a two-place answer as equal to one addition). 225, 232, 240, 244, 257, 257, 261.

Length of Practice.—Approximately 55 minutes.

Distribution of Practice.—Daily, for so long as was required to add 48 columns: from 10 down to 6 minutes as practice progressed.

Ability after Practice.—Number of one-place numbers added in five minutes.

——, ——, ——, ——, ——, ——, ——.
304, 417, 317, 400, 306, 374, 378,†

III.

Function.—Marking a's on two pages of English print.

Individuals.—Nine college students.

---

* These correspond respectively, to the ten initial abilities listed above.

† These correspond, respectively, to the seven initial abilities listed above.

Average Initial Ability on second day after one preliminary test of
two pages —In terms of time required, 527 seconds.
Average Length of Practice —2⅙ hours.
Distribution of Practice.—Daily for 17 days.
Ability after Practice,—348 seconds.

DIFFERENCES AMONGST INDIVIDUALS IN THE RATE OF IM-
PROVEMENT IN THE SAME FUNCTION

Individuals differ very greatly in the rate of improvement
in the case of every function where adequate measures are at
hand.   Kirby found that the gain in amount of addition done
(in 15 minutes) which resulted from sixty minutes' practice,
varied from below zero to over sixty 10-digit examples.   The
distribution of these gains is shown in Table 2.   The variation
was as great in the case of the individual gains in division.
Of course some of the extreme gains are due in part to a
record in the first trial that is, by sickness, misunderstanding
or some other irrelevant factor, unfairly low; or to a final
record that is, by an exceptionally favorable concatenation of
circumstances, unfairly high; or (but much more rarely) by
a conjunction of these two chances in the same individual.
If we allow generously for this, by supposing that in reality
no child would improve less than 10 per cent and that the
amendment of high records *down* is the same as this of low
records *up*, we still have a very wide variation, approximately
that shown in Table 3.

The causes of these individual differences in improvement may be considered under three heads: (1) differences
in methods of work which can be taught to one person as
well as to another, or somewhat nearly as well; (2) differences
in previous training which, at any given time, must be accepted,

TABLE 2.

INDIVIDUAL DIFFERENCES IN RATE OF IMPROVEMENT IN ADDITION (after Kirby ['13]). The Frequencies of Various Amounts of Difference between the Number of Examples Done Correctly in 15 Minutes *before* 45 Minutes of Practice and the Number Done Correctly in 15 Minutes *after* 45 Minutes of Practice: in the Case of 503 Pupils of Grades 4 and 5, the 45 Minutes Being Divided into 2, 3 or 7 Periods

A loss of 15 to 12 10-digit examples occurred in 4 individuals
" " " 11 " 8 " " " " 9 "
" " " 7 " 4 " " " " 24 "
" " " 3 " 0 " " " " 49 "
" gain " 1 " 4 " " " " 65 "
" " " 5 " 8 " " " " 72 "
" " " 9 " 12 " " " " 80 "
" " " 13 " 16 " " " " 61 "
" " " 17 " 20 " " " " 64 "
" " " 21 " 24 " " " " 17 "
" " " 25 " 28 " " " " 20 "
" " " 29 " 32 " " " " 18 "
" " " 33 " 36 " " " " 11 "
" " " 37 " 40 " " " " 9 "
" " " 41 " 44 " " " " 2 "
" " " 45 " 48 " " " " 4 "
" " " 49 " 52 " " " " 2 "
" " " 53 " 56 " " " " 0 "
" " " 57 " 60 " " " " 1 "
" " " 61 " 64 " " " " 2 "

but which could have been prevented; and (3) differences in original nature which must be accepted and allowed for. It is of the utmost importance to the educational theory of any function that the individual differences in rate of improvement in it should be referred to their specific causes along these three lines. Unfortunately, systematic measurements of individual differences in rate of improvement are few in number, and an experimental analysis of causes has hardly been begun. At present we know only that differences in original nature are responsible for much of the variation found.

TABLE 3.

INDIVIDUAL DIFFERENCES IN RATE OF IMPROVEMENT IN ADDITION.
The Facts of Table 2, after Large Allowances Are Made for Accidental Divergences of the Obtained Measures from the True Improvability of the Individuals Concerned: Approximate.

A gain of 1 to 4 examples correct occurred in 13 individuals
"   "   "   5 "   9   "   "   "   " 73   "
"   "   " 10 " 14   "   "   "   " 137   "
"   "   " 15 " 19   "   "   "   " 141   "
"   "   " 20 " 24   "   "   "   " 81   "
"   "   " 25 " 29   "   "   "   " 38   "
"   "   " 30 " 34   "   "   "   " 20   "
"   "   " 35 " 39   "   "   "   " 6   "
"   "   " 40 " 44   "   "   "   " 2   "
"   "   " 45 " 49   "   "   "   " 3   "

THE LIMIT OF IMPROVEMENT

The limit of efficiency of a mental function is, of course, rarely reached in experimental studies, save in the case of extremely 'narrow' functions, such as knowing the meaning of one or a few words, being able to repeat a poem, or typewriting a single sentence. The best illustrations of mental functions at their limit of efficiency are to be found among those occupations of work or play excellence in which is sought with great zeal and intelligence. The championship 'records' in typewriting, shorthand, telegraphic sending, golf, billiards, and the like, show approximations to the limits of improvement in the functions concerned in the case of individuals gifted by nature probably with specially high limits in the cases in question.

The feats of such experts—who can typewrite 70 words containing approximately 350 letters per minute, take down the most rapid speech without an error, send 49 words or 486 separate impacts on the telegraph key in a minute, keep four balls tossing in the air with one hand, multiply any number less than 1000 by any similar number in a few seconds, drive a golf ball over two hundred yards within an angle of ten degrees, and the like,—are doubtless beyond what the majority of men could ever achieve. Such expertness is the product of a rare native ability as well as of long, intelligent and earnest practice. On the other hand, the efficiency possible in any one such function in the case of an ordinary person, who gives enough time and interest to well-advised practice in it, is, I am convinced, often underestimated. The main reason why we write slowly and illegibly, add slowly and with frequent errors, delay our answers to simple questions and our easy decisions between courses of action, make few and uneven stitches, forget people's names and our own engagements, lose our tempers, and the like, is not that we are doing the best that we are capable of in that particular. It is that we have too many other improvements to make, or do not know how to direct our practice, or do not really care enough about improving, or some mixture of these three conditions.

It is my impression that the majority of men remain far below their limit of efficiency even when it is decidedly in their interest to approach it, and when they think they are doing the best that they are capable of. I venture to prophesy that the thousand bookkeepers in, say, the grocery stores of New York who have each had a thousand hours of practice at addition, are still, on the average, adding less than two-thirds as rapidly as they could, and making twice as many errors as they would at their limit. It appears likely that the majority of teachers make no gain in efficiency after their third year of service, but I am confident that the majority of such teachers could teach very much better than they do. Even in a game where excellence is zealously sought, the assertion that "I stay at just the same level, no matter how much I practice" probably does not often mean that the individual in question has really reached the physiological limit set for him in that function.

I cannot prove the assertions made in the last two paragraphs, since the experiment of subjecting such individuals to practice under proper conditions of methods and interest has not been made. Nor can I give the evidence that has led to the assertions, since it includes too many fragmentary facts from too wide a variety of sources. Only a few samples of the facts that seem to me to show that men in general thus fall short of their possible efficiencies can be quoted.

First, hardly any functions have ever been practiced in the course of the scientific study of mental functions, which did not improve and, provided they were of fairly narrow scope and with success and failure easily distinguishable, at a fairly rapid rate.

Second, there are striking cases of individuals who have had enormously long practice, as taken in the course of schools or trades, and who have kept at the same level of efficiency for a long time, but who, under more favorable conditions, make notable advances. For example, Aschaffenburg ['96 b.] had four experienced type-setters set type for an hour and a quarter, on each of four successive days, in their own shop, with their own type, etc. Either they held back in the early days for no intelligible reason, or they improved notably under the stimulus of an observer and the zeal to make a good showing.

The first and third were 'normal' days; on the second and fourth alcohol was administered, but not till after the first quarter-hour. The achievement, in terms of letters and spaces 'set' in the first quarter hour of each day, was as follows:

DAY		INDIVIDUAL			
	F S.	K O C.	C H.	J L.	AVERAGE
1	577	524	599	600	575
2	649	506	601	614	593
3	601	598	669	664	633
4	725	594	656	723	675

Third, a new stimulus to interest and effort, or a new method of training, often produces a similar advance in the ordinary work of the world. For example, the record in the pole-vault has risen in a score or so of years by many inches. This can only be explained by supposing that the pole-vaulters of twenty years ago could have vaulted much higher than they did, had they used better methods, or more zeal, or both. Probably the jugglers of the past thought that keeping three balls tossing and balancing a chair on one's nose were the limits to skill until some one did keep four balls tossing or balance a chair on an umbrella on his nose. They then found that they too could do likewise.

It seems to me therefore that mental training in schools, in industry and in morals is characterized, over and over and over again, by *spurious limits*—by levels or plateaus of efficiency which could be surpassed. The person who remains on such a level may have more important things to do than to rise above it; the rise, in and of itself, may not be worth the time required; the person's nature may be such that he truly cannot improve further, because he cannot care enough about the improvement or cannot understand the methods necessary. But sheer absolute restraint—because the mechanism for the function itself is working as well as it possibly can work— is rare.

CHAPTER XV

THE FACTORS AND CONDITIONS OF IMPROVEMENT

THE ELEMENTS IN IMPROVEMENT

We may start with the gross changes in efficiency as scored, and analyze them back into the elements which constitute them, or we may start with the elementary changes found in the simplest facts of learning and show how certain of these facts, when happening together in a certain way, produce the gross changes in efficiency as scored. Both procedures lead, I believe, to the same conclusion—that improvement is the addition or subtraction of bonds or the addition or subtraction of satisfyingness and annoyingness. When any function is improved, either some response is being put with, or disjoined from, some situation; or some state of affairs is being made more satisfying or more annoying. The rise of the practice curve parallels the growth of a system of habits, attitudes and interests.

The addition of bonds may be apparent in external behavior, as when the adder comes to connect $\frac{47}{32}$ directly with the thought of 79; apparent *via* the learner's report, as when the adder comes to connect $\frac{4}{8}$ directly with the thought of 20; or hidden in the nervous system, and observable only in the form of secondary consequences, as when the adder comes to get the response 'thought of 79' to the situation $\frac{47}{32}$, nine hundred and ninety-nine times out of a thousand instead of nine hundred and ninety.* So also for the subtraction of bonds; as in the cases, respectively, of one ceasing to write down the amount he has to 'carry'; of one ceasing to say to himself '— and — are —;' and of one getting the response 'thought of 79' to the situation $\frac{47}{32}$ in one second instead of eight seconds.†

Strengthening and *weakening* could have been used in the foregoing in place of 'addition of' and 'subtraction of.' Adding a bond is simply strengthening it *from zero strength up;* strengthening a bond is simply adding to it *piecemeal.* Subtracting a bond is weakening it to zero, and weakening it is subtracting from it piecemeal.

When one bond is weakened and another, to take its place, is simultaneously added, we have the common case of improvement by substituting a superior response.

The addition and subtraction of satisfyingness and annoyingness may also be apparent in external behavior, apparent *via* the learner's report, or observable only by one who had a view of the inner workings of the nervous system. When the sincere learner ceases his complaints at the task, choosing to memorize nonsense syllables rather than read the story he would before have infallibly preferred, all competent observers judge that the balance between the satisfyingness and the annoyingness of the state of affairs in question has changed. Or he may, without external signs other than speech, report to them an increase in zeal as each syllable is fixed. Or a certain conduction-unit in his brain may increase its readiness to conduct, but to so small an extent, or in connection with such other hap-

---

* The inner process here might be in whole or in part, one of subtracting bonds.

† The inner process here might be, in whole or in part, one of adding bonds.

penings, that he has no witness to the fact in the form of an observable increase in felt satisfaction at the felt state of affairs corresponding to that conduction-unit's conduction.

The physiology and psychology of welcoming and rejecting, liking and disliking, being content and being annoyed, have received little attention, and their role in improvement has been described only vaguely as the total fact that the person 'lost his aversion to the work' or 'gained zest for success' or the like. Everyone can, however, see their importance in the improvement of abilities like the production of music or writing English, a large part of which consists in being able to be satisfied by the good elements of what one produces, and so to reject the bad. Such cherishing and rejecting is potent also in adding, typewriting, playing billiards, and the like. Everywhere practice may not only bind the right response to a certain situation, but also teach us to be satisfied by their connection. In playing golf the satisfyingness of the sight of one's ball speeding down the course spreads to make the way one held and moved the club a little more satisfying as a response to the situation which provoked the stroke; and this makes for improvement as truly as does an actual strengthening of the bond between the situation provoking the stroke and the stroke. For, in playing golf, we do not necessarily meet each situation by the position or movement which has the closest bond with the situation, but select from several the one which feels right to us as we execute it. We may direct each stage in the club's swing to make it, in the expressive slang, 'feel good to' us. The same rejection of one satisfying response after another occurs in all mental production. Even in what seems to be a fluent sequence of sheer connecting without selection, all the responses being equally satisfying (as in expert adding), there will be found this same varied reaction and selection. Slight tendencies to think of other matters or to relax the wide-awakeness to 'combinations' do appear. Nipping these in the bud and being satisfied by unremitting devotion to the proper task is an element in speed, and the greater satisfaction thereat is consequently an element in improving speed.

EXTERNAL CONDITIONS OF IMPROVEMENT

The conditions of improvement may best be reviewed under four heads—External conditions, such as length of practice period, time of day, amount of food, and the like; Physiological conditions, such as dosing with alcohol or caffein or attack by certain diseases; Psychological conditions, such as interest and worry; and Educational conditions, such as the organization of the practice drills and the methods of work taught to the learner.

Of the external conditions, I shall discuss, as a sample problem, the *Distribution of Practice*—the length of the practice periods and of the intervals between.

The same total amount of exercise of a function, say ten hours, may of course be distributed in an infinite number of ways. The practice-periods may be ten of 60 minutes, or twenty of 30 minutes, or forty of 15 minutes, or five of 60 minutes followed by ten of 30 minutes, or a series running 100 min., 80 min., 60 min., 50 min., 40 min., 35 min., 30 min., 25 min., 25 min., 25 min., followed by thirteen, each of 10 min., etc. Each such division of the practice time may be made with any one of countless arrangements of the intervals between. For any given function, in a given individual, at a given stage of his general training and special advancement in the function, and under given coöperating and hindering conditions external to the function itself—the best distribution could be found. 'Best' would, it is understood, be defined as best for the immediate improvement of the function, or as best for its permanent efficiency, or as best for the total welfare of the learner in question, or in some intelligible way.

It might be that some simple laws would hold good for all functions at all stages of advancement in all individuals regardless of coöperating circumstances. Thus, it might be that period-lengths of from ten to twenty minutes were universally better, from any point of view, than longer or shorter period lengths; and that intervals of 24 to 48 hours were universally better, whatever the period-length, function, person and the like, than longer or shorter intervals. Or it might be that the optimum interval was universally one of twenty times the period length. Or it might be that the nearer a function was to its limit, the shorter the optimum period length became and the longer the optimum interval became.

The experimental results obtained justify in a rough way the avoidance of very long practice-periods and of very short intervals.* They seem to show, on the other hand, that much longer practice-periods than are customary in the common schools are probably entirely allowable, and that much shorter intervals are allowable than those customary between the first learning and successive 'reviews' in schools.†

* What period-length shall be considered 'very long' depends on the amount of variety and satisfyingness the function shows. Two hours is thus a very long period for addition or learning 32-syllable nonsense series, but perhaps not for playing golf or chess.

What interval between periods shall be considered 'very short' depends on the length of the periods themselves, and also on the character of the function. For adding practiced in twenty-minute periods, an interval of five minutes would be very short, and probably also one of five hours. The knowledge which would enable one to define the statement made in the text is lacking.

† 'PRACTICE-PERIOD' here does not refer to the entire recitation-length,

In the case of addition and division the matter of length of practice-period has been studied by Kirby ['13] for periods up to 20 minutes with some thirteen hundred children of the third and fourth grades.

The arrangement of Kirby's experiments in addition was as follows:

School Day		Group 22 1/2	Group 15	Group 6	Group 2
	1	15 min.	15 min.	15 min.	15 min.
" "	2	22½ "	15 "	6 "	2 "
" "	3	22½ "	15 "	6 "	2 "
" "	4	15 "	15 "	6 "	2 "
" "	5	....	15 "	6 "	2 "
" "	6	....	..	6 "	2 "
" "	7	....	..	6 "	2 "
" "	8	....	..	6 "	2 "
" "	9	....	..	3 "	2 "
" "	10	....	..	15 "	..
" "	11	....	..		and so on for 22 days*
" "	24	....	..	..	15 min.

The arrangement of Kirby's experiments in division was as follows:

School Day		Group 20	Group 10	Group 2
	1	10 min.	10 min.	10 min.
" "	2	20 "	10 "	2 "
" "	3	20 "	10 "	2 "
" "	4	10 "	10 "	2 "
" "	5	..	10 "	2 "
" "	6	..	10 "	2 "
" "	7	..	..	2 "
" "	8	..	..	2 "
" "	9	..	..	and so on for 20 days
" "	22	..	..	10 min.

but to that fraction of it devoted to drill in one function like the multiplication-table of nines, or the spelling of the names of the States, or speed in hand-writing, or rehearsing a ten-word vocabulary, or oral practice on the use of the article in German. The customary length for such units of learning is probably about five minutes

* The last of these practice days had a period of three minutes.

These experiments were made from the practical point of view, from which it is immaterial how much the children study the matter that is being practiced outside of the school hours. If we assume that they did so as much when the practice periods were distributed in many short periods as when they were distributed in few long periods, the results show that the shorter practice-periods, especially the two-minute periods, are much more advantageous. It must, however, be remembered that this assumption is almost surely somewhat in error, except for the one case of *no* practice at all out of school. If the children practiced themselves at all out of school, they would probably do so to a greater extent in four weeks than in one.* The gross superiority of the shorter over the longer periods may therefore be discounted somewhat, and be held subject to further investigation.

The results of these experiments were as follows:

In addition, the gains from practice in 22½-, 15-, 6-, and 2-minute periods, respectively, were in the relation 100, 121, 101 and 146½. In division, the gains from practice in 20-, 10-, and 2-minute periods, respectively, were in the relation 100, 110½ and 177.

PSYCHOLOGICAL CONDITIONS OF IMPROVEMENT

It should be an obvious consequence of the nature of improvement that the fundamental psychological conditions for it are that some chance be given for desirable bonds to be added or for undesirable bonds to be destroyed. Amplification or elimination must occur if there is to be any change.

The mere exercise of any modifiable function almost

---

* The improvement due to regular school work would also be greater for the groups who practiced for short periods and so over more days.

always results in some variations, but *whatever stimulates variation* gives the chance of a wider range of useful variations for the learner to adopt or reject. Ruger notes that in solving mechanical puzzles, good learners would occasionally manipulate the puzzle at random with the hope that some chance position of it would suggest variations in attack, or would deliberately seek to change their assumptions about the puzzle with the same end in view.

Whatever stimulates relevant, promising bonds will be still more favorable. Thus, to quote Ruger again, the efficient learner is characterized by special care in examining his assumptions so as to let only those which are themselves sound be potent in producing new bonds.

The selection of desirable bonds, once they have appeared at all, and the elimination of undesirable ones, are not at all necessary consequences of the mere exercise of a function. Many men in many functions let occasional advantageous practices lapse and perpetuate blunders with perverse zeal. When a function is so exercised that the consequences to the individual are alike when he fails and when he succeeds, when he strengthens a good bond and when he strengthens a bad one, when he works above his average rate and when he works below it—there can be only chance divergences from a confirmation of his initial status. So a poetical hermit, utterly devoid of literary taste, might write no better lyrics year after year. So, in fact, men who care nothing about the beauty of their speech and are not subjected to social pressure, say millions of words without improving in accent, timbre, syntax or style. So, in experiments in judging which of two weights, of 100 and 101 grams, is heavier, the record being kept secret and no other source of influence on the function than its own exercise being allowed, the subject cannot improve.

14

*Whatever does favor the repetition and satisfyingness of
the desirable bonds, and the disuse and annoyingness of the
undesirable bonds,* will, other things being equal, favor improvement. The most noteworthy psychological conditions
of improvement come under this head—are means of directing the forces of use and satisfaction in favor of desirable
and against undesirable bonds. Three of these—ease of
identification of the bonds to be formed or broken, ease of
identification of the states of affairs which should satisfy or
annoy, and ease of application of satisfaction or annoyance
to them—are direct consequences of the laws of learning and
may be described first. The next five, which we may call
the 'interest series'—interest in the work, interest in improvement, an active, inquiring attitude, attention, and acceptance
of the work as significant to the worker's wants—are potent
partly because they help to produce variations, still more because they produce relevant and desirable variations, but most
of all, perhaps, because they reinforce the good, and eliminate
the bad ones.

What is meant by 'ease of identification of the bonds to be
formed or broken,' 'ease of identification of the states of affairs
which should satisfy (or annoy),' and 'ease of application of
satisfaction (or annoyance) to them,' can be understood best
by illustrations. To improve in addition, subtraction, multiplication and division, is on the average, easier for the same
person than to improve in solving 'problems.' One reason
is that in the former the bonds to be made or strengthened are
(except in the case of the selection of the trial quotient
figures in long division) rigidly defined and subjected to exclusive practice as needed. Another reason is that the results
that should satisfy (accurate answers and greater speed) can
also be easily identified and accompanied by some satisfier in

the form of approval, shortened time of work, or even some extrinsic reward. In the solution of problems, the learner cannot so easily tell what particular bonds he has to form, drill himself in these alone, know in detail what connections should content him and how to make himself feel contented at them.

To improve in the formal matters of spelling, punctuation, syntax, approved usage, and the like, is easier than to improve in force, clearness and general literary attractiveness, partly because in the former the connections to be made and avoided can be known and exclusively exercised, and the activities that are theoretically desirable can be designated, recognized when they occur and made satisfying at the time to the actor. In the latter, it is hard to see just what connection in thought does the good or the harm in question, so as to make it and be glad at it, or be annoyed with it and avoid it. So great is the difference in improvability here that the greater part of the teaching of English writing in high-schools does not even pretend to improve the subtler general qualities of imagination, humor, force, and beauty. In the rare cases where definite situation-response connection making for 'style' can be identified, controlled and rewarded or punished, we do get rapid improvement in so far forth. For example, one of the greatest aids in teaching the subtler virtues in composition is a set of clear rules such as 'Do not begin a sentence with *and* more than once a month.' Stiff and restrictive as such rules are, they can create definite bonds in behavior, and definiteness of bonds favors improvement.

Typewriting is extremely improvable, while handwriting is rather repugnant to improvement. The chief reason seems to be, as before, that in typewriting the connections between letters and words and the required series of movements are more noticeable, efficient ones are more readily distinguished from inefficient, and efficiency is more readily stamped with approval.

The conditions which I have called the 'interest-series' have not been subjected to direct quantitative experiment. Consequently few new facts can be reported here about them. They have been recognized, though not measured, by the psychologists who have directly observed the process of learning, as, for example, in the following quotations.

"The development of this habit of rapt attention or interest, and the acquisition of a generally favorable feeling-tone is as important for learning as the development of any of the 'habits of manipulation' described above." [Book, '08, p. 71 f. and p. 74]

"In the experiments on ball-tossing and on shorthand writing, and typewriting, monotony was found to be an important factor in the rapidity with which skill was acquired, and the same condition was observed in this work. Periods of monotony alternated with periods of pleasure in the work, and, at times, of keen enthusiasm. While, as has been said, it is not probable that the depression associated with the monotony caused the plateaus, it seems quite reasonable that it prolonged them. Generally, though not always, this feeling of discouragement corresponded with the plateaus of the curve, and it is an interesting fact that returning pleasure and confidence sometimes prophesied a new advance." [Swift, '06, p. 309]

No one probably doubts that interest in the exercise of a function—liking to add, or typewrite, or learn nonsense series, or whatever the work may be—favors improvement at it. Such statements as those quoted above appeal to our common sense as probably true, though they have not been fully verified by actually comparing learning with and learning without intrinsic interest in the matter learned.

No one who has thought the matter out probably doubts that interest in the improvement itself—satisfaction at gain, and annoyance at backsliding—favors improvement. Such statements as the following would not be disputed:

"It seemed to be the strong desire to write with the utmost speed, strengthened in some cases by the thought of the value or worth of the experiment, that pushed the learners into these new and more economical ways of writing." [Book, '08, p. 96]

"If one continues to commit errors through ignorance of the fact that they are errors, he may retard his development by falling into habits of unsound play; but if they are noted as errors, and especially if they arouse a strong emotion, they are eliminated." [Cleveland, '07, p. 303]

"The mind is (in effective learning) attentive to success in the-thing-to-be-done." [Swift, '10 a., p. 151]

Direct evidence and measurements to verify such statements are lacking. Evidence of the potency of interest in the task and in improvement at it can be got indirectly by comparing (a) the improvement made in a function when the experiment is designed to measure improvement and the learner is thereby led to be concerned with the gain in his score with (b) the improvement made in the same function when the experiment is designed to measure the effect of drugs, of pauses of different lengths, of the curve of work, and the like, and the learner is likely to be less concerned with the gain in his score. No one has ever made such a comparison; and it cannot be made conveniently or elegantly. Making it as well as may be, we find good reason to assign a large favorable effect to interest in the function and in its improvement. For the gain seems to be very much greater in the former case.

The three remaining doctrines of the 'interest series,' I need only mention. The doctrine so brilliantly and earnestly defended by Dewey, that school work must be so arranged as to arouse the problem-attitude—to make the pupil feel needs and work definitely to satisfy these—would probably be accepted by all, at least to the extent of agreement that pupils will progress much faster if they do approach work with needs which its accomplishment satisfies, and with problems whose solutions its accomplishment provides. The general principle of modern educational theory that school tasks must be significant at the time to those doing them—that a pupil must have some aim in work to give his work meaning—would also probably be accepted by all, at least to the extent of belief that pupils will improve faster in work the nature and purport of which they comprehend, than in mere serial intellectual gyrations accomplished slavishly and mechanically. Most orthodox of all is the doctrine that the attentive exercise of a function will produce more rapid improvement than exercise of it with attention directed elsewhere.

To these five commonly accepted aids to improvement—interest in the work, interest in improvement, significance, problem-attitude and attentiveness—we may add two that would perhaps be disputed—the absence of irrelevant emotional excitement, and the absence of worry.

There is a conflict of theories and of practices with respect to the value of emotional fervor in learning. In the case of intellectual functions, the balance of opinion is that apart from the eager but quiet zest for the work itself and for success in it, all emotional excitement is distracting —that not only violent love, grief, humiliation and disgust, but also even moderate fear of onlookers, exultation at success and anger at competitors or at oneself, are to some

extent wastes of eneigy and preventives of improvement. In the case of moral functions, such as learning to work energetically, or to tell the truth, or to be just to pupils or employers, the balance of opinion is rather toward the view that appropriate emotional fervor provides a reinforcement. A violent feeling of hate, with idleness as its object, is supposed to make one form the habit of work; a soul-stirring, passionate love of truth favors truth-telling; conscious excitement over the equality of men creates justice. Certain practices in religious and moral revivalism seem even to advocate getting men emotionally stirred in any way whatever, on the chance of then directing this fervor toward good ends.

In the case of improvement in skill, the balance turns again toward freedom from all the crude emotional states and even from all the finer excitements, save the intrinsic satisfyingness of success and the firm repudiation of errors which can hardly be called exciting.

My first statement begged the question by using the phrase *'irrelevant excitement,'* the conflict between theories being precisely about what emotional stirrings *are* irrelevant. The conflict awaits experimental decision, but the evidence seems, to me at least, to show (1) that *all* emotional excitement is, *per se,* irrelevant, (2) that its only value is as a cause of, or symptom of, the satisfyingness of the improvement in question and the annoyingness of the failure, and (3) that it is inferior as a cause thereof to the same general frame of mind *minus* the emotional excitement.

The evidence seems to show, first, that we must distinguish the general disposition or set or attitude of a man—toward the response of flight, attack, avoidance, kindliness, idleness, or the like—from the emotional excitement which often does, but may not, accompany the attitude. Attention has been

called in the earlier chapters to the fact that the inner conscious perturbations may be left out without injuring the rest
of the instinctive response, and that the intensity of the former
may be a very poor measure of the vigor of the latter. In
the case of acquired habits, the fact is even clearer. The
real total attitude of zeal for, say, a game of cards—the set
of mind which makes a person study the game, make sacrifices
to play it, and the like—may be far more vigorous in a person
who feels no conscious thrills than in one who plays with an
inner tempest of felt enthusiasm. The general disposition to
avoid lying may be far stronger in a man who feels no excitement when a chance to lie profitably occurs than in a man
who on such an occasion thrills with conscious disgust or
disdain.

In the second place, the original attachments whereby, say,
'to feel rage at' does imply rejecting and 'to feel love for'
does imply welcoming, may be broken. The original correlations between the inner excitements of love, disgust and the
like and the attitudes of being satisfied and being annoyed may
be altered, so that either feature of the original behavior-
complex may exist without the other. A man may boil with
rage at idleness while idly boiling with rage and being content to idly boil. A man may, *per contra,* be so annoyed by
idleness as never to indulge in it and always try to cure it
without, in the traditional sense of the terms, feeling rage or
disgust or scorn or any other vehement inner passion.

In the third place, the mere quality of conscious excitement is astonishingly alike in all the exciting emotions, is
astonishingly irrespective of the direction of activity, and so
is, to an astonishing extent, irrelevant to learning (except on
the theory that a general diffuse indifferent stimulation is
desirable). We may not admit that excitement and depres-

sion, tension and calm, and satisfaction and discomfort, are all that there can be to an emotion on its conscious side, but we must admit that examination of emotional conditions discloses that what mostly differentiates equally vehement rage, scorn, and elation, say, is the tendency *to do different things and be satisfied by different resulting states of affairs.* What differences there are in the *merely emotional* consciousness in question turn out to be minor facts—surprisingly so to one brought up in the belief that rage, scorn, and elation, as inner states of consciousness, are as different as red, green and blue.

In the fourth place, the most expert and successful learners show least emotional excitement in connection with the exercise of the function which they are improving. Those who achieve most and advance most rapidly, whether in mathematics, science, music, painting, self-control or devotion, are, on the average, characterized by less inner turbulence at their work than those of low performance and slow progress. Moreover the same individual becomes, on the average, less excited in his work, the better he learns to work. The natural selection and elimination of methods of mental work which goes on in successful workers seems to eliminate emotional excitement.

Finally, in the cases where emotional excitement shows the greatest probability of being necessarily bound to rapidity of improvement, the excitement is not great, and seems to be produced by the interest and success rather than to produce them. Some excitement is of course produced by any mental activity, just as restraint from all activity tends to produce depression. Also both satisfyingness in general and success in particular are exciting. But being stimulated by working well is theoretically and practically a very, very different fact from working well because of emotional stimulation.

All the facts concerning the relation of emotional excitement to improvement therefore seem to be explained best by supposing that the interest in the function's exercise and improvement is the active force—emotional excitements being indirectly of value if they produce interest, and of value as symbols in so far as they are produced by it. They probably do not produce effective interest so often as has been supposed, the dynamic power of each emotion over behavior being able to exist without the crude inner excitements. When without them, the interest is less tiring and distracting, and so more efficient.

Much the same sort of arguments could be reviewed in the case of worry or tension. Other things being equal, tension or worry simply wastes energy and distracts the mind, offering so much friction to overcome. Zeal, satisfaction at success and annoyance at errors, can be present with a relieved state of mind as well as with one wrought up to tension by emulation, dread of failure and the like; better, in fact, for the independence of interest from its crude primitive tensions is even more easily shown than its independence from primitive excitements. It is true that some individuals seem to need to be made to worry in order to be led to work, but the only real and economical cure for their defect lies in arousing greater intrinsic interest by better motives rather than by more tension—in better mental nourishment, as it were, rather than an increased dose of a drug.

Active mental life in the prosecution of intellect, morality, and skill can go on with no greater excitement than its own progress provides and with no greater tensions than the cheerful alertness of quiet interest. Emotional peace and relaxation seem indeed, as I interpret the facts of behavior, to be, in and of themselves, always favorable to improvement.

EDUCATIONAL CONDITIONS OF IMPROVEMENT

Under the *Educational Conditions* of improvement all the conditions which school authorities provide might be treated. Their arrangement of the school program would then lead us back to conditions of time of day, length of practice periods and intervals and the like which have been described under *External Conditions*. Their management of heat, light, and ventilation, their isolation of children affected by contagious diseases, and the like, would lead us back to the *Physiological Conditions*. Their selection and arrangement of subject-matter and their methods of teaching would lead us back to the *Psychological Conditions* of interest, freedom from worry, easy identification of bonds and the like, which have just been described. The relation of the time-schedule and school hygiene to improvement need not be discussed here, but the relation of selection and arrangement of subject-matter and of methods of guiding the pupils' responses to their rate of improvement will give a useful review and clarification of certain principles already stated, and introduce us to a new and important one.

Assuming the acceptance of a certain aim for a pupil's exercise of a given function, the selection, arrangement and presentation of subject-matter, and the approval, criticism and amendment of the pupil's responses, are means of getting the pupil (1) to try to form certain bonds rather than others, (2) to form them in a certain order, (3) to identify more easily* the bonds he is to try to form, (4) to be more satisfied at the right bond, and more unready to repeat the wrong bonds, (5) to be more satisfied by the general exercise of the function,

* 'More easily' means throughout, 'more easily than he would have done if left to his own devices.'

and (6) to be more satisfied by general improvement in it.

Educational effort of any sort will show these six functions. I choose a few illustrations at random. The question concerning the desirability of giving the pupil lists of answers to his examples and problems in arithmetic is a case of balancing (3) and (4) against (1). If the answers are there the pupil can tell what he is to do and whether he has done it better, but he may cheat—that is, form no right bonds at all.

The main changes of the last score of years in the teaching of modern languages in this country offer one huge illustration of (1) and (2). In modern-language teaching we have changed from one selection and ordering of bonds to another—from arranging the subject-matter as *a set of general principles and paradigms in a grammatically convenient system, with minor exercises applying this system to reading, writing, and speaking,* to arranging it as *a multitude of separate usages in an order determined largely by interest and the opportunity offered for the formation of associations in the way in which they will be used.*

The various 'methods' in teaching beginners to read differ according to which bonds, and which order of bonds, they favor. The diacritical marks have been dropped from phonic drills, because it became clear that the gain from (3) the pupil's knowledge of just what bonds he was to form was outweighed by (1) the fact that the bonds formed were not nearly so valuable as bonds leading from the sight of a syllable as it appeared in ordinary print. Beginning with a real story such as the *Three Bears,* rather than with isolated words and short easy sentences, is advocated on the ground that the gain from (4), (5) and (6) outweighs the loss in (2) and (3). The acting out in movement what is read, and the statement of it by the pupil in his own words, are found profitable, not only because of the interest they add, but also because they teach the beginner (3) that reading is connecting not only sounds, but meanings, with certain black and white visual details.

The use of drills with a time-limit in arithmetic proves useful especially because of (6). The power of good reading to improve a pupil's speech and writing is a witness to (3) and (4), and also, by a connection not often recognized, to (1). The connection is through *inner speech;* since the pupil, in at least eight cases out of ten, says to himself what he reads, and says to himself what he is going to write, he is being actually drilled somewhat in good speaking and writing by his reading.

'Home' geography as an introduction in place of the proofs of the earth's oblate sphericity, was a change in (2) due to a just suspicion that (1) the bonds formed in the older introductions were often merely verbal, and that the process of making them required very remote and artificial means to (4), (5) and (6).

The educational guidance of learning emphasizes the kind of bonds formed more than does the unaided practice of the learner left to himself. The graded, propaedeutic and ancillary exercises of a good text-book in arithmetic, for example, and its variety of drills and applications, represent a range of selection and an amount of rejection of possible bonds to be formed that would surprise any one unacquainted with the experimentation in the teaching of arithmetic during the past four centuries. This emphasis on the kind of bonds is wise. There is no surer means to improvement than to learn only what is necessary for it; and no surer waste than to form with great labor useless or irrelevant bonds. Yet even a gifted learner, in even a function relatively free from false and blind alleys, will, if left to himself, often go astray.

One new principle is shown by the arrangement of subject matter as a condition of improvement, it being, of course, the principle of *order* or *sequence* of bonds. It might, perhaps, as well have been listed among the psychological conditions, but is shown more clearly by the organization of text-books and courses of study than by the procedures of learners left to themselves.

Contrast in this respect what a pupil eight years old would do if left to learn to add a series of four or five numbers like 46, 73, 17, 80 and 9, as one is left in the ordinary practice-experiment, with what he is led to do in school. In the latter case, the bonds between the words, *one, two, three* and *four,* and their meanings as names for collections of certain numbers of objects and as names for certain magnitudes in relation to certain units, are reviewed, strengthened, broadened and refined. Meanwhile similar bonds are created with *six, seven, eight, nine* and *ten,* and each successive integer is firmly associated with 'the preceding integer—and one more.' The single additions to those with 9 as the sum are learned and verified by counting. The figures (1, 2, 3, 4, etc.) are meanwhile connected with the words and used to replace them in the bonds so far formed. The meaning of *adding* and of *equal* and the use of the $\frac{4}{5}\frac{2}{3}\frac{5}{2}$ positions are given appropriate connections. The situations $\frac{3}{2}\frac{2}{1}\frac{2}{2}$, each accompanied by the addition attitude, are connected each with its appropriate series of responses.

The symbols visual and oral, *eleven, 11, twelve, 12,* etc., up to one hundred, are connected each with its meaning, as 'so many tens and so many ones.' An adequate sampling of the situations $\underset{36,}{52}\ \underset{41,}{37}\ \underset{33,}{63}\ \underset{43,}{46}\ \underset{26,}{72}$ etc., each accompanied by the addition attitude, are connected with their appropriate responses, the old single-addition bonds serving. The bonds between certain situations and the responses of writing single and two-place numbers in columns and adding them are formed, along with the bonds of the adding processes themselves. The bonds of column addition without carrying are

extended to situations like $\frac{21}{23} \frac{22}{21} \frac{11}{41} \frac{22}{11}$; and then to situations
 $^{14}_{}$ $^{34}_{}$
$\frac{21}{24}$ $\frac{22}{13}$ $\frac{11}{12}$ and $\frac{34}{21}$

like $\frac{3}{49}$ $\frac{62}{5}$ $\frac{3}{43}$ $\frac{2}{41}$ $\frac{32}{2}$ and $\frac{3}{64}$. The bond between o and
'not any, no' is formed; and then the associations: '5 and o are 5,' 'o and 4 are 4,' and the like. The bond between the sight of o in column addition and 'going ahead as if it were not there' is formed, and exercised in examples like

$\frac{20}{30}$ $\frac{50}{40}$ $\frac{20}{4}$ $\frac{26}{20}$ $\frac{10}{30}$ and $\frac{14}{40}$; and so, on and on, through the acquisition of bonds up to 18 as a sum, then of bonds with the higher decades, the responses here being largely oral.

These bonds are introduced and exercised partly by counting by 2's, beginning with o and 1, by 3's beginning with o, 1 and 2, by 4's beginning with o, 1, 2 and 3, etc. Then 'carrying' is associated with the essential element with which it belongs, care being taken that the numbers to be carried include *two* and *three* as well as *one;* and enough special bonds involving 'carrying' are formed to give the process general utility. Special bonds are made when o is to be 'written down,' and 1, 2, 3, etc. 'carried.'

The order of formation of bonds in the systematic training of schools is probably often pedantic and over-systematized; of the countless orders possible, many may be almost equally favorable to improvement; the order resulting from the unplanned trials and variations of a learner following inner impulses and outer suggestions with no guidance other than his previous learning and zeal to improve, may be more favorable to improvement than any which education has devised for the training of the function in question. These facts, however, do not contradict, but rather illustrate, the statement that the order of exercise of the particular bonds does condition improvement.

CHAPTER XVI

CHANGES IN RATE OF IMPROVEMENT

ILLUSTRATIVE CASES

Consider FIG. 43 which gives the number of additions of a one-place to a one-place number made in five minutes on each of thirty days of practice by four adults (averaged). It is clear that the gain in speed is greater for the first than for the second half of the practice. There is, in general, a *negative acceleration* shown by the parabolic form of the curve. Contrast this with FIG. 44, which gives the average practice curve for twenty-three women students in translating English text by replacing each letter by another in accordance with a specified 'key.' The gain in speed here during the last half of the practice is equal to, or a little greater than, that made during the first half. There is *zero acceleration* or a *slightly positive acceleration.*

Consider also FIG. 45 which shows the improvement in the number of letters per minute read off from the telegraph key's clicks in successive tests made during thirty-six weeks of practice. There is here a rapid gain for about twelve weeks, then a period of very little gain—a so-called *'Plateau,'*—and in the last twelve weeks a renewed rapid gain.

Consider finally FIG. 46. This shows in general a negative acceleration such as was very clear in FIG. 43, a *'long-time fluctuation'* in the shape of a change from rapid gain to very slow gain (from the 20th to the 45th hour of practice) fol-

15

lowed by a second period of rapid gain (from the 45th to the 55th hour of practice), and also many 'short-time fluctuations' or minor ups and down in the curve.   If the curves of FIGS. 43, 44 and 45 were replaced by the separate curves for the

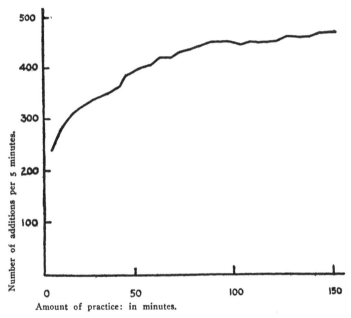

FIG. 43.   Improvement in Addition of One-Place Numbers.

single learners concerned, they too would show similar short-time fluctuations.   FIG. 47, for example, shows the four individual curves (the four highest up) of which FIG. 43 is the average.

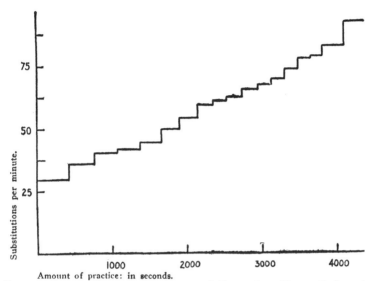

FIG. 44. Average Curve of Improvement of Twenty-three Women Students in Substituting Letters for Letters.

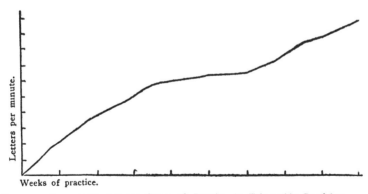

FIG. 45. Approximate Average Curve of Practice in Telegraphic Receiving.

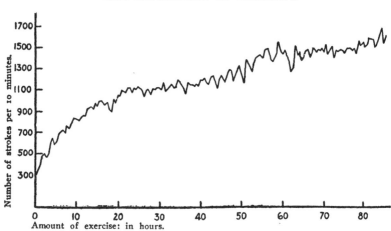

FIG. 46.   Improvement in Typewriting by the Sight Method: Subject X.   After
Book, '08, Plate opposite p. 21.

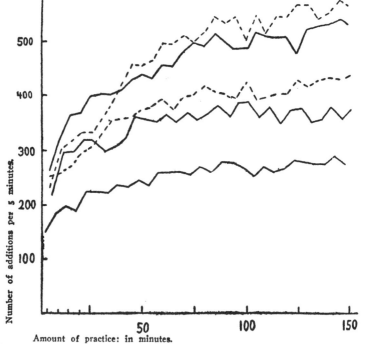

FIG. 47.   Improvement in Addition of One-Place Numbers: Five Adult Women-
After Wells, '12, Plate II, following p. 82.

These facts—that the rate of improvement changes, becoming less as practice advances, and showing long-time fluctuations such as the 'plateau,' and short-time fluctuations from week to week and day to day, appear often in experimental studies of the improvement of mental functions, and may be expected to appear often in the learning of schools, trades and professions. Such changes in the rate of improvement, that is, the form of the practice-curve, are the result of (1) the *number* of bonds, by making (or destroying) which the function is improved, (2) differences in the *ease of formation* (or destruction) of these bonds, (3) differences in the *order of formation* of the bonds, (4) differences amongst them in *effect on the score*, (5) differences at different periods of the practice, in the individual's *general power to improve the function*, (6) the *effect of the formation of one bond upon the condition of other bonds*, (7) the weakening of bonds by *disuse*, and (8) the *overexercise of bonds*. The facts can be best understood by considering certain specially arranged cases of learning.

THE CAUSES DETERMINING CHANGES IN THE RATE OF IMPROVEMENT

Case 1.

Assume: (1) that the total improvement in a function from x efficiency to the maximum efficiency is due to a given number (n) of bonds to be formed: (2) that each of these bonds is equally easy to form, requiring time t at the individual's maximum power; and (3) that each of them has an equal effect (k) in raising the score. Assume that (2) and (3) hold regardless of what order the bonds are formed in. Assume: (4) that only one bond is being formed at any one time in practice, and (5) that no effect on the score results from the formation of a bond until it is completely formed. Assume (6) that work is always done at maximum power and that 'maximum power' is a constant throughout.

Then the curve of practice will be a pure 'staircase,' with equal steps, each of k height, the number of steps being n, the total improvement nk, the total time nt. If n = 8, and the initial efficiency, $x = 4\ k$, the practice curve will be as in Fig. 48.

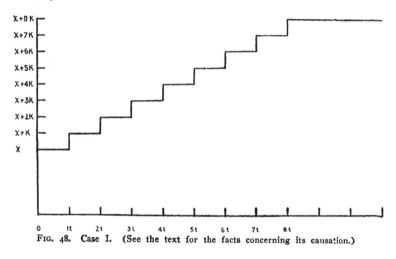

FIG. 48. Case I. (See the text for the facts concerning its causation.)

Case 1 a.

Assume as in Case 1, except that, in place of (5), it is assumed that each equal fraction of time spent at the person's maximum power upon any bond is, until the bond is completely formed, equally effective on the score. Then, the other conditions remaining the same, we have a straight-line slope till the limit is reached, as in FIG. 49.

Case 1 b.

Assume as in Case 1 a, except that any number of bonds can be being formed in the same time, the power forming one bond in time *t* being able to half form two bonds, or quarter form four bonds, or one tenth form ten bonds, etc., in an equal time. Then we still have FIG. 49.

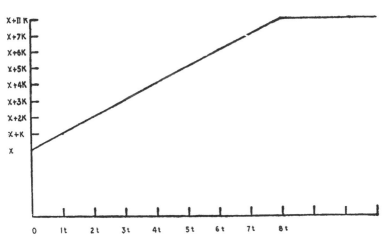

FIG. 49. Cases Ia and Ib. (See the text for the facts concerning its causation.)

Case 1 c.

Assume Case 1 a, or Case 1 b, but let *n* be infinitely large. Then we have FIG. 50, in which the straight line representing zero acceleration is supposed to extend infinitely.

Case II.

Assume Case I, except that, instead of (2), half of the bonds are each just twice as hard to form as the others, in

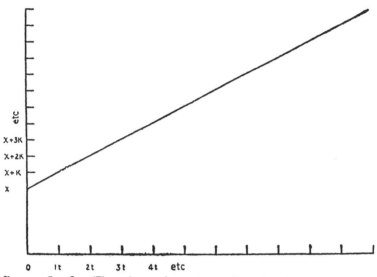

Fig. 50.   Case Ic.   (The real curve in question would continue indefinitely with the same slope.   See the text for further explanation.)

the sense of each requiring 2 *t* at maximum power while the others each require 1 *t*.   The form of the practice curve will then depend on the *order* in which the bonds are formed. The conditions assumed allow an enormous variety of orders, resulting in one particular curve for each particular order.* If the easiest bonds are all formed first, the curve will be as in FIG. 51.   If the hardest are all formed first, the curve will be as in FIG. 52.   If half of the easiest are formed first, and the other half last, the curve will be as in FIG. 53.

* Though, of course, different orders may produce identical curves.

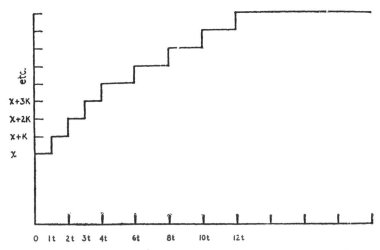

FIG. 51.   Case II: Easier Bonds First.   (See the text for explanation.)

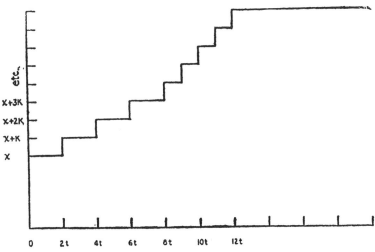

FIG. 52.   Case II: Easier Bonds Last.   (See the text for explanation.)

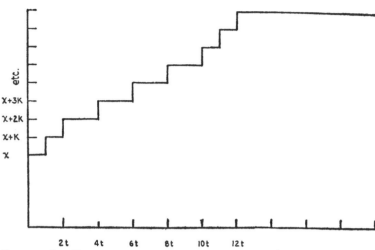

Fig. 53.   Case II: Easier Bonds First and Last.   (See the text for explanation.)

So far we have seen that, assuming the bonds to be of equal effect on the score, and assuming equal power to learn at all times in the learner, the form of the practice curve is a result of the *number of bonds,* of their *ease of formation,* and of their *order of formation.*   The number determines the limit of efficiency; the ease and order of formation determine the curve by which it is reached.   In all the cases so far used, 'equal' or 'steady' or 'even' power to improve in the function could replace 'maximum' power, and the elimination of injurious bonds could replace in whole or in part the formation of positive ones, without changing the general effect. Also, differences in ease of learning could be used in the sense that two bonds or four bonds could be formed simultaneously in say 1 *t,* as well as in the sense of their being formed separately each in half of *t* or one fourth of *t.*   These possible replacements will hold good also of all that follows in this chapter.

Now the result of a greater effect of a bond upon the score, with equal ease of formation, is the same as that of greater ease in formation with equal effect on the score. The ease of formation being kept equal, and differences in effect on the score being taken, we should get, for each order of formation of bonds, a practice curve of a given form. If the more potent bonds were learned early, there would be negative acceleration in the rate of improvement; if the least potent bonds were learned early, the reverse; and so on for all the possible orders. If the bonds differ in both ease of formation and effect on the score, we have only to estimate the net effect on the score of a unit of time spent on each bond, and then to determine the curve from the order of formation of the bonds.

For example, assume that there are 8 bonds, a, b, c, d, etc., formed in 1 t, 2 t, 3 t, 4 t, 6 t, 8 t, 12 t, and 16 t, respectively, and having, as effects on the score, 40, 20, 10, 8, 2, 4, 6 and 24, respectively. Then the effect of 1 t on the score is 40 if spent on bond a, 10 if spent on bond b, 3⅓ if spent on bond c, 2 if spent on d, ⅓ if spent on e, ½ if spent on f, ½ if spent on g, and 1½ if spent on h. Then each successive t of the practice can have its effect calculated provided the *order* of formation of the bonds is known.

By differences in the individual's general power to improve the function are meant of course differences in the time taken to form bonds which, were the individual in just the same state, would take him equal times to form. A drop in the individual's power to learn during any given time, of course, lowers the practice curve over that interval of time. If, say, by a progressive decay of interest, the power to learn was, in successive times, as 1.0, .9, .8, .7, .6, .5, .4, .3, then, in Case I, if (6) is replaced by this progressive decay in general power to learn, we should have, instead of FIG. 48, FIG. 54. If, by a progressive improvement in health or increase in interest, the power to learn was in successive times 1., 1.1, 1.2, 1.3, 1.4, 1.5, 1.6, 1.7, we should have, the other conditions being left unchanged, FIG. 55.

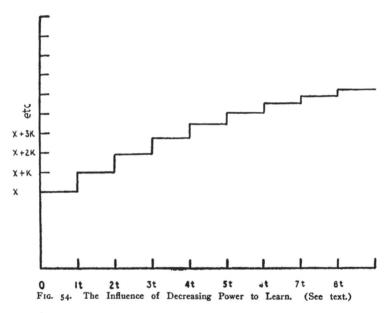

FIG. 54. The Influence of Decreasing Power to Learn. (See text.)

So far it has been assumed that the ease of formation and effect on the score of the bonds are independent of the order in which the bonds are formed. The third assumption of Case I has been left unchanged in all later cases.

In actual practice both the time taken to form a bond and its effect on the score may depend on what bonds have previously been formed. The resulting complications in the curve of practice could be calculated for any defined effect of the previous total or partial formation of any one bond or

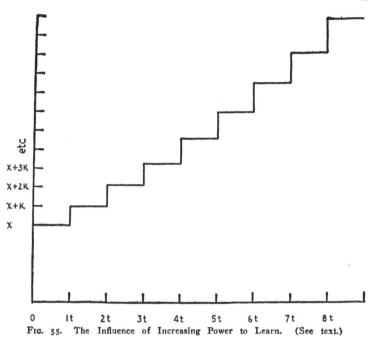

FIG. 55. The Influence of Increasing Power to Learn. (See text.)

combination of bonds upon the rest. The complications are, of course, very, very numerous.

So far, also, it has been assumed that the effect of any bond on the score appears in its totality as soon as the bond has been formed (or, in the (a) cases, that each fraction of its effect appears as soon as that fraction of its formation has been completed). But in real practice it may often occur that the full effect of a bond's formation on the score appears only after later bonds have been formed. That is, just as previously formed bonds may give an ensuing bond a greater effect than it would otherwise have had, so sequent bonds may enhance the effect on the score of those already formed. This effect of bond *b* on a preceding bond *a* could not, on its appearance, be distinguished in the gross result from an increased potency of *b* due to the preformation of *a;* but if *b* could itself, still later, be lost without the enhancement of *a* being lost, the difference between the two relations would appear.

So far, save in the last sentence, it has been assumed that after a bond is formed it retains throughout practice its full potency and requires, thereafter, zero time. But in fact some of the learner's time may be, and usually is, required to keep the bond at the condition attained; and some of the learner's time may be expended in exercising that bond to an extent not required to keep it at the condition attained—that is, in *over-learning* it. We may best consider the effects of time-requirement for retentiveness and time-waste in over-learning, separately, each in one very simple case.

Assume, then: (1) that all the work is at equal general learning power, (2) that the function improves from *x* to its limit by the addition of twenty bonds, (3) equal in ease of formation, taking 1 *t* each, and (4) equal in effect on the score, adding each 1 *k* to it. Assume (5) that (3) and (4) hold regardless of what order the bonds are formed in, (6) that only one bond is being formed at any one time, but that (7) each bond, after having been formed, *requires ½ t daily to keep it at its full strength,* and (8) that in the practice, which is of 4 *t* daily, time is spent on the older bonds so far as is necessary to keep them at their full formation. Assume (9) that each fraction of time spent on the formation or preservation of a bond has its proportional effect on the score.

Assume, for convenience in calculation, that, within the practice period of 4 *t*, the loss in old bonds is 0. Assume, that is to say, that such loss occurs only from the end of one practice period to the beginning of the next. Then:

In period 1, the learner would form bonds a, b, c and d. rising from $x + 0$ to $x + 4\,k$.

In period 2, he would spend $2\,t$ in preserving a, b, c and d, and form e and f, rising from $x + 4\,k$ to $x + 6\,k$.

In period 3, he would spend $3\,t$ in preserving a, b, c, d, e and f, and form g, rising from $x + 6\,k$ to $x + 7\,k$.

In period 4, he would spend $3\frac{1}{2}\,t$ in preserving a to g, and half form h, rising from $x + 7\,k$ to $x + 7\frac{1}{2}\,k$.

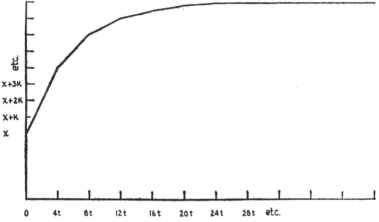

Fig. 56.   The Influence of Relearning or of Overlearning.   (See text)

In period 5, he would spend $3\frac{3}{4}\,t$ in preserving a to g and the half of h formed or, if we assume no loss by disuse until the bond is fully formed, would spend $3\frac{1}{2}\,t$ as before on a to g.   Choosing the former alternative* he learns $\frac{1}{4}$ more of h, rising from $x + 7\frac{1}{2}\,k$ to $x + 7\frac{3}{4}\,k$.

* If we choose the latter, he learns in period 5 the other half of h and rises from $x + 7\frac{1}{2}\,k$ to $x + 8\,k$.

In period 6 he would spend the entire $4\,t$ in keeping what bonds he had, and could never rise above the limit $x + 8\,k$, though bonds exist which, if any one man could hold enough of them while he formed the rest, would raise the score to $x + 20\,k$

In period 6, he would spend $3\frac{7}{8}$ t in preserving a to g and the three-fourths of h, and would form one-eighth more of h, rising from $x + 7\frac{3}{4}$ k to $x + 7\frac{7}{8}$ k. So on he would go, approaching $x + 8k$ as a limit, as shown in FIG. 56. Here we see Case I a, with a perfectly straight slope of the curve from o to the limit, turning into a case of pronounced negative acceleration, as the consequence of the expenditure of time in keeping up bonds after they are formed. And, in general, we see that, no matter how slowly bonds are weakened by disuse and no matter how time is distributed over retention of old and formation of new, the effect of the need of partial relearning will be to produce negative acceleration. Further, if there are enough bonds involved in the function, it must, for the same reason, tend to reach a limit of efficiency.*

Consider now the effect of *over-learning,* in a case where all other conditions would produce a straight-slant curve.

Assume equality of general learning power, equal ease of formation of bonds ($1t$ being required for each), equal effect on the score (1 k) regardless of order of formation, one new bond to be formed at any one time, but *one-half as much time to be spent in useless† exercise of a bond forever after it is formed* as was required to form it, fractional times spent to count proportionally on the score. Assume, that is, the conditions of Case I a, plus this *over-learning.* Then, letting each practice period be $4\,t,$ and the number of

* If new bonds of equal potency on the score were more and more easily formed as practice progressed, this tendency might, within an individual's life-time, be outweighed.

† Useless for keeping it up to its full effect, that is; not necessarily useless in general. For the over-learning might be beneficial apart from the score in the particular function during the particular practice under consideration.

bonds be any number 8 or over, we would find the following history:

In period 1, the learner would form bonds a, b, c and d, rising in score from $x + 0$ to $x + 4k$.

In period 2, he would spend $2t$ in over-learning or useless exercise of a, b, c and d, and would form e and f. His score would rise from $x + 4k$ to $x + 6k$.

In period 3 he would spend $3t$ in over-learning, and form bond g.

The future course of the practice curve would be just as in the case where half the time of formation of a bond was required to keep it up to the mark. And, in general, over-learning, in the sense of useless exercise, always disposes toward negative acceleration and reaching an unimprovable limit.

Relearning and Overlearning are, in actual practice, related in an interesting and important way. Such useless exercise of a bond as I have assumed, to make the illustration simple and its influence clear, is very rare. The over-exercise beyond what is needed to form a bond is in actual practice, up to a certain limit, the very exercise which relearns it (or keeps it from needing to be relearned)—which brings it back to its full effect (or keeps it from falling below it). There are more and less economical ways of distributing the time devoted to exercise of a bond, once it is fully formed, too much exercise at any one time being wasteful by building up something which disuse will tear down before any advantage is got from it; and too little being likely to make certain correlated bonds hard to form. The reader may well combine the assumptions of the two last described cases in a case where each bond tends to lose so much per day as a result of

16

the lapse of time; and to regain (or to be kept from losing) so much per unit of practice time as a result of a defined amount of exercise of it after it has been once formed. The general effect of relearning and over-learning, as they combine in actual practice, will be the same as the effect shown for either one of them in the artificial conditions assumed in the illustration.

We have seen how (1) the number of bonds, (2 and 3) differences amongst them in ease of formation and in effect on the score, in combination with (4) the order in which they are formed, (5) differences in the individual's general power to improve the function at different periods of the practice, (6) the relations of changed ease of formation or effect on score existing between the bonds already acquired, or those to be acquired, and any given bond, (7) the weakening of bonds by disuse, and (8) the useless over-exercise of existing bonds may produce changes in the rate of improvement, and how the kind of change that any defined state of affairs of any of these seven sorts will produce can be deduced.

Every one of these factors could almost certainly be illustrated from actual human learning. An examination of the various explanations of initial rapid rise, negative acceleration, eventual approximation to zero improvement, plateaus, and other long-time and short-time fluctuations, would, in fact, show one, or another, or some combination of two or more, of these eight facts as the condition which the author of the explanation really invoked for his particular purpose.

CHAPTER XVII

THE PERMANENCE OF IMPROVEMENT

DETERIORATION BY DISUSE

In general, as daily life abundantly shows, the disuse of a mental function weakens it, and the amount of weakening increases, the longer the lack of exercise. There have been, however, a few unfortunate statements made by psychologists to the effect that bonds perfect themselves after exercise has ceased by a process of mere inner growth or organization. So Coover and Angell ['07, p. 336] say that "the common belief in beneficial effects of incubation periods on bodily activity has been amply confirmed by numerous investigations of practice and fatigue," but give neither any evidence, nor any reference to any evidence, of the confirmation. Book, who does not himself assent to this doctrine of learning to skate in the summer and to swim in the winter, describes it as the assumption "that the associations previously formed had been slowly perfecting themselves unconsciously by some sort of neural growth process which completed itself during the interval of no practice." ['08, p. 80]

This doctrine of continuance of improvement after the cessation of practice seems to contradict the general rule announced above, and would do so if the doctrine were made general and consistent. But the advocates of learning to skate in summer and swim in the winter would in concrete cases always demand that improvement should have a certain large impetus in order to continue without further exercise, and would always admit that after a certain length of time disuse does not improve, but injures, a function's efficiency.

No one of them would expect the improvement due to a single hour's practice at skating to add an unearned increment to itself during the following summer. No one of them would expect that the gain from a hundred hours of practice at swimming, diving and other aquatic gymnastics would be found to have increased or even persisted after twenty years. The doctrine asserts the reversal of a general law of forgetting under certain circumstances, not the general truth of its opposite.

The doctrine is misleading, the real facts which in a measure excuse it being simply: (1) that an improvement in a function may be masked by fatigue, so that disuse, involving rest, produces an apparent gain; (2) that an improvement in the *strength* of desirable bonds may be masked by a decrease in their *readiness*—a drop in interest, a 'going stale,' as the athletes say—so that disuse, by doing more good to interest than it does harm to the strength of the bonds, produces an apparent improvement; (3) that unwise exercise of the function, as in worry and confusion or under misleading instructions, may form undesirable bonds, whose weakening by disuse improves the function.

We may then dismiss the doctrine of continuance of improvement after the cessation of practice as unsupported by direct evidence and contrary to all the general evidence on memory. There is always some weakening of bonds, and so, under equal conditions of rest and interest, always some deterioration of a function, with disuse. In certain cases the effect on the score may, however, be very small. Consider the very simple function in the reader of being able to tell his name when asked 'What is your name?' Even after ten years of disuse, perhaps, a slight indecision and delay might be the only observable inferiority in the function's efficiency.

RESULTS OF EXPERIMENTAL STUDIES

The functions whose deteriorations with disuse have been studied most adequately are the rather unimportant* ones of reciting at demand a certain series of nonsense syllables, and reciting at demand a certain series of sensible words forming a stanza of a poem or the like. In these cases a certain known amount of time or number of readings has produced a certain defined improvement from zero ability to the ability to recite the series once (or twice, in some of the studies); and, after certain known amounts of time have elapsed, the amount of time or number of repetitions required to restore the ability previously acquired has been measured. If, for example, a man learns 100 nonsense series, and relearns 10 of them after 1 hour, 10 after 1 day, 10 after 10 days, 10 after 30 days, 10 after 1 year, and so on, we have means of estimating certain points of the curve of deterioration or forgetting for this function in this man.

The studies in question are those of Ebbinghaus, Radossawljewitsch, Magneff and Bean.

Ebbinghaus ['85, p. 94 ff.], measuring the amount remembered by the saving of time in relearning, found that a series of nonsense syllables when studied until he could just

---

* If the curves so found could be assumed to hold good for all functions at all stages of improvement, their characteristics would be of very great importance, but, as will be shown, these curves cannot be at all generally assumed.

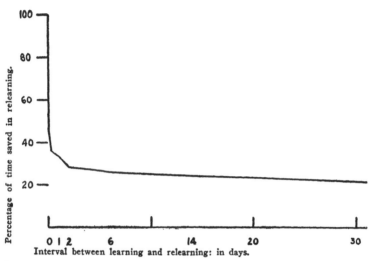

FIG. 57.   The Curve of Forgetting for Nonsense-Series Learned to the Point of One
Successful Reproduction, in the Case of Ebbinghaus.

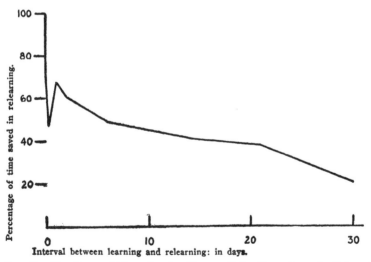

FIG. 58.   The Curve of Forgetting for Nonsense-Series Learned to the Point of
Two Successful Reproductions, as Reported by Radossawljewitsch.

repeat it correctly, left an after effect as shown in FIG. 57. At the end of *19* minutes, 42 per cent as much time was required to relearn the series as to learn it in the first place; at the end of *63* minutes, 56 per cent as much time; at the end of *8¾* hours, 64 per cent as much time; and so on. The percentages of time saved over total relearning are thus 58, 44, 36 and so on. Disuse here seems enormously potent. In a similar experiment, except that the nonsense series were learned more thoroughly—namely, until they could be repeated correctly *twice* in succession, Radossawljewitsch ['07] found the curve of forgetting to be of the same general form as FIG. 57, but with a less intense effect of disuse. His results are shown in FIG. 58.

Bean ['12, p. 19 ff.], using the learning and relearning of a series of new letters and measuring the loss in a fashion too intricate for description here, found that the loss was rapid at first and then slow, his score for the errors made at various dates in tests of knowledge of the nine letters being: one day, 3.0; four days, 4.15; seven days, 5.35; fourteen days, 5.5; twenty-one days, 5.55; twenty-eight days, 5.9. The first day's disuse thus produces as many errors as the following twenty-seven days.

Radossawljewitsch had sensible series (eight lines of poetry making about ninety syllables) learned to the point of two perfect recitals, and then relearned after a certain interval. Combining with his results those obtained by Magneff, we have, as a provisional curve of forgetting for poetry, that shown in FIG. 59.

In sharp contrast to the extensive rapid forgetting of nonsense lists and verses of poetry stand the facts found for tossing balls and typewriting by Swift, Schuyler, Book and Rejall.

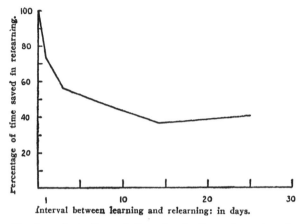

FIG. 39. The Approximate Curve of Forgetting for Poetry Learned to the Point of Two Successful Reproductions. Drawn from Data of Radossawljewitsch and Magneff.

In the case of tossing balls, the following facts are reported by Swift ['03, '05 and '10] : Subject A, having begun with a score of about 4, and having reached, in the last six days of forty-two days of practice, average scores of 50, 82, 92, 88, 68 and 105, was retested every thirty days for five months, and attained average scores of 70, 80, 140, 110, and 120. Being then tested after four hundred and eighty-one days, he attained an average score of 119. Being then tested after over four years, he attained an average score of 5; on the following day, one of 10; and on successive following days, average scores of 18, 20, 26, 35, 66, 60, 45, 100, and 160. Subject E, having begun with a score of about 10, and having reached, in the last six days of fourteen days of practice, average scores of 31, 53, 80, 105, 115 and 127, was retested every thirty days for five months,* and attained

* There was some practice with the left hand during the first thirty-days interval in the case of both A and E.

average scores of 115, 145, 155, 230, and 325. Being next
tested after an interval of 463 days, he attained an average
score of 152.

In the course of forty-five hours of practice at typewriting,
Swift had risen from a score of 350 words per hour to one of
1050. Two years and thirty-five days later he was retested,
scoring in ten hours (one per day) 700, 860, 860, 970, 1023,
1010, 1005, 1040, 990, 1100. The score of errors is not
reported, though Swift notes an "increasing liability to error."

Rejall tested the permanence of the ability to typewrite
acquired in the course of about thirty hours of practice, after
an interval of three and a half years. In the last two weeks
of the learning, he wrote at a rate of 25 words a minute with
4 errors per hundred words copied; in the memory test, he
scored, in the first five days, 18.75 words per minute with
8 errors per hundred words, 18.9 with $7\frac{1}{3}$ errors, 21 with
$6\frac{2}{3}$ errors, 22.1 with 5 errors, and 22.5 with $8\frac{2}{3}$ errors.
On continuing the practice, five hours brought him to very
nearly the same ability that thirty hours had been required
to attain originally, his average score for the six days after
five hours of relearning being 26 words per minute with $5\frac{1}{2}$
errors per hundred words.

Book found an even greater permanence of improvement in
typewriting, there being so sudden a rise in the course of the
memory test as to carry efficiency to a point beyond the best
score made in the original learning, though a year and five
months had elapsed.

The permanence of the improvement made by practice in
writing words, changing each letter to a number or a different letter, by practice in typewriting of a very simple sort (one
same sentence involving only seven letters), by practice in
checking A's or numbers, and by practice in addition, has been

measured. The permanence in these cases is much greater than that found for learning nonsense-series to the point of one or two perfect reproductions, and much less than that found for ball-tossing and typewriting. As a sample we may take the following: Six adults who had practiced adding for 150 minutes in January to April, 1910, were given two tests of five minutes each in December, 1912. Their average scores (additions for five minutes) on the first two days of the original practice were 234 and 274. On the last day of the original practice, their average score was 447. On the two days of the memory test, the averages were 343 and 375. In the number-checking, the corresponding scores were: 56 and 73 o's marked per minute in the first and second five minutes of the original learning: 107 in the last five minutes; and 74 and 80 in the first and second five minutes two and two-thirds years later.

Kirby ['13], who measured the improvement made by fourth-grade pupils by sixty minutes of practice in addition,* retested many of these pupils with a fifteen-minute period at the end of June. This was from three to twelve weeks after the last trial of the regular practice. There was no loss, or more properly, no more loss from disuse than was compensated for by the fifteen minutes of practice. He retested many of them also early in September after the vacation. In this test of fifteen minutes the pupils did not do so well as in the fifteen-minute test at the end of the regular practice or in the test at the end of June. From the first to the last fifteen-minute test of 75 minutes of practice in April and May, these pupils had gained about 15 examples. In a fifteen-minute test at the end of June they increased this

---

* Under the conditions described on page 193.

gain to about 17. In a fifteen-minute test early in September, it fell to 10.

From 20 to 45 minutes of drill in September brought the gain back to about its status at the end of the original 75 minutes of practice. The accuracy remained closely the same throughout.

In the case of division, pupils who, from the first to the last 10-minute period of sixty minutes practice, had gained 35 examples, maintained and slightly increased this gain in a test at the end of June two weeks later. In a 10-minute period early in September, this gain had fallen to 17½ examples. From 15 to 35 minutes of drill was required to bring it back.

Dr. Kirby is of the opinion that the loss between June and September is in part a consequence, not of the mere disuse of the functions in question, but of a general restlessness and unsteadiness due to the change from vacation habits to school routine.

GENERAL CONCLUSIONS

The facts of the previous section give a just picture of what has been found by investigators of the permanence of improvement. They do not enable us to give any simple comprehensive account of the rate and changes in the rate of deterioration. Indeed the reader may complain that about the only facts that they display with any unanimity and brilliancy are the apparent complexity and variability of deterioration by disuse and our lack of knowledge about it!

These facts themselves are not futile, however. What knowledge we have and what we lack may both serve to protect us against assuming, as educational practice has often done, that all learning wanes after the fashion that learning of the informational type does, and against assuming, as theorizers about practice are likely to do, that there is some magical curve of forgetting which every function at every stage will somewhat closely follow. Further, the very great difference between the effect of say a year's disuse upon one's score in typewriting and its effect upon one's score in reciting a nonsense syllable or stanza of a ·poem emphasizes certain important facts about learning.

Over-learning.—The first of these facts is that over-learning from the point of view of immediate proficiency may not be over-learning for proficiency a day or month or year hence. It is well known that in learning series of nonsense syllables and the like, more time is required to learn the series so as to be able to give it twice than to learn the series so as to just barely give it. Radossawljewitsch indulged in over-learning if learning equals "to be able just barely to give," and the greater permanence in the results of his subjects than Ebbinghaus found may be due to this. Suppose now that a series had been still further over-learned, being repeated say a thousand times. It would then have shown enormously greater permanence.

Now, roughly speaking, typewriting each new page is over-learning certain of the features of writing previous pages (writing 'the,' 'is,' 'of,' 'he' and manipulating the spacer and carriage, for example) ; typewriting at a higher rate is over-learning certain of the features of writing at a lower rate (for example, a combination of movements that, by being occasionally and slowly associated with seeing 'after that the' or 'in the midst,' raised speed to the lower level, will raise it higher by being invariably and quickly associated therewith) ; typewriting with one percent of errors is overlearning certain features of 'writing at the same rate with two percent of errors.' The practice which serves to form a few new desirable bonds results in the strengthening of many old ones in ways or to degrees that do not show in the score at the time, but do show in the length of time that these bonds will persist. Over-learning then doubtless accounts for a part of the less effect of disuse on the score in the case of the typewriting of Swift, Schuyler and Book than on the score in the case of knowledge of nonsense series, poems, and vocabularies.

Over-learning is an important fact because if the improvement of any one of the functions that have been studied in any of the last five chapters could be analyzed into its elements—into the bonds that have been added and subtracted— a very large percentage of the bonds added would be found to have been at any stage over-learned in the sense of being stronger than was needed to produce the score produced at that stage, all other bonds remaining as they were. Thus, even in a nonsense series, as ordinarily studied, the first and last syllables are a little over-learned by the time the middle members are barely learned. In telegraphic receiving, the bonds connecting certain series of clicks with words like 'is,' 'of,' 'the' and 'and' are over-learned by the time that the bonds connecting other series of clicks with rarer words are barely learned. The economical arrangement of learning depends very largely on the extent to which this is a waste avoidable by better methods of learning and, on the other hand, the extent to which it is necessary in order that the bond itself may hold until, in the future course of practice, it gets added exercise; and in order that other bonds may be more easily formed and retained.

The Possible Advantage of Direct Sensori-Motor Bonds in Permanence.—It is perhaps the case that functions whose improvement consists in responding more surely and more quickly by some movements of the muscles to some sense presentations with which the former are to be bound with few intermediaries, retain their improvement better than functions where the surety and speed of bonds from one internally initiated event in the brain to another are the main facts to be improved. Skating, dancing, swimming, typewriting in an advanced stage, on the one hand, and the recital of poems or nonsense series, knowledge of chemistry or geology, the ability to translate English into German, and typewriting at the beginning, on the other, illustrate and suggest this contrast.

It is possible that the secondary or so-called higher connections in the nervous system which correspond to the association of "ideas" are fundamentally less retentive of modification produced in them by learning than are the more primary and direct neural bonds which correspond to the association of sensory situation and motor response. Knowledge may be by the nature of man's neurones less retainable than skill. Roughly, as a matter of general observation, it seems to be.

The Relation of a Function's Organization to Permanence of Improvement.—A few illustrations will serve to show the possibility that the organization or arrangement of a function's bonds might be influential in determining the effect of disuse upon a man's score. Contrast, for example, the ability to reproduce in order a list of twelve unrelated words (say, *hereafter, president, designate,* etc.) with the ability to give these same words when the German words which they translate are presented,—supposing the series and the twelve pairings to have both been learned by mere mechanical repetition, and to be tested by the requests "Give series 23" and "Give the English meanings of .., .., .., .., etc." In each case there are twelve main bonds. In the former these are from *series 23* to *hereafter,* from *hereafter* to *president,* from *president* to *designate,* etc.; and in so far as the permanence of the ability depends on these main bonds, the failure of any one of them reduces the score from that point on to zero, the rest of the chain vanishing with the broken link. In the latter case the main bonds are independent, each being permitted to do its full service for the score. On the other hand, in the former case there are weaker subsidiary bonds between the *'Series 23'* and all the members, between each later member and all following it, and even slight bonds leading from each member to those closely preceding it.

Apparently these subsidiary bonds do not serve well enough in resisting disuse to counterbalance the gain due to independent action of each main bond. For, apparently, if a serial twelve and twelve pairs are each learned to the point of one or two perfect tests, the former will be sooner forgotten.

Contrast also the ability to *typewrite* Latin that is gained in 100 hours study by an English-reading adult with the ability to *translate* it that he gains in an equal amount of time (both having been acquired by an adult who knows English well). The actual number of bonds is perhaps greater in the former case, since each letter has acquired many different movements according to the preceding letters, and each word of many hundreds has acquired a total coordination corresponding to it, while a hundred hours of translation does not give a very wide vocabulary or knowledge of forms. But in the former case the bonds help each other out as they do not in the latter; the bonds with words are groupings and modifications of letter-habits; the various bonds leading from the same letter according to its antecedents in the copy are variants containing common elements. The organization by roots and endings does somewhat the same service for translation, but to nothing like the same extent.

It seems likely that, apart from over-learning of any one bond as a total and apart from any possible superior permanence of direct sensori-motor connections, such an organized hierarchy of bonds consisting of new combinations of, and minor modifications of, old elements, would resist disuse better than the much less closely knit set of bonds from words to meanings which a hundred hours of study of Latin secures.

Learning Not to Forget.—We may conceive of disuse as a combination of forces which attack the bonds upon which a function's efficiency depends, making breaches, as it were, in the walls which exercise has built up, or conquering certain outposts and redoubts which exercise had won. We may conceive of relearning as the repair of these breaches, the recapture of these redoubts, the restoration of what was lost during the interval of disuse. Now if the attacks of disuse are at all specialized, relearning will be profitable in proportion as it is specialized—makes repairs where needed. The mere allround equal strengthening of bonds will be less potent protection against future attacks from disuse than a special strengthening of those spots whose weakness has been shown by their surrender to past attacks. Relearning what has been forgotten will then tend to be learning what is most likely to be forgotten and consequently most needs to be learned.

Now in such practice as the typewriting or ball-tossing

there is automatically provided by the conditions of the work a rather large amount of such specialized relearning. Learning is guided by the score. The learner does strengthen his walls especially where the interval since the last practice has torn them down; for otherwise he makes less progress. He is, by the guidance of the score, protected somewhat against unnecessary over-learning.

The difference between his learning and that in the case of memorizing a nonsense series is partly that he learns not to forget by relearning what has been forgotten until it is so well learned as to withstand the disuse of at least a day or so. He guards against future attacks by unconsciously trying one remedy after another for past attacks until he becomes able to withstand them.

In learning a nonsense series that can barely be learned in five minutes, ten minutes' worth of further learning is more potent for future permanence if it is applied a day later than if it is applied at the time, and still more potent if it is applied in divisions of just enough time to relearn on successive days. There are several factors operative in producing this effect, but the application of exercise so as to regain what has been lost rather than promiscuously is almost certainly one. For the same reason the concentration of exercise in learning vocabularies upon the pairs upon which at any given test one fails is economical for future permanence.

Deterioration as a Result of Competition.—So far the effect of disuse in and of itself has been our concern. But when a function lies idle during an interval of time its situations may acquire competing bonds, either alternative or opposite to those constituting the function. The time in question is occupied somehow; and the future fate of the function

17

depends upon how it is occupied as well as how long it is. The situations composed of the typewriting 'set' of mind, being seated before the machine with copy, and the special words thereof, for example, acquire as totals no alternative bonds; also their old bonds are little interfered with by whatever bonds the words of the copy may have acquired as elements in other total situations of reading, translating, copying by hand and the like. The situations composed of the 'recalling nonsense-series set,' sitting before certain apparatus and the recall of the several syllables of designated series also acquire as totals no alternative bonds (provided no other series involving the same or closely similar syllables are learned or relearned during the interval); but their syllable elements are probably more interfered with by their occurrence in different series in reading and speech. If other nonsense series containing some of the same or closely similar syllables are learned or relearned during the interval, the interference is greater. It is obvious that, other things being equal, the less the interference, the greater will be the permanence over the same interval.

On the whole, then, the scanty and apparently inconsistent facts about the rate of forgetting and changes in it perhaps agree in revealing that the amount of forgetting, and the form of the curve of forgetting, in each case, are consequences of the nature of the bonds, the degree of over-learning of each and of each of the elements of each, their relations, and the competing bonds which whatever activities fill the interval establish. No one 'curve of forgetting' could then be expected for different functions at similar stages of advancement or for the same function at different stages of advancement much less for different functions at different stages of advancement.

CHAPTER XVIII

THE INFLUENCE OF IMPROVEMENT IN ONE MENTAL FUNC-
TION UPON THE EFFICIENCY OF OTHER FUNCTIONS

FACILITATION AND INHIBITION

The bonds whose strengthening and weakening constitute
the changes in condition of mental functions in a man are
not each utterly independent of the rest, but are related to
form the obvious dynamic unity which the intellect, character,
taste and skill of any one man displays. What happens to
any one bond makes differences to other bonds in the same
man that it does not make to those bonds in a different man.
The amount of difference made ranges from cases where a
change in one bond causes or constitutes an almost equal
change in another to cases where the change in one produces
approximately zero changes in the other. The nature of the
difference made ranges from cases where the whole effect of
the strengthening or weakening of one bond acts to produce
a corresponding effect on another to cases where the whole
effect of its strengthening is to weaken, and of its weakening
to strengthen, the other.

We may use the terms *facilitation, reinforcement, assistance* or *positive similar change* for cases where a strengthening
of one bond produces more or less strengthening in another,
and the term *negative similar change* for cases where a
weakening of one bond produces more or less weakening in

another. It is probable that a relation of positive similar change between two bonds implies the existence of the relation of negative similar change between them. We may use the terms *inhibition, opposition* or *positive opposite change* for cases where a strengthening of one bond produces more or less weakening of another, and the term *negative opposite change* for cases where the weakening of one bond produces more or less strengthening in another. It is probable that the former relation between two bonds implies the latter also. The terms facilitation, reinforcement and inhibition have been somewhat specialized in use by psychologists so that the unambiguous *similar change* and *opposite change* are the safest to use.

I shall in general restrict discussion to the positive actions, since whatever general theory accounts for them probably accounts for the corresponding effect of the weakening of the one bond upon the other.

Similar Change

The strengthening of one bond produces a similar change in another when the two are in part identical—when, that is, the two situations are in part identical and these identical elements in the situations have (*in toto* or in respect to some of their elements) identical responses bound to them.

We may distinguish the following amounts of identity:

Entire Similar Change by Composition of Totals.

The bonds A B C $\rightarrow$ 1, 2, 3, and X Y Z $\rightarrow$ 48, 49, 50, being strengthened, the bond A B C X Y Z $\rightarrow$ 1, 2, 3, 48, 49, 50 is strengthened. Thus, learning that □ is square and that a certain appearance is black facilitates the learning that ■ is a black square.

Partial Similar Change by Insertion of Totals.

The bond A B C $\rightarrow$ 1, 2, 3 being strengthened, the bond A B C X Y Z $\rightarrow$ 1, 2, 3, 48, 49, 50 is strengthened. Thus, knowing the meaning of half of a compound word facilitates the learning of the entire word's meaning.

Entire Similar Change by Composition of Elements.

The bonds A B C $\rightarrow$ 1, 2, 3 and X Y Z $\rightarrow$ 48, 49, 50 being strengthened, the bond A X $\rightarrow$ 1, 48 is strengthened. Thus, phonic drills with *sit, sat, sun, say, saw, some* and with *pick, lick, kick, Dick,* facilitate the process of learning to read *sick.*

Partial Similar Change by Insertion of Elements.

The bond A B C $\rightarrow$ 1, 2, 3 being strengthened, the bond A X Y $\rightarrow$ 1, 48, 49 is strengthened. Thus, the first half of the drills just mentioned would be beneficial alone.

In the illustrations used for these four cases, the composition out of old bonds or the insertion of an old bond is fairly easy to deduce from easily observable behavior; but such dependence of one situation-response bond upon others may be to any extent a hidden event within man's neurones.

As a consequence, there may be Similar Change of bonds due to identities that are beyond our direct cognizance; and, on the other hand, there may be a failure of similar change where our superficial observation expects it, because a similarity of result is brought about by two sets of bonds which have no identical element. As an illustration of the first of these two facts, we may take the possible case of the strengthening of the bonds productive of accuracy in judging the differences of pairs of weights by the increased strength of the bonds productive of accuracy in judging the differences of pairs of colors. If the facilitation should be found to occur, we would perhaps be at a loss to locate the identity, beyond a cryptic assignment of it to 'attentiveness to small shocks of difference.' As an illustration of the second fact, we may take the case of the bonds between the thought of, say, an elephant, a map or a certain room, and clear, vivid visual images of these things. Such bonds are found* to have very little or no favorable effect on the bonds leading from the same situations to correct judgments about, say, the elephant's external anatomy, the features of the map, or the contents of the room.

There are three cases of similar change which are of special practical importance, which we may call facilitation by *reorganization,* by *transferred set or attitude,* and by *transferred neglect.*

When the bonds acquired in learning vocabularies assist the learner in reading sentences, or when the letter habits of telegraphy and typewriting enable the learner to form the word habits, the old bonds are not compounded just as they are, nor, on the other hand, are the new bonds learned separately, as it were, on top of the old ones. The new ones use the old ones, but by *reorganizing* them through 'short-circuiting' and other forms of associative shifting, and by trying and selecting from various amalgamations and modifications of them.

It may be said in opposition that this last is not a proper case of similar strengthening, since the formation of the letter habits does not actually form the word habits, but only makes them easier to form. From a certain pedantic point of view this may be admitted, but, as has been shown, it is not wise to try to restrict the strengthening of a bond to cases where the strengthening manifests itself immediately in a change in

*For example, by the author ['07], by Betts ['09], and by Ruger ['10].

the score. Strengthening has been used in this volume to equal greater ease of formation to X strength as well as an obvious change from Y strength up—to mean nearer to X as well as further from Y. And this more catholic use is advisable.

When an animal, by experience in securing food by operating mechanical contrivances, becomes more active in the tenth puzzle-box than it was in the first, or when a man, in the course of noun-checking experiments, acquires a wary, business-like scrutiny of the lines with no halts or dawdlings, and maintains it when checking verbs or prepositions,—we have facilitation by the *transfer of a set or attitude*. Ebert and Meumann ['05] report that the mere decision to accept certain work as interesting improved it; Fracker ['08] found that the adjustment to *naming* the order of four intensities of the same tuning-fork (as 1, 2, 3, 4 for the order from least to greatest intensity, or 4, 3, 2, 1 for the reverse, or 1, 2, 4, 3, and the like) helped greatly to strengthen the bonds needed to permit the learner to give the correct order after an interval filled with another task. Ruger ['10] found that the attitude of confidence begot of success in solving puzzles aided in the solution of others, and gives other illustrations of the same general facilitation by transferred attitude or set of mind.

A large part of learning is dropping out and driving out harmful or irrelevant bonds, and the weakening of these may be of advantage not only to the particular bond in whose favor they were driven out, but to other bonds whose formation or action they would otherwise have impeded. The *transfer of tendencies to neglect* is as real as the transfer of positive action. Learning a score of series of nonsense syllables is found to facilitate learning another score, partly because the irritation and distaste which are originally bound to the task are disjoined from it by the early practice.

Opposite Change

Strengthening the bond between a given situation, or situation element, A, and the response 1, weakens the opposite bond—between A and the response 'Opposite of 1.' Both the truth and the value of this statement depend upon a definition of 'Opposite.' The statement is true, but valueless, if we mean by it the tautology that the opposite response to 1 is one whose connection with A weakens the connection of 1 with A. Yet it is hard to find any valuable universal criterion of oppositeness in bonds. When the response 1 is an observable movement of the body, the opposite response may be roughly defined as the one which *undoes the work done by* 1—as by moving the body or part of the body in the opposite direction, or by expelling forth from the mouth what has just been taken into it. In a similar way, I should define as opposite any two bonds in the neurones *of which each undoes the work done by the other.* This definition, though, in my opinion, sound and destined to be helpful, is not of much value in our present ignorance of what bonds in the neurones correspond to any given fact of behavior.*

---

* I judge that our ordinary usage extends this definition much farther and more loosely, calling any two *responses* opposite when, the conditions outside the man being the same, either undoes the work done by the other. Thus, if conditions remain the same, assent undoes the social work of dissent, though the muscular movements are not opposite as such. The thoughts, 'Subtract 2' and 'It is not black,' are thus the opposites of 'Add 2' and 'It is black,' in the sense of undoing certain intellectual work done by them. But, with this extended usage of the term, it is far from sure that any general statement of opposite change is true. A child, for example, who is taught to say, on seeing a certain

Until we know what the actual behavior is in the neurones in the case of a bond, our attempts to define the kind of bonds which will mutually annihilate each other, thus turn into uninstructive tautologies or unsafe prophecies. Meanwhile we do know concretely that certain pairs of bonds do thus produce, one on the other, opposite change,—do manifest simon-pure inhibition. Two bonds from the same situation-element to motor responses of opposite or antagonistic effect, as above described, are a stock example of such a pair. Often confused with such cases of pure contrariness are cases of *alternative bonds,* where with one situation element two or more bonds are formed, leading to different responses. Thus, if ten different nonsense series, each beginning with 'wef kob,' are learned, the 'wef kob' may not call up any one of them as well as it would have done, had only that one been learned. Thus, having sorted objects into piles by color may make one have a lower score in sorting them by size than one would otherwise have had.

It must be remembered that in such cases the alternative bonds are never from *exactly* the same total compound of situation outside and condition inside the man. There is always some difference, though it may be an unnoticed feature of the man's attitude or 'set,' between the total states of affairs leading to the two responses. This fact gives the principle of explanation for the disputes concerning whether such alternative bonds do or do not inhibit one another. So long as the bonds are attached undiscriminatingly to the situation's gross features, they do inhibit each other; but it is possible to have an arrangement for switching accurately

gray object, 'It is black; It is not black' would certainly not be left in the same condition thereby as if he had said nothing at all; nor would he have the same effect on his hearers as if he had said nothing at all.

from one set of bonds to another, according to some minor differences in the external situation or learner's set of mind, so that there is no inhibition, but even, perhaps, facilitation.

For example, if the bonds are *wef kob* of the 12 syllable series I learned Saturday' $\rightarrow$ jur, bim, etc., and *'wef kob'* of the 16 syllable series I learned yesterday' $\rightarrow$ ziz, nok, etc., the bonds may do each other no harm, the 'of the 12 syllable series I learned Saturday' firmly excluding any bonds with 'of the 16 syllable series, etc.' from influence. So a person trained to sort objects by color or by size may come to be able to sort them ten times by color and then change over to size without a tenth of a second of reduction in his speed, at the mere signal 'Size now' or the like.

In the case of alternative systems of bonds there is then often an inhibition for a time, reducing to zero as the two systems of bonds get organized in connection with two systems of mental sets or attitudes, and perhaps giving way to facilitation by reason of certain serviceable identities in the bonds.

So a man trained for an hour on a typewriter of standard keyboard might, after a second hour of practice, with the keys being changed about to the order

$$
\begin{array}{ccccccc}
a & b & c & d & e & f & g \\
h & i & j & k & l & m & n \\
o & p & q & r & s & t & u \\
v & w & x & y & z, & &
\end{array}
$$

do worse than at the beginning; but if he practiced an hour daily on each sort of machine he would not fall back to his initial score for long, would soon come to be able to turn from one to the other system of bonds at the mere sight of the machine, and would probably find that 20 hours of the two alternative systems gave greater ability at either than ten hours of practice at it alone would have given.

The mass results of the similar and opposite changes in a certain group of bonds (call it group B) which have been brought about by the strengthening and weakening of bonds in a certain other group (call it group A), appear in the improvement or deterioration in one function (B) which is due to the improvement of another function (A).

These mass results may be measured without knowledge of the particular facilitations and inhibitions of single bonds to which they are ultimately due. We may, that is, find out how far improvement in, say, checking o's, gives added ability in checking the A's on certain printed pages, without any ultimate analysis of the functions into their constituent bonds or demonstration of the relations of similar and opposite change that obtain between them. We thus secure a basis of knowledge for educational theories of the general or disciplinary value of specific practice of various sorts. Many such mass results have been obtained in the last dozen years, and with important consequences to educational theory. With some of their consequences the rest of this chapter will be concerned.

CHANGES IN EXPECTATION OF MENTAL DISCIPLINE

One of the quarrels of the educational theorists concerns the extent to which special forms of training improve the general capacities of the mind. Does the study of Latin or of mathematics improve one's general reasoning powers? Does laboratory work in science train the power of observation for all sorts of facts? Does matching colored sticks educate the senses for all sorts of discriminations?

The problem, which is clearly one of psychological fact, may be best stated in psychological terms as follows: How far does the training of any mental function improve other mental functions? In less technical phrase, How far does an ability, say to reason, acquired with data A, extend also to data $B, C, D,$ etc.?

No one can doubt that all of the ordinary forms of home or school training have some influence upon mental traits in addition to the specific changes which they make in the particular function the improvement of which is their direct object. On the other hand, no careful observer would assert that the influence upon the other mental traits is comparable in amount to that upon the direct object of training. By doubling a boy's reasoning power in arithmetical problems we do not double it for formal grammar or chess or economic history or theories of evolution. By tripling the accuracy of movement in fingering exercises we do not triple it for typewriting, playing billiards or painting. The gain of courage in the game of football is never equaled by the gain in moral courage or resistance to intellectual obstacles. The real question is not, 'Does improvement of one function alter others?' but, 'To what extent, and how, does it?'

The answer which I shall try to defend is that a change in one function alters any other only in so far as the two functions have as factors identical elements. The change in the second function is in amount that due to the change in the elements common to it and the first. The change is simply the necessary result upon the second function of the alteration of those of its factors which were elements of the first function, and so were altered by its training. To take a concrete example, improvement in addition will alter one's ability in multiplication because addition is absolutely identical with a part of multiplication and because certain other processes,—*e. g.,* eye movements and the inhibition of all save arithmetical impulses,—are in part common to the two functions.

Chief amongst such identical elements of practical importance in education are associations including ideas about aims and ideas of method and general principles, and associations involving elementary facts of experience such as length, color, number, which are repeated again and again in differing combinations.

By identical elements are meant mental processes which have the same cell action in the brain as their physical correlate. It is of course often not possible to tell just what features of two mental abilities are thus identical.

Until very recently books on education answered our questions in a manner very different from this. They extended the influence of any special form of discipline much farther, and described its manner of operation only by vague and, I think, meaningless phrases.

In place of any descriptive account I shall give a number of quotations picked fifteen years ago almost at random from all the statements about the influence of special training on general ability made in some fifty books on education.

Since the mind is a unit and the faculties are simply phases or manifestations of its activity, whatever strengthens one faculty indirectly strengthens all the others. The *verbal* memory seems to be an exception to this statement, however, for it may be abnormally cultivated without involving to any profitable extent the other faculties. But only things that are rightly perceived and rightly understood can be *rightly* remembered. Hence whatever develops the acquisitive and assimilative powers will also strengthen memory; and, conversely, rightly strengthening the memory necessitates the developing and training of the other powers. [R. N. Roark, 'Method in Education,' p. 27]

It is as a means of training the faculties of perception and generalization that the study of such a language as Latin in comparison with English is so valuable. [C. L. Morgan, 'Psychology for Teachers,' p. 186]

Arithmetic, if judiciously taught, forms in the pupil habits of mental attention, argumentative sequence, absolute accuracy, and satisfaction in truth as a result, that do not seem to spring equally from the study of any other subject suitable to this elementary stage of instruction. [Joseph Payne, 'Lectures on Education,' Vol. I., p. 260]

By means of experimental and observational work in science, not only will his attention be excited, the power of observation, previously awakened, much strengthened, and the senses exercised and disciplined, but the very important habit of doing homage to the authority of facts rather than to the authority of men, be initiated. [*Ibid.*, p. 261]

. . . The study of the Latin language itself does eminently discipline the faculties and secure to a greater degree than that of the other subjects we have discussed, the formation and growth of those mental qualities which are the best preparatives for the business of life—whether that business is to consist in making fresh mental acquisitions or in directing the powers thus strengthened and matured, to professional or other pursuits. [*Ibid.*, p. 264]

Let us now examine in detail the advantages which a person who has taken the ordinary Bachelor's degree has derived from the study of classics. Aside from the discipline of the will, which comes from any hard work, we find the following: (1) His memory for facts has been strengthened by committing paradigms and learning a new vocabulary. (2) He has been obliged to formulate pretty distinctly a regular system of classified facts—the facts which form the material of the grammar—classified in due form under chapter, section, subsection and so on. This means that he has learned to remember things by their relations—a power which can hardly be acquired without practice in forming or using such classified systems. (3) He has had his judgment broadened and strengthened by constant calls upon it to account for things which cannot be accounted for without its exercise. [E. H. Babbitt, on p. 126 of 'Methods of Teaching the Modern Languages']

The value of the study of German 'lies in the scientific study of the language itself, in the consequent training of the reason, of the powers of observation, comparison and synthesis; in short, in the upbuilding and strengthening of the scientific intellect.' [Calvin Thomas, 'Methods of Teaching Modern Languages,' p. 27]

[*Advantages resulting from the teaching of drawing.*] The visual, mental and manual powers are cultivated in combination, the eye being trained to see clearly and judge accurately, the mind to think, and the hand to record the appearance of the object seen, or the conceptions formed in the mind. Facility and skill in handicraft, and delicacy of manipulation, all depend largely upon the extent to which this hand and eye training has been fostered. The inventive and imaginative faculties are stimulated and exercised in design, and the graphic memory is strengthened by practice in memory drawing. The æsthetic judgment is brought into use, the power of discerning beauty, congruity, proportion, symmetry, is made stronger; and the love of the beautiful, inherent more or less in mankind, is greatly increased. [J. H. Morris, 'Teaching and Organization' (edited by P. A. Barnett), pp. 63-64]

We may conclude this list by quotations from a recent inaugural address at a great American college and from the reasons given by a number of presidents of colleges to the question, 'Why go to college?'

"We speak of the 'disciplinary' studies, . . . having in our thought the mathematics of arithmetic, elementary algebra and geometry, the Greek-Latin texts and grammars, the elements of English and of French or German. . . . The mind takes fiber, facility, strength, adaptability, certainty of touch from handling them, when the teacher knows his art and their power. The college . . . should give . . . elasticity of faculty and breadth of vision, so that they shall have a surplus of mind to expend. . . ." [Woodrow Wilson, *Science,* November 7, 1902]

Nathaniel Butler, President of Colby College: "It has been well said that an educated man has a sharp ax in his hand and an uneducated man a dull one. I should say that the purpose of a college education is to sharpen the ax to its keenest edge."

H. M. MacCracken, Chancellor of New York University: "He will possess a better disciplined mind for whatever work of life he may turn his attention to."

Timothy Dwight, late President of Yale University: "Such an education is the best means of developing thought power in a young man, and making him a thinking man of cultured mind."

It is clear that the common view was that the words accuracy, quickness, discrimination, memory, observation, attention, concentration, judgment, reasoning, etc., stand for some real and elemental abilities which are the same no matter what material they work upon; that these elemental abilities are altered by special disciplines to a large extent; that they retain those alterations when turned to other field; that thus in a more or less mysterious way learning to do one thing well will make one do better things that in concrete appearance have absolutely no community with it.

The mind was regarded as a machine of which the different faculties are parts. Experiences being thrown in at one end, perception perceives them, discrimination tells them apart, memory retains them, and so on. By training, the machine is made to work more quickly, efficiently and economically with all sorts of experiences. Or, in a still cruder type of thinking, the mind was a storage battery which could be loaded with will power or intellect or judgment, giving the individual 'a surplus of mind to expend.' General names for a host of individual processes—such as judgment, precision, concentration—were falsely taken to refer to pieces of mental machinery which one could once for all get into working order, or, still worse, to amounts of something which could be stored up in banks to be drawn on at leisure.

Such quotations would today entirely misrepresent the standard view. When the three papers by Woodworth and Thorndike appeared in 1901, describing the limited extent to which practice in sensory discrimination, the observation of small details, and the like, spread beyond the specific abilities trained, they aroused surprise and incredulity. At the present time, such a limited spread of training would be taken almost for granted.

The notions of mental machinery which, being improved for one sort of data, held the improvement equally for all sorts; of magic powers which, being trained by exercise of one sort to a high efficiency, held that efficiency whatever they might be exercised upon; and of the mind as a reservoir for potential energy which could be filled by any one activity and drawn on for any other—have now disappeared from expert writings on psychology.

The results of the many experiments wherein learners were tested in several functions, before and after a period of special practice with some one function, have proved them false. When allowance is made for the gain due to the practice of the 'before and after' tests themselves, there remains

18

commonly only a moderate amount of 'transfer' due to the special training, even when the functions tested are very similar to those trained. As for *general* improvement *in all* memorizing from special training in learning poetry, *general* improvement *in* keenness of observation *of all sorts* from special training in noticing colors in the kindergarten, shapes in a biological laboratory, or relations in Latin syntax, the percentage of the improvement that is 'transferred' is very, very slight. In general, the experiments have shown that, in the words of two of the earlier workers in this field,

"Improvement in any single mental function need not improve the ability in functions commonly called by the same name. It may injure it.

"Improvement in any single mental function rarely brings about equal improvement in any other function, no matter how similar, for the working of every mental function-group is conditioned by the nature of the data in each particular case.

"The very slight amount of variation in the nature of the data necessary to affect the efficiency of a function-group makes it fair to infer that no change in the data, however slight, is without effect on the function. The loss in the efficiency of a function trained with certain data, as we pass to·data more and more unlike the first, makes it fair to infer that there is always a point where the loss is complete, a point beyond which the influence of the training has not extended. The rapidity of this loss, that is, its amount in the case of data very similar to the data on which the function was trained, makes it fair to infer that this point is nearer than has been supposed.

"The general consideration of the cases of retention or of loss of practice effect seems to make it likely that spread of practice occurs only where identical elements are concerned in the influencing and influenced functions."

The experimental results, indeed, have tempted certain

writers to proceed too far toward the absurd conclusion that all practice is utterly specific in its effects—confined absolutely to just the particular situations that were met in the special training and just the particular habits that were formed.

The average opinion of competent psychologists at the present time is represented fairly by the following quotations:

"In any event it is desirable that the teacher should rid himself of the notion that 'thinking' is a simple unalterable faculty; that he should recognize that it is a term denoting the various ways in which things acquire significance. It is desirable to expel also the kindred notion that some subjects are inherently 'intellectual,' and hence possessed of an almost magical power to train the faculty of thought. Thinking is specific in that different things suggest their own appropriate meanings, tell their own unique stories, and in that they do this in very different ways with different persons. As the growth of the body is through the assimilation of food, so the growth of mind is through the local organization of subject-matter. Thinking is not like a sausage machine which reduces all materials indifferently to one marketable commodity, but it is a power of following up and linking together the specific suggestions that specific things arouse." [Dewey, '10, p. 38 f.]

"Three points will show the possibilities of benefit from special training beyond the specific line of reaction subjected to practice. 1. The habit pathways may altogether or in part be common to two or to many operations perhaps *externally* very different . . . 2. The method of procedure in a special habit may evidently be applicable to a much larger field . . . 3. Mental attitudes or ideals tend by chance variation and by suggestion to extend their sphere of action." [Rowe, '09, pp. 243-246, *passim*]

"Knowledge and training are not merely specific in their application, but they also have a general value. Their value arises through the factor of identical elements, of which there are at least three types [aim, method and content], and it declines rapidly as the similarity of the material of instruction of training decreases." [Ruediger, '10, p. 116]

"Now no small part of the discipline which comes from the effortful use of attention in any direction or on any topic is to be found in the habituation which is afforded in neglecting or otherwise suppressing unpleasant or distracting sensations. We learn to 'stand it' in short. . . . The actual mental mechanism by which this intellectual and moral acclimatization is secured, is extremely interesting but we cannot pause to discuss it. Certain it is that something of the sort occurs and that it is an acquirement which may presumably be carried over from one type of occupation to another. If each form of effortful attention had a wholly unique type of discomfort attached to it, this inference might be challenged. But such does not seem to be the case." [Angell, '08, p. 9 f.]

"Transfer of training is then possible in the ways indicated: (1) Where a single element to which a specific response is made functions under various environmental conditions because it is a common element in these various, and otherwise to a greater or less degree, dissimilar environments; (2) When a dominant mood or emotion so colors various environments that a characteristic response is obtained without identity of any one objective condition; (3) Where a single response in reality involves other and more general adjustments; (4) It is also possible, as Bagley suggests, through making the end of the activity a clearly conscious ideal. In this case the transfer takes place by a direct carrying over by consciousness not of the activity itself, but of the purpose of the activity, to another field." [Colvin, '09, edition of '10, p. 30 f.]

"One mental function or activity improves others in so far as and because they are in part identical with it, because it contains elements common to them. Addition improves multiplication because multiplication is largely addition; knowledge of Latin gives increased ability to learn French because many of the facts learned in the one case are needed in the other. The study of geometry may lead a pupil to be more logical in all respects, for one element of being logical in all respects is to realize that facts can be absolutely proven and to admire and desire this certain and unquestionable sort of demonstration. . . .

"These identical elements may be in the stuff, the data concerned in the training, or in the attitude, the method taken with it. The former kind may be called *identities of substance* and the latter, *identities of procedure.*

"Identity of Substance.—Thus special training in the ability to handle numbers gives an ability useful in many acts of life outside of school classes because of identity of substance, because of the fact that the stuff of the world is so often to be numbered and counted. The data of the scientist, the grocer, the carpenter and the cook are in important features the same as the data of the arithmetic class. So also the ability to speak and write well in classroom exercises in English influences life widely because home life, business and professional work are all in part talking and writing. . . .

"Identity of Procedure.—The habit acquired in a laboratory course of looking to see how chemicals do behave, instead of guessing at the matter or learning statements about it out of a book, may make a girl's methods of cooking or a boy's methods of manufacturing more scientific because the attitude of distrust of opinion and search for facts may so possess one as to be carried over from the narrower to the wider field. Difficulties in studies may prepare students for the difficulties of the world as a whole by cultivating the attitudes of neglect or discomfort, ideals of accomplishing what one sets out to do, and the feeling of dissatisfaction with failure." [Thorndike, '06, pp. 243-245, *passim*]

"Mental discipline is the most important thing in education, but it is specific, not general. The ability developed by means of one subject can be transferred to another subject only in so far as the latter has elements in common with the former. Abilities should be developed in school only by means of those elements of subject-matter and of method that

are common to the most valuable phases of the outside en·
vironment.   In the high school there should also be an effort
to work out general concepts of method from the specific
methods used."   [Heck, '09, Edition of '11, p. 198]

". . . No study should have a place in the curriculum for
which this general disciplinary characteristic is the chief
recommendation.   Such advantage can probably be gotten
in some degree from every study, and the intrinsic values of
each study afford at present a far safer criterion of educational work than any which we can derive from the theory
of formal discipline."   [Angell, '08, p. 14]

THE GENERAL RATIONALE OF MENTAL DISCIPLINE

There are three facts of behavior knowledge of which
will in a vague way protect one from expecting too much,
and from not expecting enough, general influence from special
training.   First, learning is essentially the modification of
connections between actual situations and the responses of the
individual to them.   Any assumption of gain in concentration,
will-power, imaginativeness, appreciation, conscience, reasoning, or the like which cannot be described as a set of changes
in the bonds between specified situations and definable responses, is extremely risky, and probably depends upon
the magic efficacy of mythical powers.   Second, although
every change must be in a specified bond, and though, as a rule,
these bonds are between concrete, particular responses,
some of these particularized bonds are of very widespread
value.   Third, there are bonds involving situations and elements of situations which are, in the ordinary sense of the
word, general.

The first of these cautions has been reiterated so often
in this volume that no more need be said of it save that nine-

tenths of the mischief done in education by the older doctrines of mental discipline was due to the failure to describe behavior in terms of its actual elements.

The second fact accounts for a large fraction of the influence which training in one exercise, study or occupation has upon the efficiency of others. Useful connections with two, three, four, red, white, green, long, short, square-yard, square-foot, in this or that particular context, are of more or less general usefulness, since they may serve as well when the two, red, square, and the like are met in very different contexts. The ability to draw a straight four-inch line, to pronounce the vernacular, or to 'carry' in addition, in whatever particular circumstances gained, may be widely used. Of special importance are the connections of *neglect.* Such bonds as *'Stimuli to hunger save at meal times—neglect them;' 'Sounds of boys at play save at playtime'—'neglect them;' 'Ideas of lying down and closing one's eyes save at bed time,—neglect them,'* and the like are the main elements of real fact meant by 'power of attention,' or 'concentration' or 'strength of will.' In so far as a certain situation is bound to the response of neglect, it is prevented from distracting one *in general.* Of special importance also are those particular bonds which represent notions, maxims, methods, ideals, responses to abstract clues, and the like. Form the connections—*'A disagreeable thing that needs to be done—I must do it;' 'The thought 'I must do X'—enduring the discomfort till X is done;' 'The essential thing in scientific work—verification;' 'Anything that happens—has a discoverable cause,'* and the like and they may turn up again and again to impel and restrain one to whom they are living creeds. Of special importance too, as just hinted, are the connections where satisfaction and discomfort are the responses. To be satisfied only when a fact to be described has been measured objectively is an identical element in very many lines of scientific work. To be annoyed by vagueness, untested opinions, futility and failure is a prime aid toward clearness, thought and achievement.

A particular bond may be with even a very abstract or subtle element of situations. In so far as many situations of things or thoughts have some common element or feature which classes them as *beautiful, ugly, true, false, desirable, undesirable, important, trivial,* and the like, and in so far as appropriate connections are made between the element in question and some response such as *attention, neglect, enjoyment, discomfort,* special training with these elements in one field may spread to many fields. How far beauty, desirability, triviality, and the like can thus acquire responses to them regardless of their concomitants in the way that *a mile, redness* or *sixness* do, is a question. They surely do so less often and less fully. The amount of training required to make a man respond by esteem to '*truth, wherever and however present,*' would be far greater than that which would suffice to teach him to respond in some one way to '*six pounds, wherever present.*' Even the latter achievement is very rare. Ordinary training would not fit one to respond properly to the 'sixpoundness' of a certain volume of air here, or of a large block of lead on the moon. And perhaps no man could be secured against such mis-response to truth of some sort, until he had been specially trained to respond to hundreds of sorts. Still, the possibility remains of more or less general utility from particular responses to very abstract and subtle features of things and thoughts.

The third caution—that there are bonds involving situations and elements of situations which are, in the ordinary sense of the word, general—rests ultimately upon the second. Ultimately every connection is between some one state of affairs and some one response. But such elements of situations as 'being alive and awake,' 'being aware that one has a problem,' 'feeling that one has done, or has not done, one's best,' and the like, are general in the sense of occurring again and again in connection with almost anything else. And to them responses do get bound. To take the extreme case, each man has tendencies to respond to *'merely being alive and awake'* which coöperate with all his more specific tendencies.

The notion that over and above the habits and powers which he displays in his life as wage-earner, citizen, friend, and member of a family, a man has certain tendencies to respond to *anything*—certain diffuse fear or courage, integrity or shiftiness, and seriousness or flippancy, for instance,—is commonly much overworked, but has always a core of truth. His past life provides every man with a set of attitudes or mental 'sets' in response to the mere fact that a statement is made regardless of what the statement is, to the mere asking of any question, to the mere presence of a conflict of interests, regardless of what or whose the interests are, to the mere fact of being alive, awake and well, with no immediate engagement. Special training can increase for any man the chance that his attitude will be to think over the statement, to seek to settle the question, to be satisfied by justice in the case of the conflict, to look about for something interesting to do in the leisure time.

These general tendencies may be outweighed by stronger bonds formed with other features of a situation. The generally thoughtful man may greedily believe a statement about his son that tickles his paternal pride; the generally just man may prefer a conventional to an equitable solution of a conflict between the sexes. They may be outweighed; but they exist and cast their weight in turn to decide the balance against certain thoughts and acts.

As a result of all these cautions the advisable course in estimating beforehand the disciplinary effect of any study, occupation or the like would seem to be to list as accurately as possible the particular situation-response connections made therein, noting especially what the study makes one neglect, be annoyed by, and be satisfied by; what connections it forms that carry vital maxims, notions of method, ideals of accuracy, persistence, verification, openmindedness and the like; and what responses it favors toward the commonest elements of intellectual and moral life such as 'a statement' or 'a question.' Prophecy beforehand should in all cases be replaced as fast as may be by measurements of the actual changes made by the 'study' in question.

Finally, it must be remembered that a very small spread of training may be of very great educational value if it extends over a wide enough field. If a hundred hours of training in being scientific about chemistry produced only one hundredth as much improvement in being scientific about all sorts of facts, it would yet be a very remunerative educational force. If a gain of fifty percent in justice toward classmates in school affairs increased the general equitableness of a boy's behavior only one-tenth of one percent, this disciplinary effect would still perhaps be worth more than the specific habits.

CHAPTER XIX

MENTAL FATIGUE

The topic of this and the next following chapter is the temporary deterioration of mental functions due to exercise without rest—its amount, rate and changes in rate, the factors constituting it, the conditions by which it is influenced, and the effect of such deterioration in one function upon the efficiency of others.

THE DECREASE IN EFFICIENCY OF A SINGLE FUNCTION UNDER CONTINUOUS EXERCISE

The term efficiency is used here to refer to the quantity and quality of the product produced. If the quantity per unit of time remains constant, decrease in efficiency is measured by the decrease in quality; with quality constant, by the decrease in quantity; with both varying, by some composite of the two changes.

The term single function is used in antithesis to 'the mind as a whole,' not to mean a function devoid of compoundness or complexity. I mean by it such functions as adding a column of figures, reacting to a signal by a movement as quickly as possible, the signal and movement being the same throughout, judging which of two weights (all close to 100 grams) is heavier, memorizing the English equivalents of German words, or multiplying a three-place number by a three-place number, nothing being allowed to be written or spoken save the two numbers themselves. Each of these functions comprises different elements, not all of which are at work all the time. Exercise is continuous only in the sense that the subject does his best to make it so.

As the sample for intensive study, I choose an experiment of Arai ['12], which has the special merit of measuring the effect of continuous exercise of a very difficult intellectual process, as free as possible from sensory or muscular work, at a stage when it was almost free from improvement by practice, over a very long period, and on four different occasions. Miss Arai says:

"The first experiment was made during February and March, 1909, at Teachers College, Columbia University. The purpose of the experiment was to ascertain: (1) the amount, rate and the change of the rate of fatigue in the special mental function exercised, and (2) the amount of fatigue transferred to certain other functions.

"The particular function tested was that exercised in mental multiplication of pairs of numbers like

2645	8324	7954		5438
5784	7384	3528	and	2347

"About one thousand different combinations of figures were used. The order of the examples being made by chance, the distribution of difficult and easy examples is random. The subject of the experiment was the writer herself. . . . On February 2nd, the subject made the first test in the following manner. Using an ordinary watch the subject set a time for starting. When the hand of the watch reached the point set, the subject looked at the first example and multiplied mentally but with the original numbers in sight. The answer was written down as soon as it was obtained and the time recorded. Then the subject immediately took up the second example and repeated the same procedure. Thus she worked from 9:30 A. M. to 3:18 P. M. with a rest of forty-eight minutes for luncheon, and obtained the answers of twenty-four examples." ['12, p. 31 f.]

On February 4, twenty-six such examples were done in the same manner; on February 7, twelve; on February 15, thirty; and on February 22, sixty. From the seven hours continuous work of February 22, it was clear that the subject could not, by even this long period of work, be brought to a condition of inability to do the work. The work was consequently made still more difficult, as follows:

"Instead of multiplying with the original figures in sight, the subject relied on memory for the figures and multiplied them mentally with closed eyes. The method was better than the earlier one, for it not only made the task more difficult, but it helped to eliminate sensory fatigue. When the subject forgot the original figures, she looked at them again, but as the time was made longer on this account, the loss of the original figures was counted against her. But this seldom occurred as the subject was careful to commit the numbers to memory." [Arai, '12, p. 35]

Her work, that is, was to look at an example such as $\frac{4962}{2584}$, cover it, memorize the two numbers, then multiply mentally 4×4962, getting 19848, then memorize this, but keeping in mind the 4962 and the 758 to be used later, then to multiply mentally 4962 by 8 getting 39696 and perform mentally the operation of adding $\frac{19848}{39696}$.

Having obtained the 416808,* she could now forget the 19848, but must not have let slip the 4962 and 75 and must

* Other methods of operation are, of course, possible, but this was the one which she used throughout the experiment.

remember the 416808. She then multiplied 4962 by 5, and remembered to count the 24810 as 2481000 in adding it to 416808. Having obtained 2897808, she could now forget all but it and the 4962 and 7 and the fact that the 7 counted as 7000 in multiplying. Multiplying mentally and obtaining 34734, she held it in mind and added 34734000 to 2897808, and could then write down the answer 37,631,808, look at her watch, record the time, look at the next example on the sheet, say $\frac{9653}{7267}$, and proceed as above.

If the reader will try this work with the far easier task of multiplying four-place by three-place numbers for even only an hour or two he will appreciate that it is far more difficult and fatiguing (in the popular sense of requiring much disagreeable effort) than all but a few of life's customary intellectual labors.

After doing 189 examples requiring about thirty-five hours (during the week February 24-March 2) by this new method, the subject reached a point where practice effect was very slight, and secured in the next four days the record to be considered here.

"On March 3, 4, 5 and 6, the subject did the mental multiplication from 11 A. M. to 11 P. M. without any pauses except the two or three seconds between the examples for recording time. But the subject had taken a heavier breakfast than usual at 10 A. M. and a light supper after 11 P. M. Her health was in good condition and she slept soundly at night. The contents of her consciousness during the experiments were very simple, all desires being completely subjected to the one desire to get true fatigue curves." [Arai, '12, p. 37] The results of these experiments are summarized in Table 4 and FIG. 60.

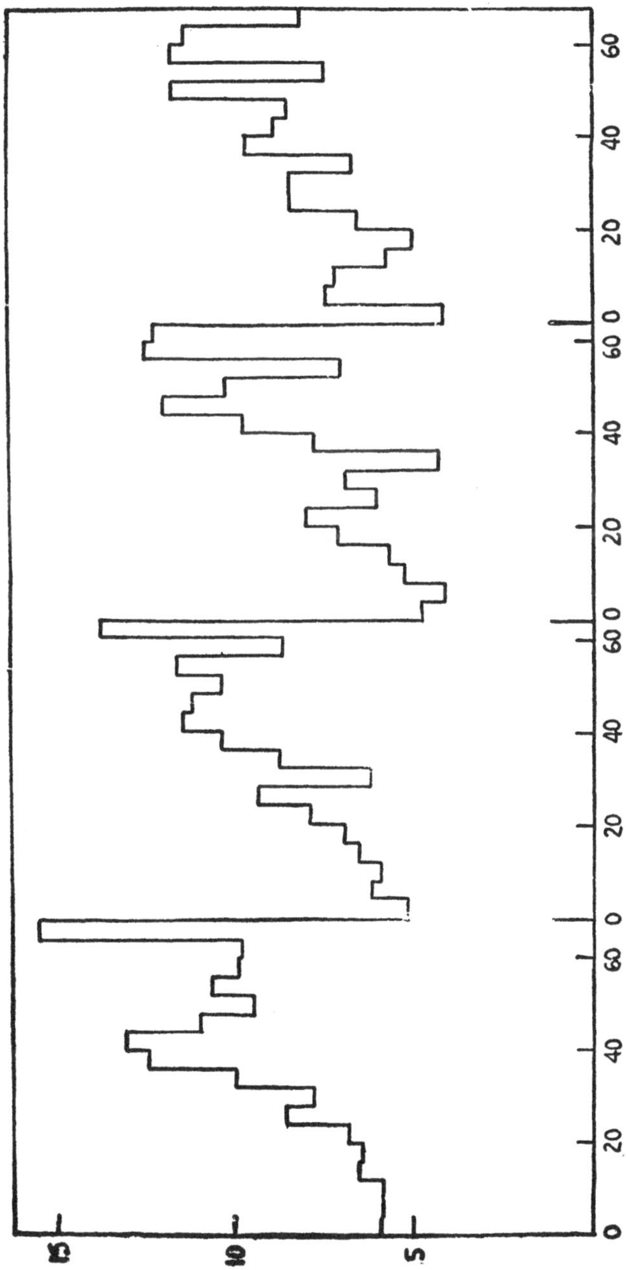

FIG. 60. Curve of Work in Mental Multiplication with Four-Place Numbers. Each inch on the base-line equals forty examples done. The height of the curve represents the time required, with allowance for errors. The rests between the end of one work-period and the beginning of the next are shown by quarter inch verticals above the zeros on the base-line.

The base line of Fig. 60 is scaled for the number of examples done, one inch equalling forty examples, each 12 hours of rest being denoted by a quarter-inch vertical line at the appropriate point on the base-line.

Above each tenth of an inch along the base line a horizontal line is drawn whose height in each case denotes the time required for the four examples in question, plus an addition for each wrong figure more than two in any answer, and a subtraction for each wrong figure less than two in any answer, of three per cent of the time required for the four examples (that is, twelve per cent of the time required per example).

TABLE 4.

FATIGUE IN THE CASE OF MENTAL MULTIPLICATION WITH FOUR-PLACE NUMBERS. After Arai, '12, p. 38 f.

Time required (in minutes), with allowances for errors, for successive sets of four examples multiplied mentally.

Set	Mar 3	Mar. 4	Mar. 5	Mar. 6	Average
1	23 6	20.7	19.3	16.5	20.0
2	23 3	24 5	16.5	29.6	23.9
3	23.2	23 5	20.9	28.5	23.4
4	26.1	25.9	22.8	23 0	24 6
5	25.8	27.8	28.3	20.2	26 8
6	27.3	31.4	31.7	26.2	29.4
7	34 3	37 3	24.0	33.6	34 0
8	31 3	24 9	27.5	33.8	29 4
9	40.0	35.0	17.1	26.7	30 9
10	49 8	41.5	31.0	38.6	40 0
11	52.2	45.8	39.1	35.6	42.5
12	43 8	44.6	48 1	34.1	44.2
13	37.9	41 8	41.0	47.0	41.4
14	42.5	46.5	27.9	29.8	36.2
15	39.7	31.1	28.3	47.1	36.6
16	39.0	52.0	50.0	45.6	40 7
17*	62.1	44.4	49.1	32.9	47.1
First eight	46.9	45.2	35.8	46.1	43.9
Last eight	101.1	96 4	99.1	78.5	93.8

* There were only three examples in the 17th set. The score was adjusted to be what it would have been for four examples done at the same speed and accuracy.

The Amount of Fatigue

The amount of fatigue is measurable by the increase in time required* as work continues, an allowance being made for practice, or by the increase of time required at the end of work over that required *at the beginning of work after full rest.* By either method we find that somewhat more than double time was required as a result of the long work without rest.

This, it must be remembered, by no means implies that the function was less than half as efficient at the end of the twelve hours of work as at the end of twelve hours of rest. On the contrary, the amount of percentile loss in absolute efficiency was probably very slight. For a person to be able to multiply a number like 9263 by one like 5748 without any visual, written, or spoken aids, even in fifteen, or for that matter in a hundred and fifty, minutes, implies a very high degree of efficiency. That a person can exert himself to the utmost at this very difficult work for ten or twelve hours without rest and still be able to do it, even if at the expense of twice or thrice as many minutes per example as at the beginning, means that the loss in efficiency by any absolute standard has been small. For Shakespeare to have required twice as long to write Hamlet as he actually did require would not have meant a loss of half the efficiency of the play-writing function! For Napoleon to have taken twenty instead of five minutes to plan a series of moves at Austerlitz would not have meant that his generalship was only one fourth as efficient!

* Here and throughout the discussion of Miss Arai's experiment *'time required'* means *'time required for work of equal accuracy.'*

19

The zero point of efficiency in the function of mental multiplication would be 'just not to multiply a number like 3 by a number like 2 in, say, ten minutes.' We do not of course know just at what point between this zero and the ability to multiply a four-place by a four-place number mentally in five minutes with only two figures in the answer wrong (as Miss Arai did at the beginning of work), we should place her ability, at the end of work, to multiply a four-place by a four-place number in eleven minutes. The reader may judge for himself. It is my impression that she could, at the end of work, certainly have multiplied a three-place by a three-place number (and probably a four-place by a three-place number) as quickly and accurately as she had multiplied a four-place by a four-place number at the beginning, and that it would be absurd to place the efficiency of her last half hour's work in each period at less than 75 per cent of the initial efficiency.

There are no other experiments with so long continued and so difficult work. There have been, however, many investigations of the effect of one or two hours of unremitting work at computation, memorizing, counting letters and the like. So, for example, Oehrn ['95] had ten individuals work each for two hours on each of six sorts of work.

Oehrn's results show that, in general, whatever fatigue there may have been was so slight as to be counterbalanced by the gain from practice including the adaptation or 'warming up' to the work. FIG. 61 shows the central tendency of the change in efficiency considering all six sorts of work together. In general that is, the subjects worked equally well throughout the entire two hours. This general result might have come from a steady improvement in some of the functions, balanced by a steady loss in efficiency in others, or from various rates of change in efficiency in the different functions. As a matter of fact, however, as FIG. 62 shows, the different particular functions follow closely the general tendency. Their slight divergences therefrom are probably due to the small number of subjects and experiments.

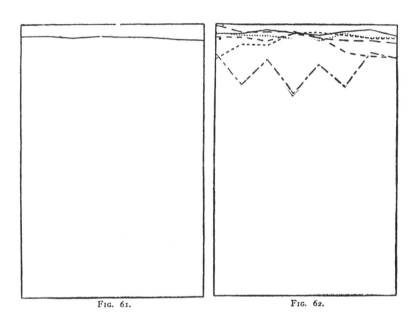

FIG. 61.   FIG. 62.

The author ['12] found with five subjects who added columns, each of 10 one-place numbers, continuously for from one and a half to two hours per day, that the difference between the last ten minutes of one day's work and the first ten minutes of the work of the next day—that is, after the rest—was, for each individual in each pair of consecutive days, as shown in Table 5. The central tendency is toward a fatigue effect of 6% (i. e., to do 6% fewer examples in the same time) from approximately 100 minutes of continuous exercise at adding.

TABLE 5. FATIGUE IN ADDING

Time (corrected for errors) required to add x rows at the end of each work period and at the beginning of the following work period. $x = 6$ for D, 2 for L, 4 for Mc, 3 for R and 6 for S. Also the per cent which the latter is of the former in each case.

	1a. At End of Work Period 1	2b. At Beginning of Work Period 2	2a. At End of Work Period 2	3b. At Beginning of Work Period 3	3a. At End of Work Period 3	4b. At Beginning of Work Period 4	2b/1a	3b/2a	4b/3a	Av. b/Av. a
D	715	565	595	620	615	580	79	104	94	92
L	975	615	590	560	545	585	63	95	107	88
Mc	543	531	579	510	511	466	98	88	91	92
R	630	545	615	545	535	495	87	88	93	89
S	897	850	842	934	779	743	95	111	95	100

Average of all per cents = 93.   Median of all per cents = 94.

The results quoted give a fair sampling of the amounts of difference found between the efficiency of a function after long exercise of it at the individual's supposed maximum exertion, and its efficiency after full rest. These differences are in general very slight. A man can work for several hours at his utmost, and at the end do nearly as well as he will after full rest. Except when the function exercised is very disagreeable, either in *toto* or in the degree of restraint which it demands, the loss during the work period is often indiscernible. Indeed there is usually a gross gain, though after full rest there is a further gain. Such statements as Binet's "Tout effort est accompagné d'une certaine fatigue" ['98, p. 302], give then a wrong impression of the amount and rate of fatigue.

Such statements have been common partly because those who have written about fatigue at all have usually been inter-

ested in it and ready to believe in its existence and magnify
its amount, partly because the gross results found for fatigue
of a muscle have misled expectations in the case of mental
fatigue, and partly because many students of this problem
begged the question by presupposing that mental work done
without rest must decrease the ability to do further work,
and partly because of one particular fallacious supposition
which requires brief comment here.

I refer to the supposition that *any decrease in the permanent improvement* (resulting from, say two hours of continuous work) *below the permanent improvement that would
have been made if the two hours had been distributed in the
best possible manner,* is to be reckoned as fatigue. This argument sounds innocent, but is essentially unsound. It confuses
a temporary deficiency which rest can cure with a permanent
deficiency which *rest cannot cure,* but which a better distribution of the practice periods *could have prevented.*

Exercise of a function without rest shows two radically
different effects. One is that the function is, at the end of
the exercise, slightly less efficient than it becomes after a
certain amount of rest. The other is that it is still less
efficient than it would have become if the exercise had been
distributed optimally so as to prevent over-learning, loss of
satisfyingness, practice at less than maximal effort, and the
like. The two effects should not be confused.

The fallacy of arguing that long use causes a temporary
deterioration because the permanent improvement is less with
it than it would have been with the same time in short periods
is much the same as in the argument that a man who had a
thousand dollars at 10 A. M., January 1, and the same amount
at 10 P. M. of the same day, must really have lost a fifth
of it, since, had he speculated successfully with it on six

or eight separate occasions during the day, he would have increased it to twelve hundred dollars.

THE CURVE OF WORK

Various notions have been entertained concerning changes in the rate of decrease in efficiency of a function in the course of continuous exercise,—that is, changes in the slope of the curve of work. For instance, we have the doctrine that at the very beginning a person tends, other things being equal, to work at a higher efficiency than ever again. This we may call the doctrine of the 'Initial Spurt.' A second doctrine is that knowledge that the end is at hand produces in the last fraction of a work-period of limited length, other things being equal, a marked rise in efficiency. This we may call the doctrine of the 'End Spurt.' A third doctrine is that for the first half-hour or so, other things being equal, efficiency increases gradually. This we may call the doctrine of 'Incitement' or the 'Warming-Up' effect. A fourth doctrine is that a slower, longer and more lasting gain exists alongside of the 'Warming-Up' effect, called Adaptation. A fifth doctrine is that any more than usually rapid decrease in efficiency, by attracting the person's attention and rousing him to greater exertion, tends, other things being equal, to be followed by a relative increase in efficiency and maintenance of efficiency at a relatively high level for a few minutes. This we may call the doctrine of 'Spurt after Fatigue.' A sixth doctrine is that slight ups and downs in efficiency come rhythmically in correspondence with fluctuations of attention, each total 'wave' being about two seconds long.

It should be noted that the terms Initial Spurt, End Spurt, 'Spurt after Fatigue,' 'Spurt after Disturbance,' 'Warming-

Up' (Anregung), 'Adaptation' (Gewöhnung), 'Rhythm of Attention,' and the like, may each be used in two meanings. They may refer to objective changes in the efficiency of the function,—that is, in the height of the curve—or to imagined causes of such objective changes. Thus, End-Spurt may mean either 'an increase in efficiency in the last five or ten minutes of work,' or 'a reinforcing potency from knowledge that the end is near.' 'Adaptation' or Gewöhnung may mean either 'a rise in efficiency, slower than the rise called Warming-up and less permanent than the rise due to practice,' or some real factor which causes this rise and is different from the factors causing 'Warming-Up' or the practice effect.

I shall in this chapter use these terms only in the former objective meanings of changes in the efficiency of the function, asking, for instance, in the case of Initial Spurt, "To what extent is a high degree of efficiency appearing in the first few minutes of work characteristic of work curves in general, or of certain individuals in certain kinds of work?"

Initial Spurt

This phenomenon is certainly not characteristic of work curves in general. In the case of the 37 work-periods of 16 subjects engaged in mental multiplication (of a three-place number by a three-place number) there was no evidence of it. In the case of five adults working at addition (each for four two-hour periods), there is no evidence of it.

I am unable to find anywhere any evidence of consistent initial spurt with any individual in all mental functions or with all (or nearly all) individuals in any kind of mental work, much less with all individuals in all kinds of work. The work curves obtained by Oehrn, ['95] Amberg, ['95]

Weygandt, ['97] Lindley, ['00] and other workers in Kraepelin's laboratory give no such evidence. Nor is it to be found in the data got by Yoakum, ['09] so far as he presents them.

Lindley's work, which was the most extensive, showed as speed ratios for successive five-minute periods at the beginning of work, 100, 98, 97, 97, and 96, using the data from all three subjects. The first five minutes, that is, differed from the second substantially only as the fourth from the fifth. Putting together Weygandt's series I find ratios of 100, 97 and 95½ for the first three five-minute periods. Hoch and Kraepelin ['95, p. 431 ff.] showed, on the whole, ratios of 100, 99, 98 and 94 for the first four five-minute periods. Miesemer ['02] showed ratios of 100, 96, 98, 97. In fact the very results of Rivers and Kraepelin, ['96] to explain which Initial Spurt was specially invoked, give as ratios (by five-minute periods) 100, 87, 99, 101, 102, 102. Clearly the fact in them to be explained is the 87 of the second five minutes rather than the 100 of the first five.

It is, I admit, very likely that some individuals in some kinds of work tend to fall off rapidly from the too exacting standard which they set themselves at the beginning, just as some tend to rise rapidly above the standard which they cautiously try at the beginning. But these idiosyncrasies must not be misinterpreted as a general law.

End Spurt

It is often the case in ordinary mental work with a time limit, that as one approaches the end of the work period, the knowledge that he is approaching it leads him to spurt. In ordinary mental work one does not work throughout at one's possible maximum, so that such a spurt is easily possible. In experimental work, when the subject is required to work throughout at maximum possible efficiency, such a spurt can come only if the subject has deliberately disregarded instructions, or if the knowledge of the approaching end releases forces over which he had no control. The latter is apparently possible, various external stimuli, such as other competing individuals, applause and the like, being apparently able to add a reinforcement beyond what a subject's own determination can summon.

On the whole, no subject who has been tested four or more times shows consistently any great end-spurt; the general tendency is to a rise, in the last five or ten minutes, of three or four per cent in the amount of work per unit of time.

Spurt after Fatigue and Spurt after Disturbance

In mental work in ordinary life a person may obviously, if he is not doing his best, at any time do a little better to make up for an observed temporary deficiency, however caused. Deficiencies due to disturbances certainly, and to fatigue, if that acted unevenly throughout a work period, might be thus noticed and counterbalanced. In a subject who is keeping his efficiency at a maximum so far as he can control it, the observation of a fall in achievement might still so act as a reinforcement.

It should be noted, however, that on general grounds the suggestion that one is doing well would seem more favorable to the efficiency of one already doing his best than the suggestion that he is doing badly, and that empirically no one has correlated the fluctuations in work curves with the incidence of disturbances of known character. The doctrine of spurt after fatigue and spurt after disturbance in the case of work done under the conditions of the ordinary fatigue experiment, is then at present a speculative hypothesis. .It was devised apparently to explain the fluctuations in efficiency, from one minute or five-minute period to another, which are found in continuous adding, cancelling letters, memorizing, or other forms of mental work.

A rise following a fall in the curve easily attracts observation and tempts readily to theorizing. A rise followed by a rise, or a fall followed by a fall, is not so striking. The explanation of a 'fall-rise' sequence by spurt after disturbance or spurt after fatigue is really unwise, however. For if the fall is caused by a disturbance, no cause is required for the rise save the ending of the disturbance; while if no external cause is known for a given fall, there is no reason why one should pretend to know the cause of its sequent rise. The wiser effort would be to seek hypotheses which would account for rise-fall, rise-rise, fall-fall, and fall-rise sequences, one and all, and, until such hypotheses could be subjected to verification, to be content with attributing them to 'accidental' variations.

Warming Up

The best definition of 'warming-up' as an objective act is that part of an increase of efficiency during the first 20 minutes (or some other assigned early portion) of a work period, which is abolished by a moderate rest, say of 60 minutes. Such warming-up should show itself clearly in individuals at or near the limit of practice, and, in others, should compound with the effect of practice to make the rise in efficiency especially rapid in the first twenty minutes of work, or the fall (supposing the function to diminish in efficiency) specially slow in this same period. What time is assigned in the definition of warming-up effect is of little consequence to the investigation so long as *some* time is assigned.

There is little or no direct evidence of warming-up in the records got by Oehrn ['95], Lindley ['oo], Weygandt ['97], Bolton ['02], Miesemer ['02], or Rivers and Kraepelin ['96]. Possible indirect evidence of it may be got from the finding of Wimms ['07] that 20 minutes of work at simple computation, but in a form involving trying control of the eye's fixations, was more efficient when done in two equal periods with a ten-minute rest between than when either no rest or a 20-minute rest was given. My sixteen subjects ['11] working at mental multiplication of a three-place by a three-place number showed signs of its presence, but not conclusively.

It seems likely, from the cruder observations of daily life, that for many individuals in many functions, there is a warming-up effect as defined, but I am unable, with the data at hand from Kraepelin's pupils or others, to separate out this temporary improvement that comes at the beginning of the exercise of a function after rest, from the more permanent improvement that comes from exercise of the function in general. I am confident that it has commonly been exaggerated. It should also be noted that intellectual warming-up in the popular sense refers rather to fore-exercise of *other functions,* in order to get materials and motives with which and by which the given function is to work, than to an intrinsic alteration of it.

There is also probably often a rapid *relearning,* with consequent rise in the score, during the first few minutes of a practice-period. This is perhaps what is meant by Warming-Up or Incitement by certain writers. It is doubtful

whether a rest of sixty minutes or so would abolish this
rise in the score resulting from relearning. And it seems more
useful to think of a rise due to relearning in the terms which
exactly describe it, rather than in the vaguer terms—Anregung,
Incitement, or Warming-Up.

Summary

The essential empirical facts about the curve of mental
work seem then to be as follows: Two hours or less of
continuous exercise of a function at maximum efficiency, so
far as the worker can make it so, produce a temporary negative
effect, curable by rest, of not over ten per cent, and in most
functions still less than that. Fluctuations of considerable
amount occur in any one work period for any one subject,
but except for a rise in achievement of approximately four per
cent near the end when the date of the end is known, no
regularity in them has been proved for any one of them for
any one subject in any one sort of work, much less for any
one subject in all sorts of work, or for all subjects in any
one sort of work. The supposed laws that the very first few
minutes and the minutes after a drop in efficiency are periods
of specially high efficiency are not supported by the facts.
A special gradual increase in efficiency in the first fifteen or
twenty minutes is not demonstrable in the case of the simple
functions such as addition, mental multiplication, marking
words of certain sorts and the like. The fluctuations in a
single day's record for a single subject are then in no sense
explained by referring them to fervor at starting, fervor after
disturbance, fervor after fatigue, incitement or adaptation.

The most important fact about the curve of efficiency of
a function under two hours or less continuous maximal

exercise is that it is, when freed from daily eccentricities, so near a straight line and so near a horizontal line. The work grows much less satisfying or much more unbearable, but not much less effective. The commonest instinctive response to the intolerability of mental work is to stop it altogether. When, as under the conditions of the experiments, this response is not allowed, habit leads us to continue work at our standard of speed and accuracy. Such falling off from this standard as does occur is, in the writer's opinion, due to an unconscious reduction of the intolerability, by intermitting the work or some parts of it.

THE CURVE OF SATISFYINGNESS

All our measurements so far have been of the quantity and quality of the product, not of the satisfyingness of the process. Of the latter, indeed, there have been only occasional and very crude reports. No one has ever made the experiment of arranging with workers that they should work at least two hours, and be given, say, two cents a minute for every minute that they continue at maximal exertion beyond two hours, being compelled to pay two cents for every minute less than two hours if they stop work. Nor has any experimenter equated the requirement of X production or the privilege of Y rest at given stages in a period of production with any measure of value whatever.

In ordinary life, such equating is of enormous importance. Having, say, a thousand sums to compute, one does them all rapidly and continuously, resting at the end; or at moderate speed, not resting at all; or rapidly at first, and then more and more slowly; or one inserts a thousand rests of two seconds; or eight or ten rests of three or four minutes; and so on through the infinite variety of ways of administering one's mental production. What one does is determined in large measure precisely by balancing the satisfyingness of money-rewards, free time, following familiar customs, and the like against the annoyingness of this or that feature of the process. John, who is annoyed by hurry, inserts his rests bit by bit. James, who is more annoyed by the lack of free time for some cherished pursuit, saves his rests till the product is complete.

Anyone who undergoes experiments in working mentally as continuously and perfectly as he can for a long period can get some rough idea of the curve of satisfyingness for his own case, with the function in question, in the circumstances of competing desires in question. In the general accounts of mental work and fatigue, the impressions obtained thus, or from the ordinary experiences of life, play a part. The notion of Warming-Up, for example, has included the diminishing annoyance of a process due to the progressive inattention to competing desires, interest in achievement, and the like. So, also, the effect of knowledge that the end is nigh in producing a spurt is attributed, and probably rightly, in part to the fact that the satisfyingness of reaching the end, and of using one's last chance to do one's utmost spreads to make the process itself more satisfying.

The curve of satisfyingness need not follow the curve of achievement. The slight amount of the decrease in efficiency, due to continued exercise of a function under the condition that one shall do his utmost throughout, may be accompanied by a very great decrease in the satisfyingness of the process. The very individual who after five or six hours, adds or multiplies more rapidly and accurately than ever, may be in a condition which would in ordinary life make him stop the work on grounds of absolute unfitness to continue. The supposed unfitness would not be an inevitable inefficiency in the function itself, but the effort, tension and misery for which its unsatisfyingness was responsible. Indeed, the less a man was fatigued in the sense of becoming unable to produce, the more he might be fatigued in the sense of finding the process intolerable.

Although little can be said about the effects of any given continued task on satisfyingness, such are of very great importance. In ordinary life the amount, rate and changes in rate of increase or decrease in the efficiency of a given function are not determined in any simple mechanical way by the amount of energy possessed at the start, the opportunity for it to be spent, and the lengths of rest periods devoted to its recuperation. Nor are they determined by mysterious tendencies, *Fervor at Beginning, Spurt after Disturbance, Anregung or Warming Up, Arbeitsbereitschaft,* and so on. They are determined, as are any responses of the animal, by its original tendencies, past experiences and present attitude, including the tendencies to be satisfied and to be annoyed by this and that state of affairs.

A man does not, by beginning to add, open a valve which releases mental energy at a rate depending on the store of it possessed. Inactivity does not necessarily restore the energy. Nor does the valve work wider and wider open by *Anregung,* or widen and contract every few seconds by the *Rhythm of Attention,* or open very wide by a strange foresight just before it is to be closed. A man's behavior during two hours of adding is a series of responses to whatever of the original situation persists plus the new elements due to each stage of the work. These responses are conditioned only slightly by such changes in the animal as can properly be likened to a lessening of a fund of energy. The appeals of ungratified

impulses as they weaken by inattention or grow stronger
the lapse of time, the loss of the zest of novelty as the sai
process is repeated, the sensory pains from strained postu
misuse of the eyes and the like—are all as truly effective
determining the work-curves of ordinary life as is the me
amount of time employed or product produced. But the
act primarily on the satisfyingness of the process and or
indirectly on the quality and quantity of the product.

CHAPTER XX

MENTAL FATIGUE (CONTINUED)

THE INFLUENCE OF CONTINUOUS MENTAL WORK, SPECIAL OR GENERAL, UPON GENERAL ABILITY

It is really idle to inquire whether fatigue is specific or general—whether, that is, continued work at one function diminishes efficiency in only it, or in all functions equally. We do not have to choose between these alternatives. The first is almost always, and the latter always, false. It is a separate problem to tell for any given loss in efficiency of any function due to its exercise without rest just what the effect upon every other function will be. Some functions will suffer little or not at all; others, much. The real questions are: *"How much* does continued work at any one or any combination of tasks diminish efficiency for any other task?" and "How does it?"

The same doctrine of transfer by identical elements noted in the case of the influence of improvement in one mental function upon the efficiency of other functions is applicable here to the influence of diminished efficiency. However, as was noted in the case of practice, we usually lack the knowledge by which to know beforehand in what respects and to what extent two functions are physiologically identical. Moreover, we lack, in the majority of cases, knowledge of how the various elements of a function share in the total loss in efficiency. Consequently, if a function, say, adding, loses one fifth in efficiency as a result of five hours of work, it is as yet impossible to prophesy the resulting loss in another ability, say, to memorize nonsense syllables, save very roughly.

The clearest cases of identical elements important in the transfer of fatigue, are the headaches and deprivations. A headache produced by five hours of mental multiplication may act equally to diminish efficiency in writing poetry. The deprivations from sleep, exercise, sociability, games and the like are common elements of very many different forms of mental work. Just as learning not to be distracted by certain impulses is a means of improvement common to many functions, so the increased urgency of these impulses due to long deprivation may be a means of decreasing efficiency in many functions. In many of the actual tasks of school, professional, business and industrial work, eye-strain is an important identical element. Factors essentially irrelevant to fatigue itself—notably, excitement, worry, sleeplessness and loss of appetite—may appear in connection with work at one task and diminish efficiency for many, or even all, other tasks.

Students of mental work and fatigue have not, however, commonly thought of the problem as a series of special problems of the influence of a given amount of work with a given function or functions upon the temporary efficiency of each of countless others. They have thought of mental work vaguely as the work of 'the mind' or 'the brain,' and have openly or tacitly accepted one or another form of the theory that continuous work reduced some supply of mental energy. They have commonly assumed therefore that any work must reduce the efficiency of the mind for all work.

They seem to have expected also that any work would reduce the efficiency of the mind *equally* for all work. The questions in their minds have been, "Does this or that work temporarily enfeeble the mind?" and "Does such and such a test measure power to work?"

There resulted about a dozen investigations each attempting to measure the effect of a more or less well defined amount of mental work upon the efficiency of some convenient sample of the mind's operations.

EXPERIMENTAL RESULTS

Samples of the facts are, briefly, as follows:

Sikorski ['79], testing the same children first before school and then after school in writing from dictation, found the average percentage of wrong letters to be for six grades :*

Before school	1.24	1.21	.72	.66	.61	.46
After school	1.57	1.45	1.03	.94	.81	.80

The central tendency is thus toward a third more errors in the late tests (.7 and .10).

I trust that the reader is not so unsophisticated as to assume that the above figures, even if taken at their face value, show an efficiency before school 1.33 times that existing after school. They as truly mean that, since about 99.3 per cent of the letters were correct in the morning, and about 99.0 per cent after school, the efficiency before school was 1.0033 times that existing after school.

Bolton ['92] reports the results of tests, arranged in coöperation with Dr. Franz Boas, to measure the number of digits that could be remembered after a single hearing (using lists of 4, 5, 6, 7 and 8) early and late in the school day. He tested 136 pupils four times in the morning, and 219

* Sikorski carelessly took no account of the speed of work, so that he did not measure the efficiency of the function at all.

pupils four times—first, late in the session; second, early the next morning; third, late in that day's session; and fourth, early the next morning. Each test comprised twelve series of figures. The 219 pupils did almost exactly as well at the end as at the beginning of the session, though the combined result of practice and novelty should have made the second and fourth tests better than the first and third. The 219 pupils also improved as much from morning to night as from night to morning, and as much as the 136 pupils used as a check improved from one test to the next. Indeed, the data show a slight apparent advantage in the late period.

Friedrich ['97] tested a class of 51 pupils of an average age of 10 years, on eleven occasions during a period of six weeks, using dictation, addition and multiplication. The last two were of the type $\frac{275831406}{694132258}$ and $\frac{27583140}{2}$ (or 3, 4, 5, or 6).

With the dictations there was an increase in the number of errors in later over earlier periods, and in the same periods without previous rest over earlier periods with rest; but as no record was kept of the speed of the work, efficiency cannot be measured. From the results of other similar tests, it is probable that the speed increased. The results as to accuracy are given in Table 14.

Friedrich gave twenty minutes time for about 206 single additions or multiplications. Consequently all but the very slowest pupils finished all the examples before the time was up, so that we have no record at all of the speed of the work after the first test, and only a very imperfect and distorted record for that. Now it is known from the results of other workers that in repeated tests with such simple additions and multiplications, a child tends to work more and more rapidly at the cost of accuracy. The number of errors is then certainly a wrong measure of efficiency. Apparently, if he had recorded the time taken, he would have found, even allowing a discount of so many as ten additions for each error, no decrease whatever in the efficiency-scores for the tests late in the school day. His gross results as to accuracy are given in Table 6.

TABLE 6

THE RESULTS OBTAINED BY FRIEDRICH CONCERNING THE ACCURACY OF SCHOOL WORK AT DIFFERENT PERIODS OF THE DAY.

Time of test	Letters, etc., written in Dictations		Figures of sums and products in Computations	
	Per-cent right	Per-cent wrong	Per-cent right	Per-cent wrong
Before 1st hour	99.8	.2	98.9	1 1
After 1st hour	99.6	.4	98 4	1 6
After 2nd hour and 8 min. rest........	99.3	.7	98.0	2 0
After 2nd hour	99 2	.8	98 0	2 0
After 3rd hour and two 15 min. rests	99 4	.6	98.1	1.9
After 3rd hour and 15 min. rest......	99 0	1.0	97.8	2.2
After 3rd hour	99.0	1 0	97.7	2.3
Before 1st hour	99.8	.2	98.1	1 9
After 1st hour	99 2	.8	97.9	2.1
After 2nd hour and 15 min. rest......	99 4	.6	97.9	2.1
After 2nd hour	98 9	1.1	97 6	2 4

(Morning Session for the first seven rows; Afternoon Session for the last four rows.)

As with Sikorski's results, so with Friedrich's, the number of errors has been carelessly taken as a direct measure of inefficiency. Binet and Henri, for example, print a diagram like FIG. 63, which gives the impression that efficiency decreases enormously with the progress of the school-day and the absence of rests. Even supposing the speed of work to have remained constant, this diagram is very misleading. Efficiency is as properly measured by the number written correctly as by the inverse of the number written incorrectly. If the former measure is used, the diagram becomes FIG. 64. FIG. 63 and FIG. 64 measure *absolutely the same fact*. The case is as if we had a man's gains and losses in trade for

consecutive hours of the day. Suppose him to have made
998 dollars and lost 2 dollars the first hour, to have made

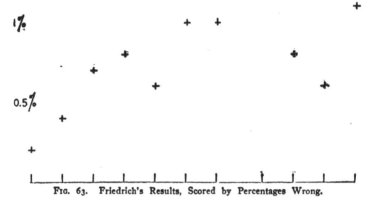

FIG. 63.   Friedrich's Results, Scored by Percentages Wrong.

996 dollars and lost 4 dollars the second hour, and so on.
Both gains and losses should figure in estimating his efficiency.
Now in the case in hand, we do not know how much more

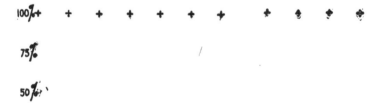

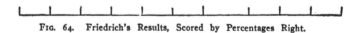

FIG. 64.   Friedrich's Results, Scored by Percentages Right.

efficiency is required to copy correctly 998 out of a thousand
letters than to copy 996. The first performance is, however,
surely not twice times as efficient.

The author ['00], eliminating the influence of both practice and novelty by the simple expedient of never giving the same test twice to any individual, found the efficiency of school children (in adding,* multiplying,† marking misspelled words on a page of print,‡ memorizing lists of 10 digits, 5 nonsense syllables,§ 10 letters and 6 simple forms,¶ and counting dots) substantially the same at near the end as at the beginning of the school session.

The children who were tested with one function early in the school session were tested with another function late in the session. Thus no child ever repeats any test, and all influence of practice and novelty is avoided. At the same time any influence upon the results from the accidental superiority of one half of the children to the other half can be detected and allowed for. The number of children taking a test varied from 240 to 700. Since all the tests were given by the author and his assistant, each one's time being equally divided between 'early' and 'late' tests, the only factor left to produce any difference is the difference of time of day,

---

* With examples, each of five four-place numbers.

† With 9 examples like $\frac{7986}{4523}$

‡ With a passage like:

After waiting some time Captain B— and myself walked acros the rice fields to the shad of a tree. There we herd the trumpett of an elephant: we reshed etc.

§ With the following:

ba ni su et ko and *ig fa tu le ro*

¶ The forms being:

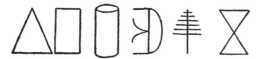

with whatever differences in amount of school work and other factors it implied.

The following facts appeared:

Experiment 1.—Those who did the multiplication work late in the session did 99.3 per cent as much and made 3.9 per cent more mistakes than those who did it early, and numbered 64 who misunderstood or grossly failed in the test against 56 among the early ones.

Experiment 2.—The test in marking misspelled words which was given early to those who did the multiplication late, and *vice versa,* shows the following results for those who took it late as compared with those who took it early. Relative amount of page covered, 99.0 per cent; relative number of words marked, 105.0 per cent; relative number of words marked improperly, 97.9 per cent. Thus the decrease in ability shown in test 1 is offset by an equal increase in the case of test 2.

Experiments 3 and 4.—Tests in memorizing figures were given to four classes early and four late. Taking both together, we find that the pupils who did the work late in the forenoon or late in the afternoon memorized almost 2 per cent more than those who had the work early. But with tests in memorizing letters and nonsense syllables, where the pupils were reversed, we find the late pupils memorized only 98 per cent as much as the early with test 4, and 99.8 per cent as much with test 7. So here again the balance is practically equal.

Experiments 5 and 6.—The test in memorizing forms was given late to only half the total group of pupils; and the set who took it early were shown by the other tests to be a little more intelligent. Here the late pupils did only 94.6 per cent as well. That this was wholly due to a difference in average ability is also witnessed by the fact that when 75 per cent of these scholars were tested in counting dots (those who memorized forms early counted dots late, and *vice versa*) the scholars taking the test *late* did much more than five per cent better.

If we take account of the conditions of the experiments and replace partial by adequate measures of efficiency, the apparent conflict between the results of Sikorski and Friedrich on the one hand, and those of Bolton and Thorndike on the other, turns out a harmony. The work in late periods is really only a little better or a little worse than in early periods. There is a general tendency of school children to increase speed at the expense of precision in repeated tests in adding, copying and the like. This fact has permitted the illusion of great deficiency and led to the fallacy of interpreting a series like "99 right, 1 wrong; 98 right, 2 wrong; 97 right, 3 wrong" as "1 wrong; 2 wrong; 3 wrong," and then as "Early Efficiency = 1; Middle efficiency = ½; Late efficiency = ⅓." It is the false inferences only that are in conflict with the result, "Efficiency approximately equal at all three periods."

The results obtained by other investigators agree substantially in showing similarly that ability to work is, in school pupils, throughout and at the close of the school session, almost or quite unimpaired.* When the effects of both novelty and practice are eliminated, no differences in achievement appear as a result of the work of the school session. Where they are not eliminated the former seems approximately

---

* Whether school pupils do, in fact, ordinarily achieve much less in late than in early periods is left as a question for educational experiments to decide. The common impression amongst teachers that they do may be to a large extent illusory.

to balance the latter. It is clear from the facts summarized that the assertions made in text-books on school hygiene that there are great and important differences between the results of tests at different periods of the school session, are quite unjustifiable. The very results referred to in support of these assertions disprove them.

GENERAL THEORIES OF MENTAL WORK AND FATIGUE

We can now return to some of the fundamental facts about mental work and fatigue. In the course of our survey of the facts known concerning mental work and fatigue we have been led to define the real questions involved so as to relieve them from vagueness and to discourage merely verbal answers to them. Instead of pretending to describe changes in mental energy available following upon energy expended, we have measured the changes in the quantity and quality of certain products when the individual produces them as incessantly as he can. The change in, say, four hours of such production can be studied by itself, or be compared with the change in four hours of production distributed in any other way. The production at the end of such a period can be compared with that after an interval of no production.

We could also measure, though this has not been done, the satisfyingness or intolerability of the process of production at any stage.

Mental work has been noted as an ambiguous term, meaning on the one hand (1) mental achievement—the production of certain products, and on the other hand (2) mental effort —the initiation or continuance or prevention or cessation of a certain response in spite of the intrinsic relative unsatisfyingness of that behavior.

Mental rest is similarly ambiguous. In thinking about it one should make clear whether he is concerned with (1) mental inactivity—the absence of mental achievement, or with (2) mental relaxation—the absence of mental effort.

The *efficiency* of a function may be defined as the quantity and quality of the product produced (1) per unit of time, or (2) per unit of time with a given amount of effort. Call the former the *gross* efficiency of the function; and the latter, its *analyzed* efficiency.

If we stick to the first meaning—the objective fact—in each case, we have a series of useful objective definitions of important facts in behavior, which may be called work, rest and fatigue, as follows:

Mental work (achievement) is the behavior of an organism whereby certain products* are produced. Continuous mental work means the behavior of an individual who is producing as incessantly as he can.

Rest (inactivity) of a single function is an interval in which the individual does nothing toward that sort of production. General rest similarly would mean an interval in which he did nothing toward production of any sort. This perfect general rest is of course only approximated.

The fatigue of a function is that diminution in its productivity or gross efficiency which inactivity† can cure.

The *'fatigue,'* so defined, due to two hours of work seems to be very small. In general, under pressure from the determination to continue doing one's utmost, the associative mechanism of the brain involved in any given mental function seems to work for a long time with a very slight decrease in

---

* Such as poems memorized, books written, problems solved, decisions made, houses planned, lessons taught or prepared, and the like.

† Either of that function or in general as may be specified.

gross efficiency. But fatigue is not necessarily, and is probably not in fact, so slight, if it is measured by the diminution in *analyzed* efficiency—in the productivity per unit of time with a given amount of effort. It may well be that in order to maintain the same degree of *satisfyingness* at the end as at the beginning of the five hours of work, the individuals referred to in the above measures would have had to relax in speed and carefulness so much as to have shown a decrease in efficiency of 30 or 40 per cent on an absolute scale; or an increase in the time required, accuracy being constant, of over 100 per cent.

The great present need in experimentation on mental work is to measure mental effort as fully as mental achievement, and so to compute the changes in analyzed efficiency—the quality and quantity of the product per unit of time with a given amount of effort.

We may distinguish the maximum power of a man's neurones to make certain connections from their readiness to do so. A man may be *able* (in the former sense) to multiply 629 by 736 as quickly as ever, at a time when the work is ten times as intolerable.

All the facts, both of experimental studies and of everyday life, support the hypothesis that the effect of continuous exercise upon *readiness* is far quicker, greater and more significant than its effect upon *maximum power*. Fatigue in the vague popular sense means that we are less willing rather than that we are less able, that the probability of achievement is decreased by the increased effort that it requires rather than that the possibility of achievement is decreased inevitably,— that the activity of the function becomes less satisfying rather than intrinsically and necessarily feebler.

The ultimate physiological explanation of the phenomena

of mental work and fatigue will therefore, I venture to prophesy, be found largely in the conditions of readiness and unreadiness of the neurones, and the main practical problem of the administration of mental work will be found to be the problem of interest.

The 'Mechanical' or 'Energy' theory and the 'Biological' or 'Response' theory

In the early discussions of mental work and fatigue, the use of the term *Work* led thinkers naturally enough to follow the train of thought suggested by physics and to conceive of mental work as the consequence of expenditure of mental energy, of fatigue as the consumption of a stock of potential energy, and of rest as an opportunity for its restoration. If left vague enough, such a mechanical theory of the operation of mental functions does no great harm, but it is almost always misleading; and, when it is at all rigorously defined, it becomes, I think, either meaningless or wrong. Some of the reasons for preferring what may be called the Biological Theories or Response Theories or Extrinsic Theories of mental work and fatigue, may be briefly mentioned.

The first reason is that the rate of change in efficiency as more and more work is done without rest is not such as should be the case by a mechanical theory. It is far too irregular. The curves of work, special or general, have no such evenness as the curve for the pressure from a reservoir whence water runs out faster than it runs in, or the curve of force of impact of a ball dropped from steadily decreasing heights.

The mechanical theories of work consequently have to invent various subsidiary forces to act in conjunction with the loss of energy so as to produce the irregular course which efficiency actually takes under continuous work. For example, the fact of a gain in efficiency in the first ten or twenty or even forty minutes of work, contrary, of course, to expectation from the loss-of-energy doctrine, is attributed to the influence of Incitement or Warming-Up or Anregung. Similarly the fact of a frequent gain in efficiency in the last ten minutes of work, provided the worker is aware that they are the last, is attributed to a tendency to Final Spurt—to an increased 'exertion of the will' due to knowledge that the end of work is near. The resort to these subsidiary factors is, of course, an admission that loss in energy is not an adequate cause of the changes in the amount of work done hour by hour as work is continued.

The second argument concerns the enormous potency of interest in maintaining, and of repugnance in diminishing, efficiency in work without rest. Consider, for example, the effect of an offer, made at the end of the tenth hour of work, to give the worker a thousand dollars for every one per cent of improvement above his last hour's score. Consider similarly the probable work-curves resulting when a devotee of the game plays chess, and when he answers undesired and unprofitable questions, in each case for five or six continuous hours. Interest does not add to, nor does repugnance subtract from, a store of energy. By the mechanical theories rest and work monopolize these two functions. Interest could, at the most, only release the energy faster. But it is a fact easily verifiable that interest *does* add to, and that repugnance *does* subtract from, the amount of work done. The amount of work done then cannot depend closely upon the magnitude of a supply of mechanically conceived energy.

Finally the nature of mental work and of decreased efficiency in it, make the hypothesis of a usable and restorable supply of energy inappropriate. Consider any representative samples of mental work—*e. g.*, addition, solving geometrical problems, writing essays, devising arguments, correcting examination papers, reading proof. The work is the production of the *right* responses to certain situations. The mere amount of movement, of consciousness, or of neurone action is irrelevant. If we are to have a physical metaphor to illustrate mental work, we may say that the work of adding 7 and 9 is not like moving a pound through a foot against gravity, but is like the work of moving a pound of lead from a given space in Boston to a given space in New York. The mere physical work of the latter varies enormously, according to the condition of the vehicle used, the condition of the roads travelled, the route taken, and the opposition encountered from fire, flood, living animals and other natural forces. There is always a *qualitative* demand and a variety of obstacles to be overcome, and a choice of ways and means.

No physical metaphor is desirable. All that is meant by mental work is getting the required responses to certain situations. All that is meant by fatigue is the temporary diminution in the efficiency in making such required connections which comes from incessantly making them. Why the diminished efficiency should be so caused is a matter for investigation, not presupposition. All that a supply of 'mental energy' could properly mean would be a supply of power to make the required connections; and since what hinders making a connection in learning is its consequences, the reasonable expectation is that what will hinder making it in fatigue will be its consequences. An animal tends to repeat a connection when repeating it brings a satisfying state of affairs, and may be expected to discontinue it when repeating it annoys him. An animal would seem likely to discontinue or decrease mental work because continuing it annoys him rather than because some inner fund of impulsion, which might be likened to physical potential energy, was running low. The more promising theory would seem to be one that explained why mental work continued without rest became less and less satisfying.

This the Biological or Response Theory tries to do. Work without rest, it maintains, becomes less satisfying (1) by losing the zest of novelty, (2) by producing ennui, a certain intellectual nausea, sensory pains and even headache, and (3) by imposing certain deprivations—for instance, from physical exercise, social intercourse, or sleep.

That these facts of behavior are found where diminished efficiency as a result of work without rest is found, is a fact subject to verification by observation and experiment. Even the advocates of a mechanical theory will hardly deny it. That they cause the loss in efficiency is shown by the gain which follows their elimination. Varying the superficial form of arithmetical drills, while exercising the same mental function, will postpone the loss in efficiency by maintaining the force of novelty. The addition of a money reward, or of a demonstration that the work is useful for some desired end, or of competition for excellence, may temporarily abolish fatigue by abolishing the ennui. The common phrase that one is 'tired of' certain work represents a certain stage of fatigue better than 'tired by' it does.

The extreme condition where the mind seems literally nauseated—will not have anything to do with the problem—may be cured similarly by an increase in the value of the answers to be got. As a fatigued muscle can be given renewed efficiency by washing out or counteracting the products created by its action, so a fatigued mind can be in part restored by washing out ennui and repugnance by in-attention or counteracting them by interest and motive. It is harder to eliminate experimentally sensory pains and head-aches, but it seems probable that if these incubi could be lifted off, efficiency would rise.

That eliminating the deprivations, or in clearer phrase, permitting the indulgence of certain impulses, increases the efficiency of work is almost a crucial experiment for decision between the two classes of theory. When a boy regains efficiency by being allowed to walk up and down the room, or when the presence of a friend to study with her doubles a girl's achievement, it is clear that the previous deficiency was but little due to a lower pressure from a lessened reservoir of energy.

The effect of mental work without rest in causing deprivations, and of rest in permitting the corresponding indulgences, has been little studied. Attention has been centred upon what happens in the function that is working in disregard of the other functions which are being denied exercise. It is the fact that we are fatigued by what we do not do as truly, and perhaps as much, as by what we do. For children *not* to run and jump and squirm and sing and laugh and talk is the essence of mental work. For us all *not* to indulge in our favorite occupations is, as hour after hour of reading legal reports, or adding columns, or what-ever the task may be, progresses, a more and more impressive feature of the task. Cases of special theoretic interest are those where the deprivation is from opportunity to do other mental work. For, in some such cases, the other work, deprivation from which fatigues, and exercises at which rests, the individual, would be rated by men in general as very

21

exhausting. By the ordinary energy-theories it would involve large expenditures of mental energy.

If one could count up all the cases where individuals have stopped mental work and could know the chief cause in each case, it seems likely that the plea of some contrary impulse for gratification, some game to be played, sensory pleasure to be enjoyed, or the like, would be by far the commonest cause. Rest, again, except when spent in sleep, is not as a rule devoted to replenishing lost mental energy. It is far oftener devoted to indulging wants which mental work proscribes. To read, to talk with one's family and friends, to hunt or fish, to play active or sedentary games, and to make or listen to music, are occupations that often require a large expense of 'mental energy,' however defined, and that almost never approximate to the mental inaction of *dolce far niente* or sleep. They rest us by relief from strain and irritation, but not by cessation of mental action.

No theory of mental work and fatigue should then fail to take account of what continued work prevents the worker from doing. The little child who complained "I am tired of not playing," expressed admirably one feature of fatigue. The strain of not giving way to certain tendencies to response is as important as the strain of continuing certain others. Work in the popular sense is distinguished from play or recreation less by the amount of positive action than by the amount of restriction. We are fatigued by what we do *not* do.

On the whole, the biological theory seems much more probable. The effect of continuous mental work may be in part to use up some store of a complex of patience, self-control, vigor and the like, which may be called mental energy, but it surely is to produce certain annoying states to which the natural response is a diminution or cessation of the activity which causes them. The behavior which results in certain products such as sums done, dictations written, paragraphs translated, and the like, is subject to the laws of all behavior, and to no others. If a continuance of the productive responses at the same speed and in such a form as to give equal quality, is satisfying to the individual concerned, he will continue them. If such continuance brings discomfort, he will tend to stop them altogether, or to intermit them, or to make them in such altered form and speed as lets them bring relative satisfaction. Stopping the work outright does not of course occur in the great majority of experimental investigations of fatigue, but is very common in ordinary mental work. Intermitting the work, dropping it, taking it up as thoughts of rewards, punishments, duty and the like, make idleness even more discomforting than the work, dropping it again, and so on, are also, in the nature of the case, rare in the experimental studies, but very common everywhere else. Relaxing speed and care and tension to such a degree that the work is less annoying than is the condition of not working (with the consequences attached thereto) is the device to which the subjects of the experiments are restricted. Whether one relaxes, intermits or stops work, the immediate reason is not that he has not the 'energy' to go on with it, but that he feels more comfortable to relax, intermit or stop it. Whatever parallel to a decreased store of energy there is, is effective chiefly by making the responses concerned in production less satisfying than they were before.

THE HYGIENE OF MENTAL WORK

Readers of this section should remember that we are

dealing with mental work—the work of the connection-system—not with either the work of the sense organs or the work of the muscles which so often accompanies it. This matter is of special importance in the case of fatigue of the sensory and motor apparatus of the eyes. So-called "mental" work in schools, business and professional life involves reading, writing or visual examination of objects to such an extent that the diminution of efficiency below what is desirable and the injuries from work are to a very large extent due to inability of the eyes to do what the mind requires and to overstrain of the eyes in the mind's service. It is well to keep sharply apart the means of increasing the efficiency of, and preventing injury from, purely mental work and the means of increasing the efficiency of, and preventing injury from, the use of the eyes. Interest, for example, rarely injures the mind, but may lead to very great harm to the eyes. Rest, in the sense of inactivity—the absence of any set task—may, through worry, depress or irritate the mind, but it is almost always good for the eyes. The theoretical and practical problems connected with the use of the eyes should form an important topic in educational hygiene, but in this book I shall not discuss them.

The practical application of the facts about mental fatigue may best be considered under the two topics—Desirable Means of Increasing Efficiency, and Desirable Means of Preventing Injury from Over-work.

Means of Increasing Mental Efficiency

Roughly we may: (1) increase the organism's mental vigor or tendency to mental activity; (2) decrease the resistance, the forces inhibiting work; (3) improve the direction and method of activity; and (4) relieve the mind from the waste of excitement and worry.

The inner responsiveness of an animal to occasions for mental work is most economically improved by improving its general health. Other more direct influences limited to the connection-system there may be, but the safest hope is the maintenance of the health of the entire bodily machine. Consider the abolition of the effects of indigestion, rickets, chorea and scarlet fever, or of insufficient oxygen, food and sleep, in the case of children; consider the abolition of the effects of malaria, tuberculosis and alcoholism in the case of adults; consider even such a very minor factor as the common 'cold.'

The resistance which blocks mental work may be diminished by supplying interest and motive. It has been shown that certain kinds and amounts of mental activity are maintained without external subsidies, but much of what has to be done creates in the doing ennui, repulsion and pain, and deprives the worker of various satisfiers. The worker is thereby impelled to decrease, intermit or abandon the work. The resistances thus caused are not, however, inevitable, and curable only by rest. The same work done with interest does not so soon produce ennui and repugnance. The denial of certain satisfiers, such as games, conversation or reverie, may be balanced by the addition of new ones, such as a money-reward, zeal to improve, or confidence that the work will profit oneself and others. The inventor, man of science or poet, working a score of hours without rest at full efficiency, is not an exception to the laws of work, but an illustration of them. The limit of work for every man is elastic at the pull of interest and personal profit.

As a muscle becomes anew responsive to the stimulus, when the toxic products of its contraction are washed out or neutralized, so a mental function may be made to continue its output by washing out the repugnance and need for effort by an interest, and neutralizing the pain of restraint by a motive. In the case of wise and experienced adults, it is often hard to thus dissolve fatigue by adding interests and motives; they perhaps have already themselves used all the available ones. But the rank and file have not thus exhausted the preventives of repugnance and distraction; and children have hardly learned to use any of them. The children of a school class may work with doubled efficiency simply from learning the significance of the work to their wants, and associating the work with sociability, cheerfulness and achievement.

Since individuals differ in their interests the proper distribution of the different pieces of work to be performed in the world will by diminishing resistance make the sum total done larger. If each man did the mental work for which he was fit and which he enjoyed, men would work willingly much longer than they now do. But if each worked only at tasks of real value and with the guidance of exact science, men could probably attain equal results though working far less than they now do. The best means of increasing efficiency are very simple ones—ceasing to learn by roundabout and stupid methods what is not so and ceasing to prepare with anxiety and pain for what will not occur. The time and effort wasted upon superstitions, pedantries and fads of which the science of the future will convict us, doubtless make the major part of our present burden.

One can hardly overestimate the value of peace and equanimity as means of increasing mental efficiency. Since nothing is done by worry or excitement that cannot be done better in their absence, there is nothing but gain in saving for achievement the time and strength now spent in ferment and ebullition. Too much of the life of home, school, industry, business, and even the professions, is still on a par with the war dances of primitive man. We need not burn down a house to roast a pig.

Means of Preventing Injury from Over-Work

A certain amount of mental work is healthful. The connection-system requires exercise as truly as food and rest. It can have too little as well as too much activity; and it maintains its 'tone' and power of resistance to mental disease better if a certain amount of its activity is 'work' in the service of remote and unselfish ends, rather than 'play' for personal and immediate gratification.

Too much work may be injurious positively, not only by direct mischief to the neurones doing the work itself, but also by producing in the system the states corresponding to over-excitement and worry. It may also be injurious negatively by depriving the animal of the joy, appetite, physical exercise, and sleep essential to health. It may be injurious in the broader sense of diminishing the value of life, by its deprivations, of whatever sort. As men and things now are, the direct injury intrinsically and necessarily consequent upon mental work, seems to be very, very much less than that due to over-excitement, worry, and the physical, intellectual and moral deprivations.

For over-excitement and worry from mental work, wise formation of habits is the preventive and cure. Mental workers should be taught that emotionality is not a measure of interest, that tension is not a measure of energy, nor over-action of strength, that anxiety is not a measure of devotion.

and that peaceful absorption is the feeling proper to achievement. Having learned to judge their efficiency, not by how they feel, but by what they get done, they should practice themselves in casting off every weight of irrelevant thought or feeling, in dismissing as unhealthy and immoral all worry over what has been done, or what one cannot prevent.

For the deprivations, the first remedies to be applied are healthful physical conditions, interest and motive. Proper air and light, proper posture and physical exercise, enough food and sleep, and work whose purpose is rational, whose difficulty is adapted to one's powers, and whose rewards are just, should be tried before recourse to the abandonment of work itself. It is indeed doubtful if sheer rest is the appropriate remedy for a hundredth part of the injuries that result from mental work in our present irrational conduct of it.

However, since for many men, for a long time to come, mental work probably will be carried on with effort against resistance, by individuals who are not properly guarded in general health, it is worth while to inquire whether there is some point or stage in the course of mental work at which a worker should allow himself, or be allowed, or perhaps required, to stop work.

For the unlearned activities and those developing out of them in a simple environment of unconquered nature and of human beings unsophisticated by ideas, there are present certain equally unlearned checks to over-activity. Mental work beyond a certain point produces ennui, repugnance, sleepiness and pain; prolonged restraint from individual or social play produces an intense impulse to its gratification. In the absence of habits of forcing oneself to work in spite of present discomfort and deprivation, these natural checks would operate freely. The animal would be protected against over-work in the same measure that he was protected against starvation or over-feeding, by unlearned impulses. These would work crudely and imperfectly, sometimes failing to check the activity aroused by hunger or the sex instincts, when rest would be preferable, and sometimes letting him rest when continued vigilance would save him. In the complicated environment created by human intellect and morals, man learns to neglect these natural checks in favor of more remote and civilized ends, and is forced by fear of punishment to work in spite of them. They may fail to operate at all, temporary zeal or long habit rendering the individual immune to all impulses contrary to the accomplishment of his work. It would perhaps be possible for not a single one of these checks to operate, no matter how long work continued, until the man, possessed by zeal for the beloved achievement, and unwarned by repugnance, sleepiness or pain, died cheerfully working to the end.

It is for the welfare of men in the long run not to obey these *natural* checks, but no one simple *rational* check can be used to replace them. It is consequently impossible to find any uniform rule for deciding when to stop work. 'Follow nature,' 'Work as long as you can,' 'Work until a decrease in efficiency appears,' or any other rule announced for all workers, is bound to be wrong. It is unnecessary for most workers to stop when they are bored and sleepy, and it is unsafe for some to work until they are. The best practical rule seems to be to make sure of adequate exercise and sleep, to divide the balance of time reasonably between the duties and pleasures of life, and to work throughout the amount of time due for work, diminishing the natural checks so far as may be by securing proper physical conditions, interest and motive, and, for the rest, disregarding them. What amount of exercise and what amount of sleep are adequate varies with age and individuality. To insure against injury, the allowance may be made generously. The essence of mental hygiene is then—interest for efficiency; and for protection, sleep.

PART III

Individual Differences and Their Causes

CHAPTER XXI

INTRODUCTION

THE PROBLEMS OF INDIVIDUAL DIFFERENCES

In describing the original tendencies of man as a species, attention was called to the fact that the original natures of individual men and women were not exact duplicates, presenting the characteristics of the human species invariably, but deviated from the type of the species in the strength of this, that and the other instinct. In describing the laws of learning or modifiability and the changes in mental functions which learning brings to pass, it was assumed that different individuals learned at different rates; and that identical natures must, if subjected to the action of different external situations or environments, become different. The reports of studies of the amount, rate and permanence of improvement gave frequent illustrations of the variability of individual men in whatever feature of intellect, character or skill we examine. It is the purpose of the remaining chapters of this volume to present the main facts concerning these individual differences and their causes.

The best means of introduction to the study of individual differences, their causes and their educational significance, will be to examine an actual first-hand study of them. For this purpose I choose certain parts of Mr. S. A. Courtis' report on the arithmetical abilities of children in the schools of New York City ['11-'12].

Mr. Courtis measured the achievements of pupils in responding to eight tests. Test 7 is reproduced below.

ARITHMETIC—Test No. 7. Fundamentals

Name................:..........*School*................*Grade*......

In the blank space below, work as many of these examples as possible in the time allowed   Work them in order as numbered, writing each answer in the "answer" column before commencing a new example. Do no work on any other paper.

Num-ber	Operation	Example	Answer	Right
1	Addition	a 25 + 830 + 122 = ... (Write answer in this column) ☞ b 232 + 8021 + 703 + 3030 = .		
2	Subtraction	a 5496 — 163 = ... b 943276 — 812102 = ...		
3	Multiplication	2012 × 213 = ...		
4	Division	158664 ÷ 132 = ...		
5	Addition	6134 + 213 + 4800 + 6005 + 3050 + 474 = ...		
6	Subtraction	73210142 — 49676378 = ...		
7 / 8	Multiplication	46508 × 456 = ...		
9	Division	27217182 ÷ 6 = ...		
10 / 11	Division	3127102 ÷ 463 = ...		
12 / 13	Addition	85586 + 69685 + 39397 + 95836 + 37768 + 69666 + 78888 + 54987 = ...		
14	Subtraction	1565431 — 5878675 = ...		
15 / 16	Multiplication	78965 × 678 = ...		
17	Division	44502486 ÷ 7 —		
18 / 19	Division	5373003 ÷ 769 —		

Consider now the results of Test 7 in a certain eighth-grade class as shown in Fig. 65. Consider also Table 7, which gives similar facts for all the eighth grade children

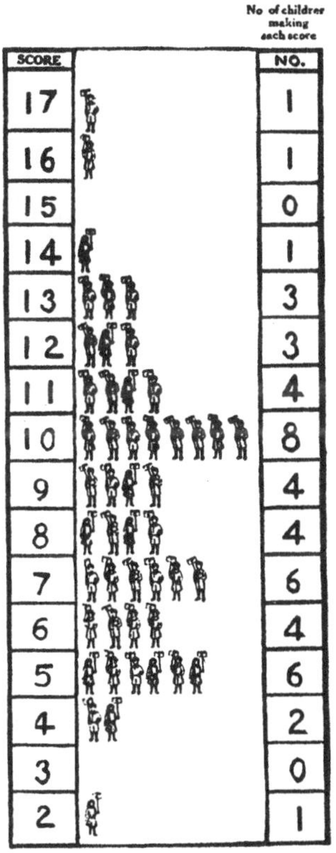

No of children making each score

SCORE		NO.
17		1
16		1
15		0
14		1
13		3
12		3
11		4
10		8
9		4
8		4
7		6
6		4
5		6
4		2
3		0
2		1

Fig. 65. The Variation in Ability within a Single Class. After Courtis, '11-'12, p. 48.

tested. The picture and this table state an important fact—the existence of great individual differences even among those of the same school grade, and so of roughly similar training in arithmetic—and suggest that differences in original capacities must play a large part in producing the differences that are actually found between one human being and another.

TABLE 7

THE VARIATION AMONG 8TH GRADE PUPILS IN ARITHMETICAL COM-
PUTATION. After Courtis, '11-'12, p. 46.

"Score" or "Quantity": Examples done correctly in 12 minutes in the case of Test 7	Number of children making each score or "Frequency": 8th grade children in New York City
19	31
18	25
17	86
16	107
15	182
14	251
13	327
12	390
11	453
10	497
9	475
8	425
7	333
6	312
5	239
4	152
3	88
2	71
1	30
0	28

Another problem in the causation of individual differences is illustrated by Mr. Courtis' tables comparing the two sexes.

I quote (in Table 8) the one for Test 6 in the 7B grade.*

It appears that in the number of examples attempted there was little or no difference between the sexes, but that in the number of correct answers the boys did somewhat better than the girls of the same grade.

The effects of sex, whether by inherited sex qualities or by the circumstances in which training differs for the sexes, have been the subject of many speculative opinions and of some few impartial investigations. They will be discussed by themselves in Chapter XXII.

The influence of remote ancestry or race could be studied similarly by comparing two groups of children of the same sex, age, and training, but different in that the one group sprang from, say, East European Hebrews and the other from, say, North American Indians.

* Test 6 was as follows:

Do not work the following examples. Read each example through, make up your mind what operation you would use if you were going to work it, then write the name of the operation selected in the blank space after the example. Use the following abbreviations:—"Add." for addition, "Sub" for subtraction, "Mul." for multiplication, and "Div." for division.

1. The children of a school gave a sleighride party. There were 9 sleighs used, and each sleigh held 30 children. How many children were there in the party?.............................

2. Two school-girls played a number game. The score of the girl that lost was 57 points and she was beaten by 16 points What was the score of the girl that won?....................

3. A girl counted the automobiles that passed a school. The total was 60 in two hours. If the girl saw 27 pass the first hour how many did she see the second?..........................

4. On a playground there were five equal groups of children each playing a different game. If there were 75 children altogether, how many were there in each group?................

And so on for twelve similar examples.

Other possible causes of differences in arithmetical achievement are:—differences in near ancestry or 'family,' differences in maturity, and differences in the length of time devoted to arithmetic in the schools, in the methods used in teaching it, or in other circumstances of training.

TABLE 8.

SEX DIFFERENCES IN A SPEED TEST IN REASONING: Boys and Girls in the 7 B Grades Compared. After Courtis, 'II-'I2, p. 138.

Quantity: Number of Examples attempted in Test 6 in I minute	Frequency in 7 B Grade		Quantity: Number of Examples done correctly in Test 6 in I minute	Frequency in 7 B Grade	
	Boys	Girls		Boys	Girls
16	I	6	16	I	
15			15		
14	I		14		
13	4	3	13		
12	7	6	12	I	I
II	7	II	II		2
10	15	18	10	6	4
9	34	21	9	10	4
8	59	52	8	23	II
7	119	88	7	50	24
6	240	216	6	110	61
5	287	273	5	197	132
4	238	230	4	245	197
3	161	172	3	245	236
2	55	65	2	201	273
I	6	6	I	113	175
0	I	I	0	33	48

In this sample study the individual differences amongst pupils have been displayed in the form of *tables of distribution*, giving the *frequency* of each degree of ability—that is, the number or percentage of individuals of each degree of ability. The main features of such a *frequency table* or *table of distribution* can be seen at once in their relations one to another, if

TABLE Q.

SAMPLE OF DISTRIBUTION TABLES.

Distribution of Progress in School among Connecticut children in 1903		Distribution of Ability in Copying Figures in 6th grade children. After Courtis, '11-'12, p 54		Distribution of Ability in Adding Pairs of One-Place Numbers in High-School Pupils. After Courtis, '11-12, p. 52	
Quantity: Grade reached at age of 10	Frequency: Number of Children	Quantity: Number of digits copied in 60 seconds	Frequency in 6th Grade Children	Quantity: Number of pairs added in 60 seconds	Frequency in High School Pupils
		0 to 9	9		
Kinder-		10 " 19	12		
garten	9	20 " 29	22	20 to 29	2
1st grade	442	30 " 39	18	30 " 39	4
2nd "	1389	40 " 49	57	40 " 49	41
3rd "	3293	50 " 59	107	50 " 59	113
4th "	4433	60 " 69	291	60 " 69	272
5th "	3200	70 " 79	536	70 " 79	235
6th "	1227	80 " 89	1274	80 " 89	196
7th "	237	90 " 99	1256	90 " 99	86
8th "	48	100 " 109	1066	100 " 109	43
9th "	4	110 " 119	494	110 " 119	2
10th "	1	120 " 129	359	120 " 129	2
		130 " 139	64		
		140 " 149	36		
		150 " 159	19		
		160 " 169	47		
		170 " 179	2		
		180 " 189	1		

it is presented in graphic form, by letting intervals along a horizontal base-line or scale denote the different scores made or degrees of ability found, and letting the height of a horizontal line over each such interval represent the number of individuals

22

possessing that degree of ability.   By joining the separate
horizontals a surface of frequency is enclosed.

Such distribution tables and the corresponding surfaces of
frequency for certain specified groups of individuals are shown
in Table 9 and FIGS. 66, 67 and 68 for the cases of *Grade
reached by Connecticut children at the age of 10, Speed of
sixth-grade children in copying figures,* and *Efficiency of high-
school children in adding pairs of one-place numbers.*

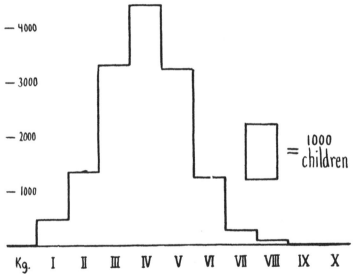

FIG. 66.   The Number of 10-year-old Children in Connecticut (1903), in Each
School Grade.

Such tables of distribution or surfaces of frequency are the
terms in which the student of individual psychology must do
very much of his thinking, both when he tries to describe, and
when he tries to account for, the variation of human beings
around the type of the species.   In the next chapter, for
example, in comparing the sexes, in respect to one or another
mental trait, we shall have to think of the surface of frequency
for men in each trait and the surface of frequency for women
in the same trait and to compare these two total surfaces of
frequency.

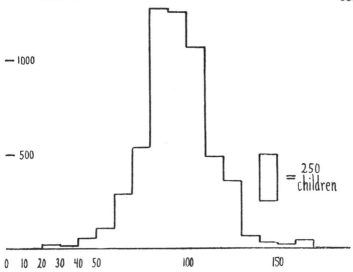

FIG. 67.   The Number of Sixth-Grade Children in New York City Copying 0-9 Digits, 10 to 19 Digits, etc., in 60 Seconds.

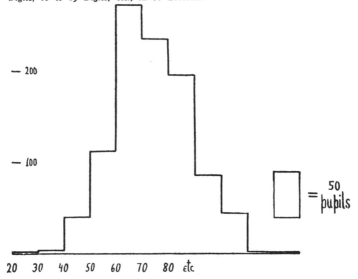

FIG. 68.   The Number of High-School Pupils Adding 20-29 Pairs of Numbers, 30-39 Pairs, etc., in 60 Seconds.

CHAPTER XXII

THE CAUSES OF INDIVIDUAL DIFFERENCES:

SEX AND RACE

SEX DIFFERENCES IN ABILITY

The ability possessed by any individual in any mental trait is the result of (1) his original nature, (2) the extent to which his original tendencies have matured by mere inner growth, and (3) the circumstances of his life and training. His original nature is determined partly by sex, partly by his remote ancestry or race, partly by his near ancestry or family, and partly by the unknown causes of variation whereby children of the same parents receive differing inheritances. We have then to study the influence of *sex, remote ancestry, near ancestry, maturity* and *environment.*

By way of preface to an account of sex differences it is well to note that their existence does not necessarily imply in any case the advisability of differences in school and home training, and, on the other hand, that even if the mental make-up of the sexes were identical it might still be wisest to educate them differently. It is true that a difference of two groups in a mental trait will theoretically involve differences in treatment, but practical considerations apart from that of developing the highest efficiency in that trait may outweigh the advantages of the differential treatment. For instance, consumptives theoretically need a different mode of life from people with healthy lungs, but it might in some cases be wiser to leave a consumptive to his ordinary habits rather than to cause in him consciousness of his disease and worry concerning it. On the other hand, two boys might be identical in mental structure, yet their education might best be very different if we wished to make one of them a chemist and the other a psychologist.

Let us note in the second place that the existence of differences need not imply the need of different training, because those very differences may have been due to the different training actually received and might never have appeared had training been alike in the two classes. It is folly to argue from any mental condition in an individual or class without ascertaining whether it is due to original nature or to training.

The chapter should properly be devoted exclusively to the differences necessarily produced by sex. Those produced by virtue of the adventitiously different training which boy and girl undergo belong in Chapter XXV. So far as may be, such a separation of differences due to sex-nature from those due to our traditional treatment of the sexes is in fact made. But in many cases where the amount of the difference that is to be credited to training is doubtful, the difference will be described in the present chapter, the discount to be made being left to the reader's judgment.

An adequate comparison of men with women, or of boys with girls of the same age, requires that the two tables of distribution of surfaces of frequency for the two sexes in the ability in question be shown, as was done in Table 8 on page 336 and as is done in Figure 69 (the dotted line being for girls). Such tables or surfaces show the whole fact, including the extent to which the two groups are alike or *overlap* as well as the extent to which they *differ.*

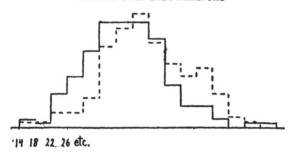

'14 18 22 26 etc.

Fig. 69   The Number of A's Marked in 60 Seconds by 12-year-old Boys and by 12-year-old Girls   The continuous line encloses the surface of frequency for boys; the dash-line encloses the surface of frequency for girls.

The essence of any such pair of tables of distribution or surfaces of frequency may, however, be stated in a single quantity—the *percentage of one group that reaches or exceeds the medium* of the other group*.   For example, if the two groups differ as shown in Fig. 70, the percentage of one group

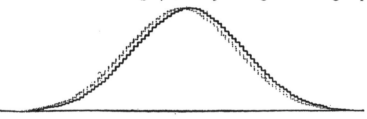

Fig. 70   The amount of difference between two groups when the per cent of one group reaching or exceeding the median of the other group is 45 or 55.

reaching or exceeding the median ability of the other group is 45 or 55.   45 per cent of the 'dotted line' surface lies to the right of the median of the 'heavy line' surface; and 55 per cent of the 'heavy line' surface lies to the right of the median of the 'dotted line' surface.   If the two groups differ as shown in Fig. 71, the percentage of the 'dotted line' group reaching or exceeding the median ability of the 'heavy line' group is 40.

* The *median* or *median ability* is the *mid-ability*, the point on the scale in question which divides the groups in question into an upper and a lower half.

The reverse comparison gives 60 per cent. If the two groups differ as shown in Fig. 72, the percentage of one group reaching or exceeding the median ability of the other is 25 or 75. If the two groups differ as shown in Fig. 73, the percentages are almost or quite 0 and 100.

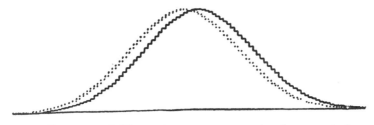

FIG. 71 The amount of difference between two groups when the per cent of one group reaching or exceeding the median of the other group is 40 or 60.

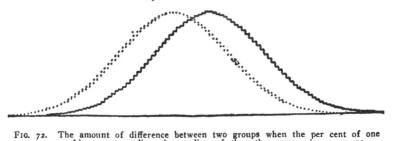

FIG. 72. The amount of difference between two groups when the per cent of one group reaching or exceeding the median of the other group is 25 or 75.

Conversely, when we are told that 60 per cent of men reach or exceed the median ability of women in a certain test of ingenuity, we may infer that the difference between men and women in this trait is approximately as shown in Fig. 71, the heavy line being taken to represent the men. If we are told that in industry only 28 per cent of men reach or exceed the median amount for women we may infer that the difference between men and women is nearly, but not quite, as great as that shown in Fig. 72, the dotted line being here taken to

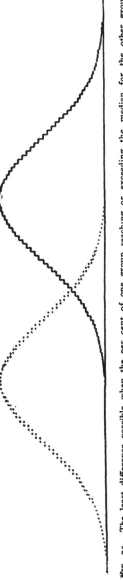

FIG. 73.   The least difference possible when the per cent of one group reaching or exceeding the median for the other group is 0 or 100.

represent the men. A single percentage then, when taken in connection with these diagrams, gives a serviceable comparison of the abilities of the two groups in the trait in question.

I shall use such percentages in what follows. It will be remembered that for practical purposes of school education any percentage between 40 and 60 represents a very small difference with very great 'overlapping.'

The percentages of males reaching or exceeding the median ability of females in such traits as have been subjected to exact investigation are roughly as follows:

In speed of naming colors and sorting cards by color and
    discriminating colors as in a test for color blindness   24
In finding and checking small visual details such as letters   33
In spelling   33
In school 'marks' in English   35
In school 'marks' in foreign languages   40
In memorizing for immediate recall   42
In lowness of sensory thresholds   43
In retentiveness   47
In tests of speed and accuracy of association   48
In tests of general information   50
In school 'marks' in mathematics   50
In school 'marks' (total average)   50
In tests of discrimination (other than for color)   51
In range of sensitivity   52
In school 'marks' in history   55
In tests of ingenuity   63
In accuracy of arm movements   66
In school marks in physics and chemistry   68
In reaction time   70
In speed of finger and arm movements   71

The most important characteristic of these differences is

their small amount. The individual differences within one sex so enormously outweigh the differences between the sexes in these intellectual and semi-intellectual traits that for practical purposes the sex difference may be disregarded. So far as ability goes, there could hardly be a stupider way to get two groups alike within each group but differing between the groups than to take the two sexes. As is well known, the experiments of the past generation in educating women have shown their equal competence in school work of elementary, secondary and collegiate grade. The present generation's experience is showing the same fact for professional education and business service. The psychologists' measurements lead to the conclusion that this equality of achievement comes from an equality of natural gifts, not from an overstraining of the lesser talents of women.

SEX DIFFERENCES IN TRAITS NOT MEASURED OBJECTIVELY

We have now to turn from fairly satisfactory studies of sex differences in sensory, motor and intellectual capacities, to a looser discussion of the life of feeling, action and general achievement. Here objective and precise measurements will seldom be at our service.

There are two studies which do report such differences quantitatively, but the data given are subject, unfortunately, to whatever errors of prejudice or custom teachers, physicians, and German women of intellectual interests make in rating individuals, and to possibly important errors due to the existence in their minds of different standards for the two sexes.

Karl Pearson ['04], in securing data on the resemblances of children of the same parents, had children rated by their teachers for various qualities—as quiet or noisy, shy or self-assertive, and the like.

On calculating the probable percentages of boys reaching or exceeding the degree of each trait that is reached or exceeded by half of the girls, we have:—

61% of boys are as athletic as or more athletic than the median girl.

62% of boys are as noisy as or more noisy than the median girl.

42% of boys are as shy as or more shy than the median girl.

57% of boys are as self-conscious as or more self-conscious than the median girl.

46% of boys are as popular as or more popular than the median girl.

40% of boys are as conscientious as or more conscientious than the median girl.

56% of boys are as quick-tempered as or more quick-tempered than the median girl.

47% of boys are as intelligent as or more intelligent than the median girl.

43% of boys write as well as or better than the median girl.

Heymans and Wiersma ['06, '07 and '08] studied mental differences of the sexes by means of estimates of individuals made by other individuals who knew them more or less intimately. The report covered 90 topics, some of which included several traits. The individual was graded very coarsely—*e. g.,* as emotional or not emotional; or as a drunkard, an habitual drinker, an occasional drinker, or a total abstainer. Such reports are, as has been noted, inferior evidence, since the person making them may use different standards for men and for women. Thus the same degree of emotionality might be called emotional in the case of a man and not emotional in the case of a woman, or *vice versa.*

On the whole, the results of the ratings, though very inferior to objective measurements, are probably superior to the mere opinions which one could give from reflection on the common facts of life and his own narrow circle of acquaintances. They may at least serve to make the reader critical of whatever such opinions he has.

I have therefore calculated from them the probable per cent of men reaching or exceeding the median woman in respect to each trait, counting the ratings by men and those by women as of equal weight. The differences so estimated I have arranged roughly in the order of their magnitude. The largest difference is that :—

Only 15 per cent of men are as much more interested in persons than in things as the median woman is.

The next largest differences are that :—

In accurate and orderly retention of what is read........	73% of men equal or excel the median woman.
In industry	28% " " " " " " " "
In adroitness in manual work.	28% " " " " " " " "
In love of sedentary games of skill.....................	71% " " " " " " " "
In emotionality..............	30% " " " " " " " "
In temperance in the use of alcoholic drinks....30% (or less)	" " " " " " " "
In independence.............	70% " " " " " " " "
In zeal for money making.....	69% " " " " " " " "
In desire for change..........	32% " " " " " " " "
In impulsiveness.............	34% " " " " " " " "
In quickness of recovery from grief.....................	66% " " " " " " " "

Then come the following:

In activity (of the aimless sort)	36%	of men equal or excel the median woman.							
In dissatisfaction with oneself.	36%	"	"	"	"	"	"	"	"
In religiousness	36%	"	"	"	"	"	"	"	"
In excitability	37%	"	"	"	"	"	"	"	"
In sympathy	38%	"	"	"	"	"	"	"	"
In patience	38%	"	"	"	"	"	"	"	"
In love of sports	62%	"	"	"	"	"	"	"	"
In humor	61%	"	"	"	"	"	"	"	"
In risibility	39%	"	"	"	"	"	"	"	"
In talkativeness	40%	"	"	"	"	"	"	"	"
In gaiety	40%	"	"	"	"	"	"	"	"
In vanity of person	40%	"	"	"	"	"	"	"	"

There are very slight differences as follows: men are a little oftener reported as critical, attached to opinions once formed, given to ambitious plans, given to contradiction, sensible, decisive, gifted in mathematics, gifted in literature, specific, of good memories, fond of eating and drinking, fond of distinction, strict, and also easy-going, in discipline with children, kind to subordinates, widely read, and punctual. They are a little less often reported as good-natured, anxious, easily reconciled after anger, insistent on immediate results, good judges of human nature, practically resourceful, narrow, gifted in languages, gifted in music, good observers, thrifty, domineering, kind and careful in discipline with children, active in philanthropic work, demonstrative, honest about money, fond of intercourse with social superiors, timid, well posted about the affairs of acquaintances, polite, attentive, tidy, and courageous in sickness.

In the following traits there is still less difference reported or no difference observable: Trustfulness, tolerance, inconstancy in sympathies, devotion to old memories, quickness in comprehension, superficiality, stupidity, ability in drawing, acting, mimicing, ear for music, patriotism, naturalness, straightforwardness, truthfulness, kindness to animals, snobbishness, courage, and pleasure-seeking.

It would be desirable in any such study that the sex differences in the instinctive acts, interests, aversions and emotional responses should be studied apart from the differences in similar traits that have been produced by circumstances. Two instincts are worthy of special attention. The most striking difference in instinctive equipment consists in the strength of the fighting instinct in the male and of the nursing instinct in the female. No one will doubt that men are more possessed by the instinct to fight, to be the winner in games and serious contests, than are women; nor that women are more possessed than men by the instinct to nurse, to care for and fuss over others, to relieve, comfort and console. And probably no serious student of human nature will doubt that these are matters of original nature. The out-and-out physical fighting for the sake of combat is pre-eminently a male instinct and the resentment at mastery, the zeal to surpass and the general joy at activity in mental as well as physical matters seem to be closely correlated with it. It has been common to talk of women's "dependence." This is, I am sure, only an awkward name for less resentment at mastery. The actual nursing of the young seems likewise to involve equally unreasoning tendencies to pet, coddle, and "do for" others. The existence of these two instincts has been long recognized by literature and common knowledge, but their importance in causing differences in the general activities of the sexes has not. The fighting instinct is in fact the cause of a very large amount of the world's intellectual endeavor. The financier does not think merely for money nor the scientist for truth nor the theologian to save souls. Their intellectual efforts are aimed in great measure to outdo the other man, to subdue nature, to conquer assent. The maternal instinct in its turn is the chief source of woman's superiorities in the moral life. The virtues in which she excels are not so much due to either any general moral superiority or any set of special moral talents as to her original impulses to relieve, comfort and console.

A SAMPLE STUDY OF RACIAL DIFFERENCES

Mayo ['13] secured the academic records of 150 negroes* who entered the high schools of New York City since 1902. For each such record he got a white pupil's† record selected under the same conditions. It is impossible to tell exactly whether and how far the two groups of pupils thus taken represent dissimilar samplings of the two total groups, negroes and whites in New York City. In my opinion the samplings are closely similar. There are no measurements of the extent to which residence in New York selects the more scholarly of negroes from the country, or of the extent to which entrance to high school selects differently from the negroes in New York than from the whites. In general, selection by entrance to the public high schools is narrow but democratic; and in Mr. Mayo's opinion and my own the high school gets a somewhat, but not much, higher selection from the colored than from the white youth. That is, in our opinion, the superiority of the colored in high school to the colored outside is greater, but not much greater, than the superiority of the whites in high school to the whites outside.

*A negro being defined as an individual reported as a negro by school officers. Mulattoes are of course frequent.

† A white pupil being defined as an individual reported as such by school officers. There may in rare cases have been some slight mixture of negro blood.

Whatever be the difference in the selection of the two groups, colored beginners in high schools in New York City differ from whites in their careers there as follows:

(1) On the average they are seven months older, only 36 per cent of them being as young as the median white.

(2) They continue in the high school longer.

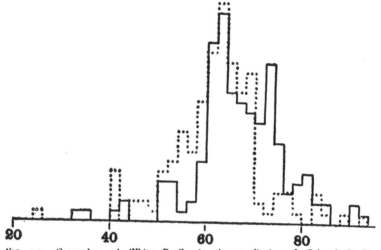

FIG. 74. Comparison of White Pupils (continuous line) and Colored Pupils (dotted line) in respect to Scholarship in the High School. The horizontal scale is for the median of all marks obtained by an individual except those obtained in courses repeated because of failure. The marks in these schools are on a 0 — 100 scale.

(3) In achievement in the different studies they are somewhat, but not very much, inferior. The general tendency is for only three-tenths of them to reach the median record for whites.

(4) The difference is greatest in the case of English, in which only 24 per cent of the colored pupils reach or exceed the median for whites.

Fig. 74 presents Dr. Mayo's results in the case of general scholarship.

The greatest difference between races so far found is that between European whites and Negritos in a simple test of intellect. The facts are shown in Figs. 75 and 76. In general, differences between races in original capacities are small in comparison with the range of differences within either race, and the amount of overlapping is great.

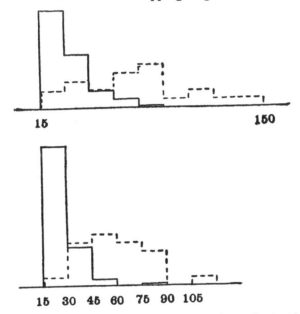

FIG. 75 (upper diagram). Comparison of whites (continuous lines) and Negritos (dotted lines) in respect to time taken to put variously shaped blocks in holes to match. The horizontal scale is for time in seconds, first trial.

FIG. 76 (lower diagram). As in FIG. 75, except that the records in the third trial were used.

CHAPTER XXIII

The Influence of Immediate Ancestry or Family

The problem naturally resolves itself into two,—the measurement of the resemblance of individuals of like ancestry and the subtraction of a proper allowance for their likeness in training. Or, more exactly, we have to measure the amount by which the likeness of individuals of like ancestry surpasses the likeness of individuals of different ancestry, and subtract from it the amount due to their greater likeness in training than that found in the case of individuals of different ancestry. Measurements of the greater *differences* of *un*related individuals with an allowance for the greater differences in their training would serve the same end. But the effect of differences in ancestry in producing differences in intellect and character is more easily measured by the effect of similarity or identity in ancestry in decreasing such differences. The facts to be considered are then measurements of resemblance and allowance for like training.

THE VARIABILITY OF INDIVIDUALS OF THE SAME SEX AND ANCESTRY

Resemblance, not repetition, is to be measured. To say that a man's original nature depends upon his ancestry does not mean that it is an exact facsimile of any one or any combination of his ancestors. There is no reason to believe that four sons of the same parents and consequently of the same total ancestry will have the same original natures. Indeed we know they will not, save by chance. For twins who have presumably in some cases identical or nearly identical antenatal influences and nurture may vary widely in both physical and mental traits. What ancestry does is to reduce the variability of the offspring and determine the point about which they do vary.

Take, for instance, the capacity to form intelligent habits or associations amongst sense impressions, ideas and acts. The number of associations between situation and act, the number, that is, of things an animal can do in response to the multitude of conditions of life, varies tremendously throughout the animal kingdom. The free swimming protozoa studied by Professor Jennings had in addition to the common physiological functions hardly more than a single habit. The sum of the life of *Paramoecium* is to eat, breathe, digest, form tissues, excrete, reproduce, move along in a steady way, and when passing from certain media into others to stop, back, turn to the aboral side and move along again as before. At the other extreme is a cultivated human being whose toilet, table manners, games, speech, reading, business, etc., involve hundreds of thousands of associative habits.

If now we take a thousand descendants of human beings and count up the number of associative habits displayed by each we shall of course find a great variability. Some of our thousand human offspring will learn fewer things than some dogs and cats. Some of them may learn many more than any of the parents from whom they sprang. But on the whole the offspring of human beings will vary about the human average instead of about the general animal average, and the average deviation of the human group will be far less than that of the whole animal kingdom.

To illustrate again, the children of parents who are, say, 3 inches above the average of the general population in stature will vary not about the general average, but about a point 2 inches above it; and will differ one from another only about ten seventeenths as much as one adult of the general population differs from another.*

Immediate ancestry will then, when influential, cause children to deviate from the general average toward the condition of their parents and to vary less among themselves than would the same number of unrelated individuals.

It might seem at first sight that two individuals of the same sex, race and parentage, two brothers or two sisters, should, if ancestry counted at all, have identical original natures and differ only in as far as different environmental forces affect them. Common observation shows this to be false, but common thinking does not always or often understand that it is false just because immediate ancestry does count. If ancestry did not count, either all men would by original nature be identical, or the variations among them would all be miracles. If ancestry did not count, two brothers might well be identical in original nature, for all human males might be. But if ancestry is a force, it is certainly a variable one, the germs produced by any one parent being somewhat different among themselves for the same reason that the germs produced by all parents together vary still more. If the germs differ at all, the differences are likely to be less amongst the germs of any one human being than amongst an equal number from all men, but the differences are not at all likely to be reduced to zero.

In all thought of inheritance, physical or mental, one should always remember that children spring, not from their parents'

*This illustration is based on the data reported by Galton in *Natural Inheritance.*

bodies and minds, but from *the germs of those parents.* The qualities of the germs of a man are what we should know in order to prophesy directly the traits of his children. One quality these germs surely possess. They are variable. Discarding syntax and elegance for emphasis, we may say that the germs of a six-foot man include some six-feet germs, some six-feet-one germs, some six-feet-two, some five-feet-eleven, some five-feet-ten, etc. Each human being gives to the future, not himself, but a variable group of germs. This hypothesis of the variability of the germs explains the fact that short parents may have tall sons; gifted parents, stupid sons; the same parents, unlike sons. We have to measure the amount of resemblance, not the frequency of identity.

The amount of resemblance between a thousand fathers and sons, pair by pair (or mothers and sons, or brothers and sisters, or uncles and nephews), is best measured by a so-called *coefficient of resemblance or coefficient of correlation.* This is a quantity varying from 1.00 (which means identity or perfect resemblance in the trait in question), through 0 (which means no more resemblance than any one person taken at random bears to any other one person of the same age and sex taken at random), to -1.00 (which means the likeness, or rather the unlikeness, that would be found if the two thousand individuals were so paired as to have within the pairs the least possible resemblance).

MEASUREMENTS OF RESEMBLANCE IN RELATED INDIVIDUALS

Before describing the similarities of closely related individuals in mental traits I shall present the results of studies in the case of some physical traits which will prove that heredity is a *vera causa,* since, in them, similarity of training is out of the question as a cause of the similarities found.

The coefficient of correlation between brothers in the color of the eyes is, according to Pearson, .52. But parents could not, if they would, exert any environmental influence upon the color of their children's eyes. The fraternal resemblance must be due to the resemblance in ancestry.

In height Pearson finds the coefficient of correlation between father and son to be .3, and that between brother and brother to be .5. In other words, a son, on the average, deviates from the general trend of the population by .3 the amount of his father's deviation, a brother by .5 the amount of his brother's. Now no one can imagine that tall fathers try especially to make their sons tall. Nor will the class 'men two inches above the average height' feed their children any more than men one inch above it.

The coefficient of fraternal correlation in the case of the cephalic index (ratio of width to length of head) is, according to Pearson, .49. Here it is utterly incredible that fathers do anything to their children that would tend to produce in them similar indices.

Finally take color of hair. Fraternal correlation is, according to Pearson, .55. Here again home influence could not cause one whit of the resemblance.

Immediate ancestry can and does, apart from any other force, cause in whole or in part the abmodality, or deviation from the C. T. of his race, of an individual in the case of stature, cephalic index and eye color. There is no reason to suppose that the brain is less influenced by ancestry than are the tissues that cause height, or the shape of the skull bones that causes cephalic index, or the deposits of pigment that cause eye color. Immediate ancestry is thus a probable cause for original mental nature. And when there is doubt as to the choice between it and the environment as the cause of differences in mental traits of individuals at any age, it must not be forgotten that the influence of the latter is, after all, largely a matter of speculation, while the influence of ancestry is in physical traits a demonstrated fact.

Deafness may be considered a physical trait because it is due to physical causes, but so are all mental traits. The real difference is that we know more about the causes in the one case than in the others. The manifestation and results of deafness are certainly mental traits.

The brother or sister of a person born deaf is found to be deaf in 245 cases out of 1,000, almost one case out of four. The number of deaf persons amongst 1,000 brothers and sisters of hearing individuals is not known exactly, but it is certainly less than 1, probably much less. That is, a person of the same ancestry as a congenitally deaf person is at least 245 (probably many more) times as likely to be deaf as a person of the same ancestry as a hearing person. The child of two parents both of whom were born deaf is at least 259 (probably many more) times as likely to be deaf as the child of two hearing parents [Fay, '98, p. 49]. In this case, as with the physical traits described, there is no reason to impute any efficacy to training. Parents born deaf would take pains to *prevent* deafness in their children.

Mr. E. L. Earle ['03] measured the spelling abilities of some 600 children in the St. Xavier school in New York by careful tests. As the children in this school commonly enter at a very early age, and as the staff and methods of teaching remain very constant, we have in the case of the 180 pairs of brothers and sisters included in the 600 children closely similar school training. Mr. Earle measured the ability of any individual by his deviation from the average for his grade and sex and found the coefficient of correlation between children of the

same family to be .50. That is, any individual is on the average 50 per cent as much above or below the average for his age
and sex as his brother or sister.

Similarities in home training might theoretically account
for this, but any one experienced in teaching will hesitate to
attribute much efficacy to such similarities. Bad spellers
remain bad spellers though their teachers change. Moreover,
Dr. J. M. Rice in his exhaustive study of spelling ability ['97]
found little or no relationship between good spelling and any
one of the popular methods, and little or none between poor
spelling and foreign parentage. Yet the training of a home
where the parents do not read or spell the language well must
be a home of relatively poor training for spelling. Cornman's
more careful study of spelling ['01] supports the view that
ability to spell is little influenced by such differences in school
or home training as commonly exist.

These facts make it almost certain that immediate ancestry
does count somewhat in producing the likenesses and differences found amongst men in mental traits. In the measurements now to be reported, the influence of family training
enters as a more probable alternative cause of the resemblance.
I shall in each case give the measurement of resemblance made
and the allowance for likeness in home training suggested by
the author.

The first serious study of the inheritance of mental traits
was made in the 60's by Francis Galton and reported in
Hereditary Genius ['69, '92]. He examined carefully the
careers of the relatives of 977 men each of whom would rank
as one man in four thousand for eminent intellectual gifts.
They had relatives of that degree of eminence as follows:—
fathers 89, brothers 114, sons 129, all three together 332;
grandfathers 52, grandsons 37, uncles 53, nephews 61, all four

together 203. The probable numbers of relatives of that degree of eminence for 977 average men are as follows:—fathers, brothers, and sons together, 1; grandfathers, grandsons, uncles and nephews all together, 3. Galton argues that the training due to the possession of eminent relatives can not have been the cause of this superior chance of eminence in the relatives of gifted literary men and artists.

He says: "To recapitulate: I have endeavored to show in respect to literary and artistic eminence—

1. That men who are gifted with high abilities—even men of class E—easily rise through all the obstacles caused by inferiority of social rank.

2. Countries where there are fewer hindrances than in England, to a poor man rising in life, produce a much larger proportion of persons of culture, but not of what I call eminent men. (England and America are taken as illustration.)

3. Men who are largely aided by social advantages are unable to achieve eminence, unless they are endowed with high natural gifts."

Galton demonstrates that the adopted sons of popes do not approach equality in eminence with the real sons of gifted men. He so orders his studies of men eminent in other fields as to leave very slight basis for one who argues that training and opportunity rather than birth caused the eminence attained. Finally, Galton's own opinion, that of an eminently fair scientific man based upon an extensive study of individual biographies, may safely be taken with a very slight discount. He says:—"I feel convinced that no man can achieve a very high reputation without being gifted with very high abilities."

Dr. Frederick Adams Woods has reported in *Mental and Moral Heredity in Royalty* ['06], a work which appeared first in the Popular Science Monthly in 1902 and 1903, measurements of the resemblances in intellect and in morals of many individuals chosen from the royal families of Europe. Dr. Woods gave to each person of the 671 studied a rating from 1 to 10 on a scale for intellect—1 representing feeble-mindedness or imbecility; 10 such gifts as those of William the Silent, Frederick the Great and Gustavus Adolphus; and 2, 3, 4, 5, etc., steps at equal intervals between, in his opinion. These ratings represented Dr. Woods' impressions from reading the statements of historians and biographers about these individuals. He gave similar ratings for morality.

The ratings assigned by Dr. Woods are, of course, not accurate. No one man's ratings of nearly seven hundred historical personages could be. The effect of this chance inaccuracy would be to make all his measurements of resemblance lower than the real resemblance. He may also have erred from an unconscious prejudice by rating as too much alike individuals who were closely related. This error would tend obviously to make his estimate of resemblance too high. His ratings are given in full and so far nobody has proved or even suggested that they are thus biased.

There is still another **chance** for error. The reputation of a prince may be a peculiarly **unfair** measure of his ability. A son whose gifted father has brought the nation's affairs into a prosperous condition may thereby get, in histories and biographies, an unduly high rating; whereas a son who must strive against the unfavorable conditions produced by a stupid father, may thereby incur an undeserved repute of inefficiency. This is, however, no more plausible a supposition than the opposite one that a moderately gifted son would be rated too low by contrast with a gifted father and too high if his predecessor had been a marked failure. On the whole Dr. Woods' ratings seem little subject to error other than chance inaccuracy, so that the resemblances calculated from them are probably too low rather than too high.

The general tendency to resemblance he finds to be :—
In intellect :—

> Offspring and fathers, $r = .30$;*
> Offspring and grandfathers, $r = .16$;
> Offspring and greatgrandfathers, $r = .15$

In morals :—

> Offspring and fathers, $r = .30$
> Offspring and grandfathers, $r = .175$

Dr. Woods thinks that little or no allowance need be made for greater similarity of environment for son and father or grandfather than existed for sons of royal families in general. He says that, while educational opportunities have been unequal, the "advantages and hindrances must have always been of an accidental character, depending on various causes, and their distribution would occur largely at haphazard throughout the entire number of collected persons (832); and could not account for the great group of mediocrity and inferiority, like the houses of Hanover, Denmark, Mecklenburg, and latter Spain, Portugal and France." ['06, p. 284.]

So also the advantages of high military or political office have been, in his opinion, distributed "at random throughout the entire number and could not produce the grouping by close blood relationship found throughout this entire study." ['06, p. 285.]

He tests one environmental influence by the facts, namely, the advantage of succession to the throne.

"There is one peculiar way in which a little more than half of all the males have had a considerable advantage over the

---

* r is used as a symbol for the coefficient of correlation or resemblance.

others in gaining distinction as important historical characters. The eldest sons, or if not the eldest, those sons to whom the succession has devolved, have undoubtedly had greater opportunities to become illustrious than those to whom the succession did not fall by right of primogeniture. I think every one must feel that perhaps much of the greatness of Frederick II, of Prussia, Gustavus Adolphus, and William the Silent, was due to their official position; but an actual mathematical count is entirely opposed to this view. The inheritors of the succession are no more plentiful in the higher grades than in the lower. The figures below show the number in each grade who came into power by inheriting the throne.

Grades	1	2	3	4	5	6	7	8	9	10
Total number in each Grade	7	21	41	49	71	70	68	43	18	7
Succession Inheritors	5	14	26	31	49	38	45	23	12	4
Per cent	71	67	63	64	69	54	67	54	67	57

It is thus seen that from 54 to 71 per cent inherited the succession in the different grades. The upper grades are in no way composed of men whose opportunities were enhanced by virtue of this high position. Thus we see that a certain very decided difference in outward circumstances—namely, the right of succession—can be proved to have no effect on intellectual distinction, or at least so small as to be unmeasurable without much greater data. The younger sons have made neither a poorer nor a better showing." ['06, pp. 285-286.]

His conclusion is:—"The upshot of it all is, that as regards intellectual life, environment is a totally inadequate explanation. If it explains certain characters in certain instances, it always fails to explain as many more; while heredity not only explains all (or at least 90 per cent) of the intellectual side of character in practically every instance, but does so best when questions of environment are left out of the discussion. Therefore, it would seem that we are forced to the conclusion that all these rough differences in intellectual activity which are susceptible of grading on a scale of ten are due to predetermined differences in the primary germ-cells." ['06, p. 286.]

In 1905 the author published a report [Thorndike, '05] of measurements of the resemblances of fifty pairs of twins in marking A's on a printed page of capital letters (A test), marking words containing certain combinations of letters (a-t and r-e), marking misspelled words on a sheet containing 100 words (misspelled word test), addition, multiplication and writing the opposites of a set of words. I quote or summarize the essential facts.

The resemblances of twins, resemblance meaning any greater likeness than would be found in a pair of children of the same age and sex picked at random from the school population of New York City, are:—

In the A test	R = .69
In the a-t and r-e tests	R = .71
In the misspelled word test	R = .80+
In addition	R = .75
In multiplication	R = .84
In the opposites test	R = .90

If now these resemblances are due to the fact that the two members of any twin pair are treated alike at home, have the same parental models, attend the same school and are subject in general to closely similar environmental conditions, then (1) twins should, up to the age of leaving home, grow more and more alike, and in our measurements the twins 13 and 14 years old should be much more alike than those 9 and 10 years old. Again, (2) if similarity in training is the cause of similarity in mental traits, ordinary fraternal pairs not over four or five years apart in age should show a resemblance somewhat nearly as great as twin pairs, for the home and school conditions of a pair of the former will not be much less similar than those of a pair of the latter. Again, (3) if training is the cause, twins should show greater resemblance in the case of traits much subject to training, such as ability in addition or in multiplication, than in traits less subject to training, such as quickness in marking off the A's on a sheet of printed capitals, or in writing the opposites of words.

On the other hand, (1) the nearer the resemblance of young twins comes to equaling that of old, (2) the greater the superiority of twin resemblance to ordinary fraternal resemblance is, and (3) the nearer twin resemblance in relatively untrained capacities comes to equaling that in capacities at which the home and school direct their attention, the more must the resemblances found be attributed to inborn traits.

The older twins show no closer resemblance than the younger twins, and the chances are surely four to one that with an infinite number of twins tested the 12-14-year-olds would not show a resemblance .15 greater than the 9-11-year-olds. The facts are :—

The Resemblances of Young and Old Twins Compared

	Twins 9-11	Twins 12-14
1) A test	66	73
2) a-t and r-e tests	81	62
3) Misspelled word test	76	74
4) Addition	90	54
5) Multiplication	91	69
6) Opposites	96	88
Averages	83	70

I have measured the resemblances between siblings (children of the same parents) a few years apart in age only imperfectly, and only in the A test, a-t test and opposites tests. The resemblances are between .3 and .4, or less than half the resemblance found for twins.

The variations in the closeness of resemblance of the twins

in the different traits show little, and possibly no, direct correlation with the amount of opportunity for environmental influences. The traits most subject to training (addition and multiplication) do show closer resemblances than the traits least subject to training (the A, a-t and r-e test); but on the other hand show less close resemblances than the traits moderately subject to training (the misspelled word test and opposites test).

The facts then are easily, simply and completely explained by one simple hypothesis: namely, that the natures of the germ cells—the conditions of conception—cause whatever similarities and differences exist in the original natures of men, that these conditions influence body and mind equally, and that in life the differences in modification of body and mind produced by such differences as obtain between the environments of present-day New York City public school children are slight.

We must be careful, however, not to confuse two totally different things: (1) the power of the environment,—for instance, of schools, laws, books and social ideals,—to produce differences in the relative achievements of men, and (2) the power of the environment to produce differences in absolute achievement. It has been shown that the relative differences in certain mental traits which were found in these one hundred children are due almost entirely to differences in ancestry, not in training; but this does not in the least deny that better methods of training might improve all their achievements fifty per cent or that the absence of training, say, in spelling and arithmetic, might decrease the corresponding achievements to zero.

The argument is limited entirely to the causes which make one person differ from another in mental achievements *under the same general conditions of life at the beginning of the twentieth century in New York City as pupils in its school sys-*

tem. If the resemblance of twins has been measured in the case of a group made up partly of New York City school children and partly of children of equal capacity brought up in the wilds of Africa, the variability of the group in addition and multiplication would have increased and the correlation coefficients would rise. They would then measure the influence of original nature plus the now much increased influence of the environment.

CHAPTER XXIV

THE INFLUENCE OF MATURITY

No competent student doubts that in certain mental traits maturity or inner mental growth causes one individual to differ year by year from his former self, irrespective of all training. The same force necessarily accounts for some of the differences found between children of different degrees of mental maturity. If by a miracle a hundred children could be found who were alike in sex, ancestry and training, but who were divided into two groups by a difference in the extent to which the original impetus to mental development had run its course, the groups would differ, in at least certain traits, in accordance with this difference in stage of growth or maturity.

About the magnitude of the influence of maturity there is, however, a wide range of opinion, from that which would expect children in the same stage of growth to be all closely alike and all very different from children in a later stage of growth, regardless of differences in their ancestry and training, to that which would expect children of the same ancestry and training to be all very much alike, regardless of differences in stage of growth.

The study of the facts is made difficult by the absence of any exact measure of maturity, that is, of the extent to which the original impetus to mental development has run its course. Length of life is the measure which has been used, but chronological age is not identical with physiological maturity and neither of these two is identical with mental maturity. An individual's degree of mental maturity cannot be inferred from his age. On the average, however, sixteen-year-olds will differ from six-year-olds because of the effect of ten years of inner growth plus the effect of the average amount of training that accompanies that growth. And if we could separate out the effect of mere growth from within from the effect of the training that accompanies it, we could measure each of the two. Such separation is, however, well-nigh impossible with present knowledge.

Consider, for example, the facts given by Gilbert for the ability of ten-year-old boys and seventeen-year-old boys in discriminating weights. The median error made by the ten-year-olds was 8.6 grams; the median error made by the seventeen-year-olds was 6.0 grams. Just what can be inferred about maturity's effect upon the power to discriminate weights from these measurements?

It is clear that an alteration in any mental trait in any individual with age might be due to the mere maturing of some characteristic of original nature or might be the creation of some environmental force. The educational inferences would be exactly opposite in the two cases. In the former we should say: This change comes as a gift from nature which we may not be able to refuse without damaging general growth. It is given as the partial basis and starting point for education. We do not have to try to get it. In the latter case we should say: This change comes as the earnings of training. It is a product of education. With a different training it might be absent. We may lack or possess it as we choose.

Moreover, in the case of many measurements of mental traits, for instance those quoted, the change due to an individual's age would be possibly due not only to the maturing of the

trait or the influence of training upon it, but also to the influence
of both maturity and training upon the ability to understand
and the wish to follow instructions and the ambition to do well
in tests.

As a matter of fact all three of these factors are involved in
most of the changes of mental traits with age. Even if the
changes are due directly to outside forces, in the form of the
experiences of life and training, maturity may still count as a
force co-operating with these or furnishing the conditions in
the individual which permit their action on him to produce the
mental changes in question. On the other hand, mere inner
growth, no matter how potent, requires usually some stimuli
from without. A child grows mentally in some kind of a
world of experience, forming some habits. Only in thought
can the contribution of his inner impulsions be separated off
from the contribution of the outside stimuli by which the inner
impulsions are roused to action. Furthermore, a mental test
with children almost always measures somewhat general
powers of comprehension as well as the special power of sensation, memory or the like that is its ostensible object.

So far upon the supposition that by changes in mental
traits with age, we mean changes in the same individual
measured at different ages. The average change would then
be the average of the changes in all the individuals studied.
But in the studies that have been reported, the difference
between the figures for, say, ten and eleven years, is not the
average of the changes of all the individuals studied and need
not in any real way describe them.

For (1) the difference between the average of a group at
ten and of the same group at eleven years does not describe the
real individual changes; and (2) when we measure ten-and
eleven-year-olds as we find them in school or elsewhere, we

can not be sure that the eleven-year-olds represent what the ten-year-olds will become.

The first point will be made clear by the following illustration. Suppose that eighteen boys showed at the age of ten and a half years the abilities in some mental trait denoted by the measures in the first column and made the gains during the next year shown by the figures in the second column, their consequent records at eleven and a half years being given in the third column. (Case 1.)

CASE 1			CASE 2		
Ability at 10½	Change	Ability at 11½	Ability at 10½	Change	Ability at 11½
2	5	7	2	0	2
2	5	7	2	0	2
3	4	7	3	1	4
4	3	7	4	0	4
4	4	8	4	1	5
5	4	9	5	3	8
5	1	6	5	1	6
6	3	9	6	1	7
6	3	9	6	1	7
6	1	7	6	3	9
6	1	7	6	3	9
7	1	8	7	1	8
7	3	10	7	4	11
7	1	8	7	4	11
8	0	8	8	3	11
9	1	10	9	4	13
9	0	9	9	5	14
11	0	11	11	5	16
Avg. 5 94	2 22	8 16	Avg. 5 94	2 22	8.16

If instead of this complete record we had simply the figures: 10½ years, Av. 5.94; 11½ years, Av. 8.16; Change in average ability, 2.22, we should lack the essential features of our fact; viz., (1) the variability of the changes and (2) the antagonism between ability at ten and a half years and growth during the next year. There is an almost inevitable tendency, when a single figure is given to represent change, to fancy that all children show exactly or nearly that amount of change. This is of course never true. Rate of change as well as absolute ability is variable. And it is precisely in relating the different degrees of progress found in individuals to their original capacities and individual circumstances, that educational insight will accrue. The real individual changes may often prove to be a partial function of the amount of ability already acquired, as in our illustration. The mere change in average ability given above could have come as well from a condition, shown in Case 2, just opposite in this respect to that of Case 1.

Our second point was that the eleven-year-olds tested need not represent what the ten-year-olds would become. The average changes stated in the quotations at the beginning of this chapter were obtained from facts like the following: Ten-year-olds *A, B, C, D, E, F, G, H,* etc., give an average *x;* eleven-year-olds, *L, M, N, O, P,* etc., give an average *y.* The change in average ability is $y - x$. The individuals of the two groups not being identical, the chance is given for the fallacy of selection to run riot. The eleven-twelve-year-olds certainly represent only those ten-eleven-year-olds who will live; in any test given in schools they represent only the ten-eleven-year-olds who will continue in that type of school. Now if one measures a mental trait in elementary school children he gets for different ages something like the following figures :—12-year-olds, 100; 13-year-olds, 90; 14-year-olds, 70; 15-year-olds, 30.

Nobody can imagine that the fifteen-year-olds here would give anything like a fair sampling of what the twelve-year-olds would become. The brightest twelve-year-olds pass out of the grammar school before they are fifteen. Some mental defectives leave for special institutions. Some moral defectives leave for reform schools or the free life of thievery and tramp-dom. Some children leave school to go to work. If we fill up our quota of fifteen-year-olds by adding 70 from high school pupils we jump from the frying pan into the fire, for these are a selection of the brighter, the more ambitious, and the more intellectually inclined.

I conclude, therefore, that the development of mental traits with age has not been and can not be adequately measured by such studies as those quoted. To measure it we must repeat measurements upon the same individuals and for all purposes of inference preserve intact each of the individual changes. In connection with each of them account must be taken of the training which the individual in question has undergone.

What measurements we do have may serve, however, to correct two errors of common opinion. The notion that the increases in ability due to a given amount of progress toward maturity are closely alike for all children save the so-called "abnormally precocious" or "retarded" is false. The same fraction of the total inner development, from zero to adult ability, will produce very unequal results in different children. Inner growth acts differentially according to the original nature that is growing.

The notion that maturity is the main factor in the differ-ences found amongst school children, so that grading and methods of teaching should be fitted closely to 'stage of growth,' is also false. It is by no means very hard to find seven-year-olds who can do intellectual work at which one in twenty seventeen-year-olds would fail. Although the influence of inner growth in causing individual differences cannot be measured from the data at hand, an *upper limit* for it can be set. Take discrimination of weight as a sample case. Since early age differences are in part due to training and since train-

ing acts here in the same direction as does maturity, the average
inner growth from, say, ten to seventeen must produce *less* than
the average difference found between ten-year-olds and seventeen-year-olds. Since, in Gilbert's study, the seventeen-year-
olds and ten-year-olds both come from school pupils, including
pupils in the high school, the seventeen-year-olds represent at
least as high ranking pupils in mental respects as the ten-year-
olds would become. So the effect of average inner growth

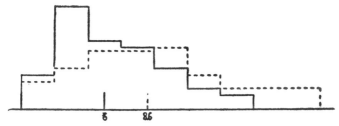

FIG. 77. The Magnitude of Age Differences in Comparison with Range for
Individuals of the Same Age. This drawing is imaginary, for Gilbert does
not give the necessary detailed data However, any detailed data that satisfied his
facts for the variability of 10-year-olds and 17-year-olds would show as great
a disparity as does this drawing between the differences due to seven years
and that due to causes acting on children of the same age.

from ten to seventeen has as its upper limit a reduction of 3
grams in the error made (from 8.6 to 6.0 grams), and is
probably much less than this. But this is (as shown in Fig. 77)
small relatively to the individual range within either group,
this topmost limit for the average effect of seven years of inner
growth being roughly less than one sixth of the effect of the
extreme differences in ancestry and training upon children of
the same age.

CHAPTER XXV

The Influence of the Environment

DIFFICULTIES IN ESTIMATING THE AMOUNT OF INFLUENCE OF THE ENVIRONMENT

The questions suggested by the title of this chapter include the effects on individuals of every environmental force, including all the agencies for intellectual and moral education. Precise quantitative answers can be given to hardly any of them.

Theoretically, there is no impossibility. Once we have estimated the original nature of a man or group of men, we have simply to note the mental changes consequent upon this or that change in climate, food, school training, friendship, sermon, occupation, etc. Practically, the complexity of the action of physical and human influences upon intellect and character hampers scientific study and favors guesswork. The environment includes a practical infinitude of different causes; these act differently upon different types of original nature and at different ages and with different co-operating circumstances; in many cases their action is very complex and must be observed over long intervals of time. Indeed it has been common to deny even the possibility of a science of the dynamics of human nature and to remain content with the haphazard opinions of novelists, proverb makers and village wise men.

Moreover, it is only by the utmost ingenuity and watchfulness that studies of changes in human nature can be freed from a characteristic fallacy—that of attributing to training facts which are really due to original nature or to selection. For instance, college graduates are found to have a much greater likelihood of being elected to Congress than other men have. Therefore it is said that a college education causes to some extent political success. But it is clear that even before they went to college the group of youth who did go were different from those who did not. Their later election to Congress may as well have been due to the mental traits which they possessed by birth or otherwise and which caused their inclusion in the class 'boys who go to college' as to any changes produced in them by the college training itself. In other words, that they were the class *selected* by the college is as important a fact as that they were the class trained by it.

Again it is said: "Who can doubt the enormous disciplinary value of the study of Latin and Greek when we see the admirable intellects of the men so trained in the English universities?" But being born from the class whose children go to the university of itself ensures to an individual uncommon mental ability.

To avoid this confusion of causes which train with those which select is extremely hard. Any class of individuals studied because they have been subjected to a certain training is almost sure to be a class not only trained by but also selected by that training. Suppose that one wishes to study the influence of a high-school course, or that of the classical as opposed to the scientific course, or that of training in independent research, or that of immoral surroundings. High school graduates are but one-fifth of grammar school graduates; and no one would claim that they represent an entirely random picking therefrom. They are surely selected for better birth, better abilities and better ideals. Again, in most high schools the graduate of the classical course represents not only a different training, but also a different selection, commonly a superior selection.* So also scientific men are a class resulting not only from the training given by research work, but also from the selection of those eager to do and fitted to do that work. Children brought up in a morally bad environment are almost sure to be of morally inferior ancestry. The ordinary arrangement of social and educational careers rarely presents us with convenient cases of similar natures, some with, some without, the form of training under consideration.

The difficulty of eliminating the influence of selection is no excuse for its neglect. Yet one may hunt through thousands of pages of discussions of the influence of certain studies, school systems, schemes of culture, religious beliefs, etc., without finding a hint of its recognition.

Either because of the general complexity of environmental influences upon any mental trait and the mixture of selective with formative influences or because of the infrequency of scientific habits and ideals in students of sociology and education, there are few facts of sufficient security and precision to be quoted. Only rarely has educational science progressed beyond the reasoned opinions of more or less capable judges. We have our beliefs about the causal relations between a hot climate and indolence, necessity and invention, lack of parental control and crime, religious training and morality, etc., but we can not be said to know these influences with adequate surety or to have any knowledge whatever of their precise amount.

A refusal to believe insecure opinions about the influence of differences in training in producing differences in human individuals does not at all imply disbelief in their influence. Such would be absurd. When the original natures are the same,

*This apparently is becoming less common every year.

every difference that the individuals later show must be due to differences in the outside forces operating upon them. And any difference in outside forces always has its effect. No man is left unchanged by even the very least of the environmental forces that act upon him. Men are the creatures of circumstance. But they are creations whose final patterns are determined in part by sex, race, ancestry and conditions of origin. Circumstances alter natures, but the alterations vary with the nature altered. It is precisely because common opinions have thought verbally in terms of *'man-training-product of training,'* instead of concretely in terms of *'men-training-products,—each of an individual's nature in interaction with his training,'* that a sound science of the influence of the environment has hardly been begun.

One of the best services such a science can render is to guard its students against such verbal plausibilities. For example, knowledge is not proportional to opportunity in the sense that an individual's degree of knowledge can be foretold from his degree of opportunity. Wealth does not create wealth in the sense that what a man will have can be estimated from what he now has. A good home does not make good children in the sense of doing so always and in proportion to its goodness. Being treated like slaves may not debase all and never debases all alike. The product of the environment is always a result of two variables, it and the man's nature.

Two of the corollaries of this axiom are of special significance. The first is that the environmental stimulus adequate to arouse a certain power or ideal or habit in one man may be hopelessly inadequate to do so in another. Washing bottles in a drug-shop was, if a common story is true, adequate to decide Faraday's career, and the voyage on the Beagle is reputed to have made Darwin a naturalist for life. But if all the youth of the land were put to work in drug-shops and later sent on scientific expeditions, the result would not be a million Faradays and Darwins, or even a million chemists and naturalists.   All that one man may need to be free is a vote; but even a long education in self-direction may be inadequate for another. Being told a few words suffices to secure the habit of reading in one child, while the child beside him remains illiterate after two years of careful tuition.   The amount of stimulus required in some cases is so infinitesimal that the power seems to spring absolutely from the man himself.   In other men no agency is found potent enough to arouse a trace of the desired result.

The second corollary is that each man in part selects his own environment.   The boy turns his eyes from the book.   Even if his eyes attend to it, his mind does not.   Even if for the time he lets it move him, it may be disregarded in memory. That connection which brings satisfaction to one man and is thereby given power over him, may disgust another nature and so be repudiated by it.   As this world's nature selects for survival those animals which are adapted to live in it, so any individual selects, by action, attention, memory and satisfaction, the features of the environment which are to survive as determinants of his intellect and character.

Common opinion and the older literature of sociology and education neglected the differential action of the environment in accord with the nature it acted on, but it would be possible for a student, enamored of the simplicity of the explanation of all men's differences by differences in their original make-up, to neglect equally obvious facts of another sort.   He might be tempted to claim that, since the features of civilization,—the acts, words, books, customs, and institutions of men,—have been invented and perpetuated by human natures, and since consequently the environment in all important respects is itself due to original nature,—therefore original nature is at bottom the cause of almost all of human destinies. "A people gets as good government as it deserves; a race has the environment its own nature has found and chosen: a man in essential matters is treated as his nature decides." So he might carelessly claim.

Many important features of the environment are thus due to the original nature of the human race as a whole, but no one man's nature and, under modern conditions, no one nation's or race's is similarly responsible for the particular environment that it meets. Forces set in motion by others play upon it. At the best it can select only negatively by disregard, and at the worst it may be molded directly against nature.

Even when it is known, and with some precision, that a given difference is due to some difference in training, there may be doubt or total ignorance as to what difference in training caused it. And even when it is known that a given difference in training has been operative and has produced an effect, there may be doubt or ignorance about what the effect is.

Illustrations of the former case are abundant in history. History is in fact largely a record of unexplained changes in human nature. Nearly all the intellectual and moral differences between the modern English, French, or Germans and their barbarous ancestors of two thousand years ago are due to differences in environment. The original natures of the stocks may have altered somewhat during that time, but surely not much. Our thoughts and ways of thinking and our habits, customs and ideals have been and are being made very unlike those of our ancestors by some outside forces. But what the forces were and how each contributed to the result is not known.

Illustrations of the latter case form a large proportion of the facts studied under the vague rubric of education. Such and such children have gone to school, they have been taught by such and such teachers, using this and that method, at a cost of so many dollars, with aid of a material plant worth so much; but what has come of it all, no cautious thinker would dare say. What has been and is being done to children in schools is more or less well described in official and private records, but what happens in children as its consequence is largely unknown.

So much for the attitude in which a student of human nature must approach the problems of the effect of different environments on identical natures, of the effect of the same environment on different natures, and of the effect of the endless different co-operations of environments and natures.

MEASUREMENTS OF THE INFLUENCE OF THE ENVIRONMENT

I shall report three samples of studies of the influence of the environment upon intellect and character. The first is Galton's *History of Twins* ['83], a study of the amount of its influence in comparison with that of original nature. The second is Rice's study of the effect of different school environments upon ability in spelling. The third is a study of the effect of changing environment upon the choice of a profession by scholarly youth.

Galton collected reports from parents concerning twins who were closely similar in infancy but whose environments differed, and twins who were in infancy notably unlike, but whose environments were in all important features identical. The increase of differences in the former case and of resemblances in the latter gives a measure of the influence of the environment. The persistence of similarities in the former case and of differences in the latter gives a measure of the influence of original nature.

The evidence in the case of the twenty pairs in the second group shows no exceptions to the rule that no weakening of inborn differences by similarities of nurture is observable. The following are representative parental observations:—

1. One parent says:—"They have had *exactly the same nurture* from their birth up to the present time; they are both perfectly healthy and strong, yet they are otherwise as dissimilar as two boys could be, physically, mentally, and in their emotional nature."

2. "I can answer most decidedly that the twins have been perfectly dissimilar in character, habits, and likeness from the moment of their birth to the present time, though they were nursed by the same woman, went to school together, and were never separated till the age of fifteen."

3. "They have never been separated, never the least differently treated in food, clothing, or education; both teethed at the same time, both had measles, whooping-cough, and scarlatina at the same time, and neither had any other serious illness. Both are and have been exceedingly healthy and have good abilities, yet they differ as much from each other in mental cast as any of my family differ from another."

5. "They were never alike either in body or mind and their dissimilarity increases daily. The external influences have been identical; they have never been separated."

9. "The home-training and influence were precisely the same, and therefore I consider the dissimilarity to be accounted for almost entirely by innate disposition and by causes over which we have no control."

The two lines of evidence taken together justify, in Galton's opinion, the following general statements:

"We may, therefore, broadly conclude that the only circumstance, within the range of those by which persons of similar conditions of life are affected, that is capable of producing a marked effect on the character of adults, is illness or some accident that causes physical infirmity. . . . The impression that all this leaves on the mind is one of some wonder whether nurture can do anything at all, beyond giving instruction and professional training. There is no escape from the conclusion that nature prevails enormously over nurture when the differences of nurture do not exceed what is commonly to be found among persons of the same rank of society and in the same country." [*ibid*. pp. 168 and 172.]

Dr. Rice's study is quoted at some length because it was the first of a series of studies of the actual results of school work, still few in number, but destined to increase rapidly with increasing scientific interest in school administration.

Dr. Rice ['97] tested the spelling ability of some 33,000 children in twenty-one schools representing a great variety in spirit, methods, time given to spelling and in other respects. He then compared the conditions in schools where the pupils did well in spelling with those in schools where they did badly. He notes first of all the slight differences between schools, only 6 out of the 21 schools being outside the limits 73.3 and 77.9, and the decrease in variation amongst schools as we pass from lower to higher grades (see Table 9), facts which show that the differences in spirit or method that characterize schools can not make much difference in achievement. Of school systems where mechanical methods are in use as compared with more progressive systems he says:

"Indeed, in both the mechanical and the progressive schools the results were variable; so that while, in some instances, the higher figures were secured by the former, in others they were obtained by the latter; and the same is true of the lower figures. For example, School B, No. 11, in which the best average (79.4) was obtained, belongs to a very progressive system; while School A, No. 12, which made only 73.9, belongs to one of our most mechanical systems. And it is a peculiar incident that, in both these cities, the results in the only other school examined are exactly reversed, although the environment is about the same."

He eliminates the possibility that home reading or cultured parents or English rather than foreign parentage is the cause of the differences amongst schools by making the comparisons of Table 10.

Dr. Rice further tabulated the results in accordance with the methods of instruction used in the different schools, interviewing some two hundred teachers for that purpose. He does not give the detailed results, but assures us that there is no reason to believe that there is any clear choice between oral and written spelling, writing isolated words and writing sentences, the sight or flash method and its absence. Phonic reading does not make bad spellers, nor do written language work and wide general reading make good spellers. "In brief," says he. "there is no direct relation between method and results. . . . The results varied as much under the same as they did under different methods of instruction."

That the amount of time given is not the cause of success in teaching spelling is shown by the facts of Table 9. Schools giving 15 or 20 minutes daily to spelling do as well as those giving 40 or 50.

After this admirable array of facts Dr. Rice jumps rather hastily to this speculative conclusion: "The facts here presented, in my opinion, will admit of only one conclusion, viz., that the results are not determined by the methods employed, but by the ability of those who use them. In other words, the first place must be given to the personal equation of the teacher, while methods and devices play a subordinate part."

This statement should have been based upon a demonstration of a high coefficient of correlation between the measure of a class in spelling and the measure of its teacher in ability, or of a great increase in variability in spelling ability as we pass from the children taught by one teacher to the children taught

25

TABLE 9.

Averages for Individual Schools in Spelling.

City	School	School Av., Sentence-Test	8th Year Sentence-Test	8th Year Composition-Test	8th Year Minutes Daily	7th Year Sentence-Test	7th Year Composition-Test	7th Year Minutes Daily	6th Year Sentence-Test	6th Year Composition-Test	6th Year Minutes Daily	5th Year Sentence-Test	5th Year Composition-Test	5th Year Minutes Daily	4th Year Sentence-Test	4th Year Composition-Test	4th Year Minutes Daily
1	A	77.1	—	—	—	76.7	—	25	77.2	—	20	79.6	—	45	B 67.6	—	—
1	B	75	82	—	—	—	—	—	77.7	98.8	—	72.6	97.4	50	A 61.8	96.8	50
	C	77.6	86.1	99.6	20	78	98.7	40	71.5	98.2	50	81.8	98.4	35	B 71	96.7	45
7	A	75.2	85.8	99	30	73.1	99.4	30	64.2	97.8	40	73.6	97.8	20	B 77	95.9	30
7	B	77.9	84.9	—	30	—	—	15	73.4	98.6	20	79.4	98.3	15	A 68.6	97.5	40
7	C	—	—	99.4	35	77.2	—	40	71.1	—	40	75	—	30	B 64.5	97	—
9	A	76.6	87.2	99.4	30	81.1	98.7	30	80	97.8	45	81.1	97.6	40	B 75.8	97.9	20
9	B	77.7	86.7	99.3	15	—	99.2	50	—	99.1	50	—	98.6	—	A 70.8	97.5	35
9	C	77.9	—	99.4	—	85.6	—	60	66.5	—	35	71.3	—	15	B 66.6	97.4	40
10	A	76.2	83.5	99.2	20	86.5	99.4	20	72.8	98.7	45	74.8	97.6	45	B 66.4	96.1	—
10	B	—	82.5	99.1	—	84.7	99.2	20	73.2	98.4	40	76.8	97.9	—	A 68.4	96.8	40
11	A	72	86.4	—	40	76	—	30	63.4	90.2	25	70.4	98.6	25	A 63.6	98.3	25

Small b indicates first half and small a second half of school year.

TABLE 9. (Continued).
AVERAGES FOR INDIVIDUAL SCHOOLS IN SPELLING.

City	School	School Av., Sentence-Test	8th Year Min. Daily	8th Year Comp.-Test	8th Year Sentence-Test	7th Year Min. Daily	7th Year Comp.-Test	7th Year Sentence-Test	6th Year Min. Daily	6th Year Comp.-Test	6th Year Sentence-Test	5th Year Min. Daily	5th Year Comp.-Test	5th Year Sentence-Test	4th Year Min. Daily	4th Year Comp.-Test	4th Year Sentence-Test
11	B	79.4			86.7 / 86.3			80	30	98.5	74	25	97.9 / 98.5	74.6 / 81.8	35	96.3 / 97.9	b 76.4 / a 79.8
12	A	73.9	40	99.1	90.2 / 90.3	40	98.8	78.3	9		75 / 75.7			66.4			b 53.2 / a 63.1
12	B	79.0			94.6 / 83.9			90		97.7	73.1 / 78.4	18	96.8	73 / 74.4	18		b 53.3 / a 67.2
15	B	73.4	12	99 / 99.4	87.2 / 86.2	12	98.3 / 98.7	76.7 / 83.3	20	98.1	57 / 71.5	10	97.4	79		97	b — / a —
15	D	78.8			88.6			74.7			63.3			73 / 73.4			b 74.3 / a 66.2
15	E	77.3	20	99.2	89.4 / 89.9	20	98.7	84	20	98.5 / 98.1	72.7 / 72.8	20	97.8 / 98.3	81.6 / 83.6	20	96.6	b 70.8 / a 67.2
15	H	77.9	20		89.4 / 84	20		80.6 / 81.4	20	98.1	69.6 / 69.8	20		74.4 / 79.4	15		b 69.1 / a 62.6
16	A	72.0	25	99.1 / 99.4	89.9 / 81.2	25	98.2 / 98.8	71.1 / 72.8	25	97.6 / 98.7	76.2 / 61.9	25	98.5 / 98.6	76.2 / 79.1	20	97.4 / 97.9	b 59.2 / a 68.4
16	B	72.7	6	98.9 / 99.2	80.2 / 84.3	20	98.5	71.3 / 75.3	15	98.1	68.7	15	98.5	73.6 / 76.4	20		b 65 / a —
19	A	73.8	5		85	10		78 / 84	35		68.8 / 72	20		70.6 / 74.4	20	97.9	b 57.4
19	B	73.3			86.8	30	99.3	69.5 / 84	30	97.7	61.3 / 69.5	40	98.5 / 98.2	66.8 / 76.6 / 73 / 78.2	40		a 68.4

Small b indicates first half, and small a second half of school year.

TABLE 10. (Table 3 of the original account).

Grade	No. of Cities	No. of Classes	No. of Pupils	General Average	Children of Foreign Parentage	Average	No. of Children Hearing Foreign Language at Home	Average	Children of Unskilled Laborers	Average
SENTENCE TEST Fourth ..	4	27	821	64 7	155	65.2	159	64.9	129	62 5
Fifth....	4	29	829	76.	153	77.4	157	76 7	129	74.5
Sixth....	4	22	778	69 7	185	69 6	165	70 3	119	70.4
Seventh .	4	18	566	78 8	81	82 5	52	81 5	55	76.8
Eighth...	4	19	528	83 1	72	83 2	64	83.2	76	85

by 10 or 20 different teachers. I calculate that if the reliabil-
ities of Dr. Rice's eighth grade averages are what they would
seem to be from tests made in eighth grades by myself and my
students,* the differences amongst them are not much greater
than we would expect by the law of chance if the teaching
were in all cases equally efficient. The average deviation from
their mean of the 12 eighth grade classes which were tested in
the first half of the year is 1.9; that of the 13 tested in the last
half of the year is 2.6; the average deviation by pure chance
of 12 eighth grade classes of 40 students each would be 1.9,
the variability of individuals being 12.2. So, in the case of the
eighth grades, we may need no cause at all for the differences
amongst schools save the inaccuracy of the averages due to
the small number of cases.

The third sample of studies of the influence of the environment is not of major importance, but is distinctive in that its
facts cannot be accounted for by any force other than the
environment. The facts are the changes in the careers of
scholarly college graduates from the class of 1840 to that of
1895, comprising 5283 members of the honorary society, Φ B K,

---

*These give a variability of 12.2 amongst the individuals of the grade.

admission to which was substantially a recognition of superior scholarship in college.

The four professions, law, medicine, teaching and the ministry, have, together, attracted almost exactly the same proportion of scholarly men in each decade. The per cent of Φ B K graduates entering some one of these four professions was 65 in 1840-59, 65½ in 1860-69, 65 in 1870-79, and 64 in 1880-1894.

Among the professions, however, there have been marked changes, as shown in Table 11. In twenty years the law doubled its attractiveness to scholarly men and then, in half that time, lost two-thirds of its gain. Medicine was, in the last decade of the period, becoming more attractive. The table shows a very rapid rise in the popularity of teaching from 1840 to 1860 and again from 1870 to 1895.· The years from '60 to '65 show an opposite tendency. The law was then gaining rapidly and the ministry was holding its own. The most striking change was the decrease in the proportion of scholarly men making the ministry their life work. The decrease would be even more marked if those who entered the ministry but gave up its regular work for that of teaching were included. The incomplete records available in the Φ B K Catalogue of 1900 give only 5½ per cent of clergymen amongst those graduating from '95-'99; and even with later additions the per cent for 1900 is probably under 10.

Roughly, it may be said that three-fourths of the scholarly young men who entered the ministry in 1850 would have gone into teaching or the law if they had happened to be born a half century later. The same original natures choose differently because the social and intellectual environment has changed.

The near future will doubtless see a rapid increase in the number and improvement in the quality of studies of the enviro_nmental causes of individual differences in mental traits. Rice's investigation of the differences due to different features of administration and teaching has been followed by similar studies by Cornman ['o2], Stone ['o8], Courtis ['o9 and later] and Thorndike ['10]. Experts in education are becoming experimentalists and quantitative thinkers and are seeking to verify or refute the established beliefs concerning the effects of

TABLE II.

PERCENTAGES OF SCHOLARLY YOUTHS MAKING THEIR LIFE WORK THAT OF:—

	Law	Medicine	Teaching	Ministry
1840—1844	14		9 4	37 5
1845—1846	14	6	11.6	40
1850—1854	9.3		13 7	36 5
1855—1859	10.5		16.4	34.5
1860—1864	· 15.2	5 5	17 2	27 5
1865—1869	19.7	4	13 9	28 5
1870—1874	19.8	5 5	16 4	22.5
1875—1879	22.5	4	17.6	22
1880—1884	16.4	4 5	21 4	19 5
1885—1889	14.4	7.5	25.5	16
1890—1894	19	7	25.4	14

educational forces upon human nature. Students of history, government, sociology, economics, ethics and religion are becoming, or will soon become, quantitative thinkers concerning the shares of the various physical and social forces in making individual men differ in politics, crime, wealth, service, idealism, or whatever trait concerns man's welfare.

To the facts presented in these three sample studies and in previous chapters, we may add certain very significant measures of the effect of equal amounts of exercise of a function upon individual differences in respect to efficiency in it. The argument is as follows: In so far as the differences in

achievement found amongst a group of men are due to differences in the quantity and quality of training which they have
had in the function in question, the provision of equal amounts
of the same sort of training for all individuals in the group
should act to *reduce* the differences. Suppose, for example,
that eleven individuals showed efficiencies of 10, 11, 12, 13,
14, 15, 16, 17, 18, 19 and 20 respectively in the number of
words that they could typewrite per minute. Suppose that this
variation had been entirely caused by a corresponding variation
in the amount of time they had spent in practicing typewriting,
say 5, 6, 7, 8, 9, 10, 11, 12, 13, 14 and 15 hours. Then giving
each individual 10 hours more of practice, so that the range in
respect to amount of practice would be from 15 to 25 hours,
should result in reducing the relative differences. The person
who now had had 15 hours of practice should by the hypothesis
show an efficiency of 20, while the person with 25 hours of
practice would not be expected to be beyond 30. Whereas the
limiting scores were as 2 to 1 (20 to 10), they should not now
differ more than as 3 to 2 (30 to 20).*

If the addition of equal amounts of practice does *not* reduce
the differences found amongst men, those differences can not
well be explained to any large extent by supposing them to have
been due to corresponding differences in amount of previous
practice. If, that is, inequalities in achievement are not reduced
by equalizing practice, they cannot well have been caused by
inequalities in previous practice. If differences in opportunity
cause the differences men display, making opportunity more
nearly equal for all by adding equal amounts to it in each case
should make the differences less.

*The exact expectation would, of course, depend upon the form of the
practice-curve in question for the function in question and the cooperating
factors in the learners; the illustration is made arbitrarily simple.

The facts found are rather startling. Equalizing practice *seems to increase differences.* The superior man seems to have got his present superiority by his own nature rather than by superior advantages of the past, since, during a period of equal advantages for all, he increases his lead.

The following table (Table 12) giving the initial and final scores in practice at the mental multiplication of a three-place by a three-place number, speaks for itself. The same effect appears, though less emphatically, in the case of Whitley's nine individuals in a similar experiment ['11]. The four who were most efficient at the start made a greater average gain from equal practice than the four who were least efficient.

TABLE 12.

The Effect of Equal Amounts of Practice upon Individual Differences in the Mental Multiplication of a Three-place by a Three-place Number.

			Amount done per unit of time.				Percentage of correct figures in answers.		
			Hours of Practice	First 5 Examples	Last 5 or 10 Examples	Gain	First 5 Examples	Last 5 or 10 Examples	Gain
Initial highest five individuals			5 1	85	147	61	70	78	18
"	next	five "	5.1	56	107	51	68	78	10
"	"	six "	5 3	46	68	22	74	82	8
"	"	six "	5 4	38	46	8	58	70	12
"	"	five "	5 2	31	57	26	47	67	20
"	"	one individual	5 2	19	32	13	100	82	-18

Using the multiplication of a three-place by a one-place number Starch ['11] got results showing the same effect. Of his eight subjects, the three best averaged 39 examples per 10

minutes in the initial test and gained on the average 45 in the
course of doing 700 examples. The three lowest, who averaged
25 examples per 10 minutes in the initial test, gained only 26
in the course of doing 700 examples, in spite of the fact that
700 examples represented for them a much greater amount of
practice, measured in time spent.

In the case of addition [Thorndike, '10], the initially highest individuals of nineteen adults showed this same greater gain
in amount done at equal accuracy per unit of time when all
nineteen were given approximately equal practice. The facts
are given in Table 13. Similar results have been obtained by
Wells ['12], Kirby ['13], Hahn and Thorndike ['14] and
others.

TABLE 13.

THE EFFECT OF EQUAL AMOUNTS OF PRACTICE UPON INDIVIDUAL DIFFERENCES
IN COLUMN-ADDITION OF ONE-PLACE NUMBERS.

	Average number of additions per 5 minutes corrected for errors			Average time spent in practice from mid-point of first test to mid-point of last test (in minutes)
	First test	Last test	Gain	
Initially highest 6 individuals	297	437	140	40
Initially next highest 6 individuals	234	345	111	49
Initially lowest 7 individuals	167—	220+	54	46

These experiments concerning the effect of practice upon
individual differences in mental multiplication, addition, marking A's on printed sheets of capitals and the like are too restricted in scope and in the amount of practice to justify any
general application of their results. In other mental functions

the achievements of a man in comparison to his fellows may be more a consequence of his advantages and less a consequence of his own nature. So far as they go, however, experiments in practice have given no support to the common assumption that differences in external conditions are responsible for the bulk of the variation found among men of the same race and general social status.

THE METHOD OF ACTION OF DIFFERENCES IN ENVIRONMENT

We may summarize the methods whereby different environments act upon intellect and morals as :—

1. Furnishing or withholding the physiological conditions for the brain's growth and health.

2. Furnishing or withholding adequate stimuli to arouse the action of which the brain is by original nature or previous action capable.

3. Reinforcing some and eliminating others of these activities in consequence of the general law of effect.*

According to this description we should look upon the mental life of an individual as developing in the same way that the animal or plant kingdom has developed. As conditions of heat and food-supply have everywhere been the first requisite to and influence on animal life, so the physiological conditions of the brain's activities are the first modifiers of feeling and action. As the stimuli of climate, food, unknown chemical and electrical forces and the rest have been the means of creating variations in the germs or of stimulating to action the inner tendency of

*In all animals capable of profiting by training any act which in a given situation brings satisfaction becomes thereby more closely associated with that situation, so that when that situation recurs the act will recur also An act that brings discomfort becomes dissociated from the situation and less likely to recur.

the germs to vary, and so have rendered possible the production of millions of different animal types, so the sights and sounds and smells of things, the words and looks and acts of men, the utensils and machinery and buildings of civilization, its pictures and music and books, awaken in the mind new mental varieties, new species of thoughts and acts. In a score of years from birth the human mind, like the animal world, originates its universe of mental forms. And as, in the animal kingdom, many of these variations fail to fit the conditions of physical nature and die after a generation or two, so in any one of us many of the mental forms produced are doomed to a speedy disappearance in consequence of their failure to fit outside events. The elimination of one species by others in the animal world is again paralleled by the death of those thoughts or acts which are out of harmony with others. Species of thoughts, like species of animals, prey upon one another in a struggle in which survival is the victor's reward. Further, just as species of animals fitted to one environment perish or become transformed when that environment changes, so mental forms fitted to infancy perish or are transformed in school life; mental forms fitted to school life perish in the environment of the workaday world; and so throughout the incessant changes of a mind's surroundings. In mental life resulting pain or discomfort is the cause of the extinction of a species. The condition of a man's mind at any stage in its history is then, like the condition of the animal kingdom at any stage in the history of the world, the result not only of the new varieties that have appeared, but also of a natural selection working upon them. The tale of a human mind's progress is the tale of the extinction of its failures. Possibility of existence, stimuli to variations, selection by elimination: these words that describe the action of the environment on animal life are equally competent to tell the record of a human life.

The influence of any environmental agency, physical or social, varies with its avoidability. Oligarchies lose in influence if there is a democracy to which men may emigrate. Customs do not make men so infallibly if there is a radical party, however small, which offers an alternative mode of life. Music's charms to soothe obviously are not so universal if men can close their ears. A creed loses authority as soon as one disbeliever seeks converts. Social environments, institutions, beliefs and modes of behavior are nearly omnipotent when undisputed; for to be the first man to revolt means either that one is a mere eccentric and so sure to be a failure, or that one is a genius and so very rare. But once a revolt is started and advertised, it may much more easily attract those whose original natures it fits. And they may be the more attracted by it for having been exposed to the opposite force. So a given environmental force may even act as a stimulus toward just the opinions, interests or acts that it is designed to thwart.

There are many differences in thought and conduct which are nearly equally tolerated by all original natures. To wear a hat or not to wear a hat, to express requests and opinions in English or to express them in German, to learn astrology or to learn the Ptolemaic astronomy or to learn the Copernican astronomy—to all original natures these are nearly indifferent issues. Which is done depends almost exclusively on environment. In general this is true of all the 'whats' of knowledge and technique. *How many* and *how hard* things a man can learn or do are largely decided by original nature, but, within these limits, *what* he learns or does is largely a matter of what he is stimulated to do and rewarded for doing. On the other hand, there are many features of original nature each of which acts to produce nearly the same effect in spite of such differences in outside forces as different men can meet in modern civilized countries.   In such countries it seems possible for any one to be a poet, or to be a political leader, or to be a money-maker, if his nature so orders.   Original nature in general is not irrepressible, and no form of it is absolutely irrepressible; but some forms of original nature seem to be nearly irrepressible by any of the environments a man in this country today is likely to have.

THE RELATIVE IMPORTANCE OF ORIGINAL NATURE AND ENVIRONMENT

It is impossible at present to estimate with security the relative shares of original nature, due to sex, race, ancestry and accidental variation, and of the environment, physical and social, in causing the differences found in men.   One can only learn the facts, interpret them with as little bias as possible, and try to secure more facts.   This interpretation is left to the student, but with certain cautions in addition to or in amplification of those already explained.

Many of the false inferences about nature *versus* nurture are due to neglect of the obvious facts:—that if the environments are alike with respect to a trait, the differences in respect to it are due entirely to original nature; that if the original natures are alike with respect to a trait, the differences in respect to it are due entirely to differences in training; and that the problem of relative shares, where both are effective, includes all the separate problems of each kind of environment acting with each kind of nature.   Any one estimate for all cases would be absurd.

Many disagreements spring from a confusion of what may

be called absolute achievement with what may be called relative achievement. A man may move up a long distance from zero and nevertheless be lower down than before in comparison with other men: absolute gain may be relative loss. One thinker may attribute differences in achievement almost wholly to nurture while another holds nature to be nearly supreme, though both thinkers possess just the same data, if the former is thinking of absolute and the latter of relative achievement. The commonest error resulting is that of concluding from the importance of sex and ancestral heredity that education and social control in general are futile. On the contrary, as I have elsewhere said, such studies as those of Chapters XXII, and XXIII merely prove the existence of, and measure certain determinants of, human intellect and character and demonstrate that the influences of the environment are differential, the product varying not only in accord with the environmental force itself but also in accord with the original nature upon which it operates. We may even expect that education will be doubly effective, once society recognizes the advantages given to some and denied to others by heredity. That men have different amounts of capacity does not imply any the less advantage from or need of wise investment. If it be true, for example, that the negro is by nature unintellectual and joyous, this does not imply that he may not be made more intelligent by wiser training or misanthropic and ugly-tempered by the treatment he now receives. It does mean that we should be stupid to expect the same results from him that we should from an especially intellectual race like the Jews, and that he will stand with equanimity a degree of disdain which a Celt would requite with dynamite and arson.

To the real work of man for man,—the increase of achievement through the improvement of the environment,—the influence of heredity offers no barrier. But to the popular demands from education and social reforms it does. For the common man does not much appreciate absolute happiness or absolute betterment. He does not rejoice that he and his children are healthier, happier and more supplied with noble pleasures than were his ancestors of a thousand years ago. His complaint is that he is not so well off as some of those about him; his pride is that he is above the common herd. The common man demands *relative* superiority,—to be above those of his own time and locality. If his son leads the community, he does not mind his real stupidity; to be the handsomest girl in the county is beauty enough. Social discontent comes from the knowledge or fancy that one is below others in welfare. The effort of children in school, of men in labor and of women in the home is, except as guided by the wise instincts of nature or more rarely by the wisdom of abstract thought, to rise above some one who seems higher. Thus the prizes which most men really seek are after all in large measure given or withheld by original nature. In the actual race of life, which is not to get ahead, but to get ahead of somebody, the chief determining factor is heredity.

But the prizes which education *ought* to seek are all within its power. The results for which a rational mankind would strive are determined largely by mankind itself. For the common good it is indifferent *who* is at the top,—*which* men are achieving most. The important thing for the common good, for all men, is that the top should be high—that much should be achieved. To the absolute welfare of all men together education is the great contributor.

Another caution is not to make false inferences about moral responsibility from the fact that individual differences are in large measure due to nature; nor to use such false inferences to discourage acceptance of evidence in support of this fact.

It is from time to time complained that a doctrine which refers mental traits largely to original make-up, and consequently to ancestry, discourages the ambitions of the well-intentioned and relieves the world's failures from merited contempt. But every one is agreed that a man's free will works only within limits, and it will not much matter for our practical attitude whether those limits are somewhat contracted. If the question is between original nature and the circumstances of nurture it is rather more encouraging to believe that success will depend on inherent qualities than to refer it entirely to advantages possessed during life, and contempt is merited more by him who has failed through being the inferior person than by the one who has failed simply from bad luck. Whether or not it is merited in either of the two cases we shall decide in view of our general notions about merit and blame, not of our psychological theories of the causes of conduct.

On the whole it seems certain that prevalent opinions much exaggerate the influence of differences in circumstances and training in producing the intellectual and moral differences found in men of the same nation and epoch. Certain natures seem to have been made by certain environments when really the nature already made selected that environment. Certain environments seem to eliminate certain traits from an individual when really they merely expel the individual *in toto*.

Thinkers about the organized educational work of church, library and school need especially to remember three facts.

First.—For the more primitive and fundamental traits in human nature such as energy, capability, persistence, leadership, sympathy and nobility the whole world affords the stimulus, a stimulus that is present well-nigh everywhere. If a man's original nature will not respond to the need of these qualities and the rewards always ready for them, it is vain to expect much from the paltry exercises of the schoolroom.

Second.—The channels in which human energy shall proceed, the specific intellectual and moral activities that shall profit by human capacities, are less determined by inborn traits. The schools should invest in profitable enterprises the capital nature provides. We can not create intellect, but we can prevent such a lamentable waste of it as was caused by scholasticism. We can not double the fund of human sympathy, but we can keep it clear of sentimental charity.

Third.—Morality is more susceptible than intellect to environmental influence. Moral traits are more often matters of the direction of capacities and the creation of desires and aversions. Over them then education has greater sway, though school education, because of the peculiar narrowness of the life of the schoolroom, has so far done little for any save the semi-intellectual virtues.

The one thing that educational theorists of today seem to place as the foremost duty of the schools—the development of powers and capacities—is the one thing that the schools or any other educational forces can do least. The one thing that they can do best is to establish those particular connections with ideas which we call knowledge and those particular connections with acts which we call habits.

CHAPTER XXVI

THE NATURE AND AMOUNT OF INDIVIDUAL DIFFERENCES IN SINGLE TRAITS

For the purpose of the following discussion, let a 'single trait' be defined as one whose varying conditions in men can be measured on one scale. A combination of traits requires two or more scales. For example, in so far as the difference between John and James in reaction time to sound can be measured as so many thousandths of a second on one scale, reaction time to sound is a single trait. The difference between John and James in temperament, on the contrary, can be stated only in terms of several scales, such as quick . . . . . slow, intense . . . . . superficial, broad . . . . . narrow, and the like. So temperament is to be regarded as a combination of traits.

Individuals may be compared with respect to one trait at a time, or with respect to certain combinations of traits. We naturally take up first the simpler case.

THE CONTINUITY OF MENTAL VARIATIONS

Continuity of variations means two things,—the absence of regularly recurring gaps, such as those between 2 petals, 3 petals, 4 petals, and the like, and the absence of irregularly recurring gaps, such as those between mice and rats, between rats and squirrels, and the like.

That continuity* of variations in a mental trait taken

*Of course continuity is not taken here in the sense of infinite divisibility. There are doubtless ultimately unit-factors which either act or do not act, singly is the rule can best be realized by trying to find exceptions to it.   Such there may be, but I am not aware that any mental trait varying in amount has been shown to vary by discrete steps.   A misleading appearance of regularly recurring gaps often arises from inadequate measurements.   In a test of memory, for example, 12 nonsense syllables being read, individuals may appear in the scores as 5, 6, 7, 8 and 9 without

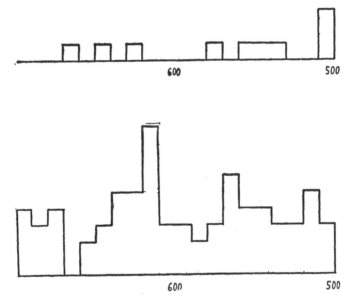

Fig. 78.   The distribution of the cases falling between 500 and 700 seconds in adding 48 columns each of 10 one-place numbers, when, in all, 37 individuals were measured (upper diagram); and when, in all, 200 individuals were measured (lower diagram).

and which consequently increase the amount of the trait by either zero or a certain amount.   But the discrete steps are exceedingly small like the steps of increase of physical mass by atoms.   Intelligence, rate of movement, memory, quickness of association, accuracy of discrimination, leadership of men and so on are continuous in the sense tha mass, ampèrage, heat, human stature and anemia are.

any 5.5's, 6.75's and the like.   But if four such tests are made and the average is taken, there will be 5.5's and 6.75's.

A misleading appearance of irregular discontinuity often arises from the insufficient number of cases measured.   If only a few individuals are measured in a trait or if the scale is a fine one, there will of course be divisions on the scale or amounts of the trait unrepresented in any individuals.   FIG. 78 gives an illustration of such a misleading appearance of discontinuity.

It should be unnecessary to warn the reader against the absurdity of deliberately changing continuous variations into a few groups by coarse scaling; next assuming that the central part of one of these coarse divisions really measures all the individuals therein; and finally imagining that, because the continuous series, varying from a to $a + b,$ has been called, say, Poor, Medium, Good and Excellent, there are really gaps within it!   Unfortunately ever gifted thinkers are guilty of this error.

THE RELATIVE FREQUENCIES OF DIFFERENT AMOUNTS OF

DIFFERENCE

FIG. 79 shows the relative frequencies of the different amounts of the trait in the case of six mental traits.   These six distributions illustrate the statement that 'variations usually cluster around one central tendency.'   This statement is not, however, universally, or even commonly, accepted.   On the contrary the common opinion is that the distribution of individuals with respect to the amount of a single trait is multi-model, as in FIG. 80A, or even a compound of entirely distinct species, as in FIG. 80B.   There would then be many small differences and many large differences with few cases of medium differences.   This may be called the 'multiple type'

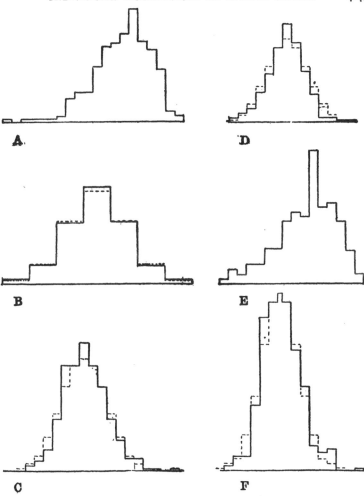

FIG. 79. Samples of the Forms of Distribution Found in Mental Traits.
A. Reaction time: 252 college freshmen
B. Memory of digits: 123 women students
C. Efficiency in marking A's on a sheet of printed capitals: 312 boys from 12
       years o months to 13 years o months
D. Efficiency in giving the opposites of words: 239 boys from 12 years o months
       to 13 years o months
E. Accuracy in drawing lines to equal a 100 mm. line: 153 girls from 13 years
       o months to 16 years o months
F. Efficiency in marking words containing each the two letters a and t: 312 boys
       from 12 years o months to 13 years o months
    In all six cases the left end of the scale represents the lowest abilities—that is,
the longest times in A, the fewest digits in B, etc. The continuous lines give
the distributions. The broken lines are to be disregarded for the present.

theory. For instance, in the case of intellect we find the terms genius, normal, feeble-minded, imbecile and idiot used as if the geniuses were separated by a clear gap from the normal individuals, these again from the feeble-minded, and so on. So also visualizers and non-visualizers, or men of normal color

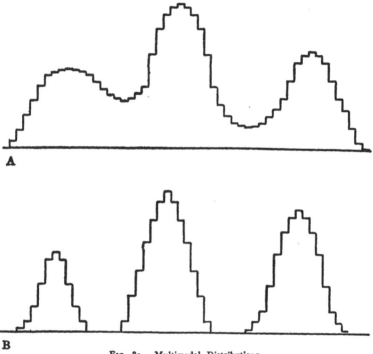

Fig. 80. Multimodal Distributions.

vision and the color blind, are spoken of as if those in each group were all almost identical and all much unlike all in the other group.

Multimodality is to be expected in traits the amount of which may be greatly increased or decreased by some one cause (or number of causes commonly acting together). If, for instance, reading Aristotle added enormously to anyone's intellectual gifts, we should expect to find men divided into two distinct surfaces of frequency on a scale for intellect, the higher ranking species being made up almost exclusively or even entirely of those who had taken the Aristotelian dose.

In certain traits, such as knowledge of a certain language, or ability to play a certain game, there are two species. One includes those who have had no opportunity to get the knowledge or ability and whose knowledge or ability is consequently o; the other is made up of those who have had some opportunity to get the knowledge or ability and who range in it from o or near o to a large amount. Understanding of spoken English, or ability to play chess or whist or golf, or ability to typewrite or to navigate a ship by the compass, would, of course, give such groups, if measured in adults the world over. Here the cause does not produce a uniform amount of the trait, but the world is so arranged that on many persons the cause does not act at all.

Many such causes may act in the case of particular habits, knowledges and skills. Since, for example, some Germans are, and some are not, subjected to the action of enforced military service, there may well be two modes to the surface of frequency of knowledge of the manual of arms, one group all knowing it very well, the other group knowing hardly anything about it. Apprenticeship to a certain trade, or enrollment in a certain kind of school, may thus lead to extreme and uniform amounts of knowledge of, say, plastering or typewriting or medicine, so as to divide human nature sharply into an ordinary and an expert class. How far this happens is not known.

If sex made a great enough difference in the amount of any trait, there would be two modes in the surface of frequency for the trait in question in the two sexes combined. But observable bimodality as a result of mixture of the sexes does not in fact appear, because the sex differences are so small. In traits in which race makes a great difference there will tend to be a mode for each racial type if two extreme races are mixed. If, however, all races or a random selection of races, were mixed, the resulting surface of frequency would not show a distinct mode for each, or probably for any one. Even so great a difference as that between the whites and the colored in scholarship in the high school is shown in the combined distribution only by a flattening of the surface of frequency as compared with that of either race alone (see Fig. 81).

The common opinion that there are distinct species of

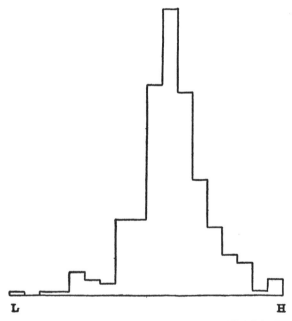

L   H

FIG. 81   The Relative Frequencies of Different Degrees of High-School Scholarship in a Group Composed of 150 Whites and 150 Negroes   The lowest grade of scholarship is at the left, the highest grade at the right, end of the scale. The two separate distributions, here combined, are shown in FIG. 74.

individuals, with more or less pronounced gaps between, does not, however, limit itself to presupposing such multimodalities as those made by men and women, by Germans and Bushmen, by five-year-olds and fifteen-year-olds, by the ordinary population and the blind in respect to vision, by plumbers and non-plumbers in respect to skill in plumbing, by those who never tried to learn chess and those who did, in respect to ability at playing chess, and the like. It knows little or nothing of the effect of various combinations of causes upon the form of distribution of a trait and it thinks of men as divided off into sharp classes in mental traits chiefly because it has not thought properly about the question at all. It merely accepts the crude adjectives and nouns which express primitive awareness of individual differences, as representatives of corresponding divisions in reality; neglects the existence of intervening grades; and does not even attempt to estimate the frequencies grade by grade. How strong this tendency to verbal thinking is can be beautifully illustrated by the firm conviction of even long-trained men of science that people are either markedly right- or markedly left-handed, are either 'normal' in color vision or far removed from the 'normal' in color weakness or color blindness. Until recently the superstition that a great gulf separated children of normal intellect from the imbeciles and idiots was also very strong in many scientific men. The multiple-type theory does not refer to the separation of individuals into groups by the presence or absence of some one cause, or closely interrelated group of causes. It simply vaguely fancies that individuals, even of the same sex, race, age and training, somehow naturally fall into distinct classes or 'types.'

In such a form it is surely almost always, if not always, wrong. A group of such individuals does not, as a rule, show a separation into two or more groups, all in one being much like each other and little like any of those in the other group, or groups. Here again the rule may be verified by searching for exceptions to it. I know of no such. It is indeed a question whether there are any 'types' that are distinct enough to really deserve the name.

CHAPTER XXVII

The Nature and Amount of Individual Differences in Combinations of Traits: Types of Intellect and Character

One feels a bareness and paltriness in such piecemeal descriptions of human beings and their differences one from another as have been given in the last chapter. The actual varieties of human nature do not stand out when one trait at a time is measured. Why, it may be asked, does psychology not take actual whole natures and state how they differ? Why does psychology not describe human minds as zoology describes animal bodies, by classifying them into families, genera and species, and by stating the differences between the different sorts of minds found?

It is true that zoology does not measure all animals in length, then in weight, then in color, then in number of organs, then in number of bones, and so on through a list of particular traits. It began with types or sorts apparent to common observation, such as worms and fishes, and described their essential features and the characteristic differences of one sort from another. And it is true that psychology might try to do likewise. If there were types or sorts of minds equally apparent to common observation, it would surely be worth while to start a description of human nature's varieties with them. But there are no sorts or types of minds that stand out clearly as birds, fishes and worms do amongst animal forms.

A SAMPLE PROBLEM : INDIVIDUAL DIFFERENCES IN IMAGERY

As a sample of the problems and their treatment we may take the natures of individuals in respect to type of imagery, that is, in respect to the combination of :—vividness of visual images, fidelity of visual images, frequency of visual images, vividness of auditory images, fidelity of auditory images, and so on, through the list.

Early in the history of the scientific study of imagery it was noted that certain individuals were able to recall in memory presentations to one sense with a high degree of vividness and fidelity, but lacked this power in the case of presentations to some other sense. The existence of persons who, for instance, could get before the mind's eye vividly and with full detail a mental photograph, as it were, of a scene, but could not thus reproduce from within a melody, an itching nose, or a blow, naturally gave rise to the notion of the 'visualizing type.'

Such cases, of notable ability to get one sort of images and notable inability to get other sorts, were then carelessly assumed to be the rule. It was supposed that a high degree of vividness, fidelity and frequency in images from one sense tended to exclude an equally high degree in images from other senses. People were called visualizers, audiles, motiles, etc., with the meaning that the visualizers had more vivid, faithful and frequent visual images than other people and less vivid, faithful and frequent images from other senses, and similarly for the audiles, or motiles. In graphic form this view would give FIG. 82.

But the actual examination of individuals showed such exclusiveness or predominance of one sort of imagery to be the exception rather than the rule. To even superficial examination it was evident that human natures did not fit into the

scheme of FIG. 82 at all well. Even those who believed unhes-
itatingly that human natures must be distributed around fairly
distinct types in respect to imagery could not, try as they might,
distribute individuals around these types. Meumann in fact
admits that in all his studies of children he never found one
such pure type. "How rare the pure types [of imagery] are

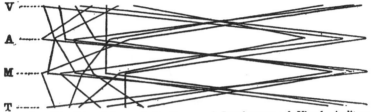

FIG. 82.   The Interrelations of the Degree of Development of Visual, Auditory,
Motor, and Touch Imagery according to the Theory of Pure Types. Imaginary
horizontal lines at V, A, M and T are scales for the degree of vividness, fidelity
and frequency of visual, auditory, motor and touch imagery respectively. The
lowest degree is in each case at the left. 12 individuals are represented, each
by a line crossing each of the scales at the point representing the individual's
ability.

amongst children is witnessed by the fact that in our extensive
investigations of children at Zurich we have never found a
perfectly pure type. Also I know of no case in the entire literature of the subject in which sure proof is given of the existence
of a pure type in the case of children." ['07, I, p. 494]   So
new intermediate types, such as the auditory-motor, visual-
motor, auditory-visual, or even visual-auditory-motor-intellec-
tual (!) [Segal, '08], were introduced. There the matter
remained until Betts ['09] actually measured a sufficient number of individuals in respect to the vividness and fidelity of non-
verbal images from the different sense-fields, so that such
cross-lines as those of FIG. 82 could be located by fact instead
of by opinion.

The pillars of the doctrine were the separation of men into
types according to the predominance of images from one sense,
and the existence of inverse relations between the different

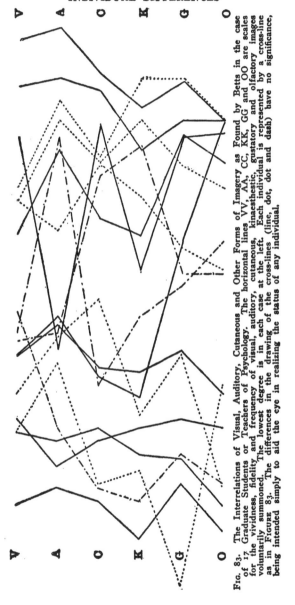

FIG. 83. The Interrelations of Visual, Auditory, Cutaneous and Other Forms of Imagery as Found by Betts in the case of 17 Graduate Students or Teachers of Psychology. The horizontal lines VV, AA, CC, KK, GG and OO are scales for the vividness, fidelity and frequency of visual, auditory, cutaneous, kinaesthetic, gustatory and olfactory images voluntarily summoned. The lowest degree is in each case at the left. Each individual is represented by a cross-line as in FIGURE 83. The differences in the drawing of the cross-lines (line, dot, dot and dash) have no significance, being intended simply to aid the eye in realizing the status of any individual,

sense-spheres in respect to the extent and perfection of imagery. Fact showed opinion to have been grossly in error as a result of its assumption that distinct types of some sort there must be. The contrary is true. Instead of distinct types, there is a con-tinuous gradation. Instead of a few 'pure' types or many 'mixed' types, there is one type—mediocrity. Instead of antagonism between the development of imagery from one sense and that from other senses there is a close correlation. Fig. 83 is a fair sample of the facts found.

This case is instructive because the fate of many theories concerning distinct types of human nature in combinations of traits is likely to be the same as the fate of the doctrine of types of imagery according to the sense involved, with inverse rela-tions between the development of imagery from one sense-field and that from other fields. In the case of temperament, for example, we have the same history. Extreme cases are given names and made into types. Verbal contrasts are supposed to have real existence. Supplementary types are invented to help out the discrepancies between the imagined types and the real distribution of individuals. And it is highly probable that, when actual measurements are made, mediocrity—a tempera-ment moderately sanguine, choleric, phlegmatic, and melan-choly; moderately slow, quick, shallow, intense, narrow and broad; moderately slow-shallow, slow-intense-narrow; moder-ately *everything,*—will be found to be the one real type.

THE THEORY OF MULTIPLE TYPES AND THE SINGLE-TYPE THEORY

The sample problem shows well two extreme views which may be taken of the varieties of human natures, of the same sex, race and degree of maturity, in respect to any combination of traits. On the one hand is the theory of multiple types, a theory which separates men more or less sharply into classes, and describes a man by naming the class to which he belongs. On the other hand is the theory of a single human type, a theory which joins all men one to another in a continuity of variation and describes a man by stating the nature and amount of his divergences from the single type.

By the theory of a single type, one make-up can be conceived such that from it all individuals would differ less than they would from any other one make-up, and such that, the greater the divergences, the rarer they would be. By the theory of multiple types, no such single true central tendency would exist. By the theory of multiple types, if a number, K, of 'typical' natures or make-ups are most favorably taken and if divergences of all individuals are measured from, in each case, that nature which the individual most resembles, the total sum of divergences is enormously reduced below what it would be if they had been measured all from some one nature. By the theory of a single type, this reduction in the sum of divergences due to measuring each individual's divergence from any one of K natures, is much less.

These two doctrines can be made clear by graphic illustrations. Let the amount of each trait in the combination be scaled, as by our custom, horizontally, the center always representing the mode. Let the nature or make-up of each individual be represented by the points where a cross-line denoting him cuts the scale lines. The theory of multiple types then gives something like Fig. 84, and that of one type something like Fig. 85. All the cross-lines of Fig. 84 can be represented as minor divergences from five typical cross-lines, far better than can all the cross lines of Fig. 85. Those of Fig. 85 can be far better represented by one typical cross-line than can those of FIG. 84.

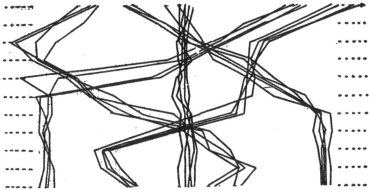

FIG. 84. A Graphic Representation of the Multiple-type Theory in the case of Combinations of Traits. The 11 horizontal dotted lines (drawn only at the extremes) represent scales for 11 traits. Each cross-line represents, by its location, the amounts of the 11 traits in one individual.

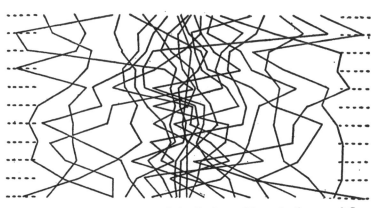

FIG. 85. A Graphic Representation of the Single-type Theory in the case of Combinations of Traits. The 11 horizontal lines represent scales for 11 traits. Each cross-line represents the amounts of the 11 traits in one individual.

It is not necessary to try to decide between these two theories, or to determine just what compromise is the true one. It is better to accept frankly our ignorance of just how individuals do differ in combinations of traits until they have been measured in respect to all the traits involved.

Since, however, many writers about human nature openly or tacitly assume the truth of the multiple type theory in a pronounced form, and are governed by it in their methods of research, of interpretation and of practical control, it will be useful to consider briefly some of the arguments in favor of the single type theory.

The first is the fact that, in proportion as exact measurements have been applied, evidence expected to favor the multiple type theory has turned out in favor of the single type theory. It is true that such cases are very rare, and that, until they are much increased in number, little should be inferred from them. But the fact remains that the single type theory arose from exact measurements, while its opposite came from speculative prepossessions.

The second is the rarity of the inverse correlations between desirable traits upon which so many of the supposed multiple types are based. We know that eye-minded and ear-minded, quick and careful, broad and deep, sensorial and intellectual, men of thought and men of action, and the like do not really represent human nature's varieties in the combinations referred to. If two horizontal scales are drawn for 'ability to learn through the eye' and 'ability to learn through the ear,' and the crosslines are drawn for a thousand individuals, they will not go as in Fig. 86 but as in Fig. 87. So also for scales for quantity of work and quality of work, and so on through the list.

The third is the fact that investigators who are strongly in favor of the multiple type theory and accustomed to interpret facts in harmony with it, yet find so few actual cases of it. Meumann, for instance, ['07, vol. I] clearly accepts the theory *in general* and demands that educational practice should give much attention to the classification of pupils under distinct types. But in concrete particulars he rarely illustrates it.

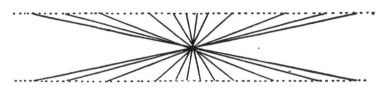

FIG. 86. A graphic representation of the condition of individuals in a combination of two traits, if these are very antagonistic or inversely correlated. The general scheme of the diagram is that used in FIGS. 82 to 85.

He says ['07, vol. I, pp. 331-332] : "By establishing types we orient ourselves in the endless possibilities of individual differences, and if we can place an individual under a type . . . . in any respect we thereby have pointed out a group of universal characters in his mental life. which he in general shares with some individuals and by which he is in general

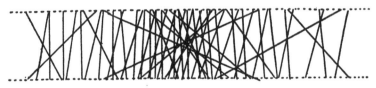

FIG. 87. A graphic representation of the condition of individuals in a combination of two traits, if these are closely and positively related.

distinguished from others." But he does not establish such types. The majority of the differences which he does report as 'typical' are differences between two extremes of the same trait. Intermediate conditions are in some of these cases demonstrably, and in all cases probably, more typical than the supposed types. And this, indeed, Meumann, in some cases, admits.

Lastly, I may mention the fact that satisfactory proof of the existence of a distribution of human individuals after the fashion demanded by the multiple type theory has never been given in a single case, and that the evidence offered by even the most scientific of the theory's adherents is such as they would certainly themselves consider very weak if they were not already certain that types of some sort there must be. Thus a fair-minded perusal of Stern's *Psychologie der Individuellen Differenzen*, designed to be a description of the types into which human nature falls, is an almost sure means of stimulating a shrewd student to the suspicion that intermediate conditions are more frequent than the supposed types, and that there are far more simply ordinary people than there are of all the 'types' put together.

Thus Stern says, "We know the enormous gap which exists between the unmusical and the musician in the discrimination of pitch, between the perfumer and the ordinary person in the recognition of odors, between the painter and the bookworm in the delicacy of color perception." On the contrary, between the keenest of the non-musical and the dullest of musicians in the discrimination of pitch there is no enormous gap, but an enormous overlapping (see Spearman, '04 b, pp. 90 and 92). Stern himself later points out that a little special practice bridges the 'enormous gap.'

Stern mentions (p. 46) "the types of the external observer (the experimental scientist, possibly) and of the introspective thinker (the mathematician or metaphysician, possibly)." But these are not distinct, contrasting types. The experimental scientist is far more likely to be a good mathematician than is the ordinary man. Mathematical ability and interest are in no sense confined to the metaphysicians. The good external observer may be excellent at introspection, and the man with a strong interest in his inner life of thought is much more likely than the average man to have a strong interest in external facts.

INDIVIDUAL DIFFERENCES IN THE AVERAGE AMOUNT OF A COMBINATION OF TRAITS

There are many combinations of traits which can be reduced to single traits by abstraction from some of their particulars. Suppose, for example, that A and B are measured in respect to efficiency in marking A's, in marking words containing each the two letters a and t, in marking hexagons on a sheet of various simple geometrical forms, in marking grays of a certain intensity on a sheet with 200 squares of grays of five intensities, and in marking misspelled words on a sheet containing a passage with 100 out of 500 words misspelled. Suppose the results to be:

	A	B
Marking A's	—1.1	+1.0
" a — t words	—1.4	+0.7
" hexagons	—.6	+1.2
" grays	.0	—.2
" misspelled words	—1.7	+1.4

B — A equals 2.1, 2.1, 1.8, —.2 and 3.1 respectively.

If we abstract from the particular differences and ask only concerning the condition of A and B, and their difference, in *average efficiency in marking these five sorts of visual objects,* the result is that A= —.96 (—4.8 divided by 5), B=+.82 (+4.1 divided by 5), and B — A = 1.78.

Such abstraction from certain particulars of each of a combination of traits can be, and is, in both ordinary and scientific thinking, carried so far as to unite in a single trait very diverse features of intellect and character. From the combination of all the accuracies of discrimination with this and that length, color, weight and the like, may be got the one trait, *accuracy in sensory discrimination.* From the quickness of formation of each of a thousand habits, is derived the single trait, *rate of learning.* Accuracy, quickness, efficiency, permanence, amount of improvement, rate of improvement, and acceleration or retardation in the rate of improvement, are important cases of the measurement on one scale of some feature of an individual's condition in a group of traits. Originality, courage, timidity, suggestibility, scholarship, judgment, interest and curiosity are samples from a long list that could be made of terms, each used with comparatives to denote, though very crudely, a man's position on a single scale. This position or amount would, however, be the resultant of many manifestations of what would have to be scored as a combination of many traits, if represented in full, concrete detail.

For all such one-scale representations of combinations of traits, the entire theory of single traits given in Chapter XXVI holds good. In particular, the single type theory holds of them with fewer exceptions. For some one large cause will much less often act upon a man with the same effect in all the traits of a combination than in some one of them. So, whereas, in discrimination of the tastes of wines or teas or the like, men may be divided into an ordinary and an expert class, they will not be, in respect to accuracy of sensory discrimination in general. Similarly, though, in knowledge of the Latin language, men may fall into two groups,—an ignorant group and a group varying around some knowledge,—in knowledge of languages in general, they do not.

Bibliography of References Made in the Text

Acher, R. A..........'10   *Spontaneous Constructions and Primitive Activities of Children Analogous to those of Primitive Man.* A. J. P., vol. 21, pp. 114-150.

Amberg, E. ....'95   *Ueber den Einfluss von Arbeitspausen auf die geistige Leistungsfähigkeit.* Psychologische Arbeiten, vol. 1, pp. 300-377.

Angell, F., and
Coover, J. E..........'07   *General Practice Effect of Special Exercise.* A. J. P., vol. 18, pp. 327-340.

Angell, J. R..........'04   *Psychology.* References are to the third edition, '06.

Angell, J. R..........'08   *The Doctrine of Formal Discipline in the Light of the Principles of General Psychology.* Educational Review, vol. 37, pp. 1-14.

Arai, T. ....'12   *Mental Fatigue.* Teachers College, Columbia University Contributions to Education, No. 54.

Aschaffenburg, G. ....'96   (b) *Praktische Arbeit unter Alkoholwirkung.* Psychologische Arbeiten, vol. 1, pp. 608-626.

Bagley, W. C. ....'05   *The Educative Process.*

Barker, L. F.........'01   *The Nervous System and its Constituent Neurones.*

Bean, C. H..........'12   *The Curve of Forgetting.* Archives of Psychology, No. 21.

Betts, G. H. ....'09   *The Distribution and Functions of Mental Imagery.* Teachers College, Columbia University Contributions to Education, No. 26.

Binet, A., and
Henri, V. ....'98   *La fatigue intellectuelle.*

Bolton, T. L.........'92   *The Growth of Memory in School Children.* A. J. P., vol. 4, pp. 362-380.

Bolton, T. L.........'02   *Ueber die Beziehungen zwischen Ermüdung, Raumsinn der Haut und Muskelleistung.* Psychologische Arbeiten, vol. 4, pp. 175-234.

423

Book, W. F. ....'08   *The Psychology of Skill: with Special Reference to Its Acquisition in Typewriting.* University of Montana Pub.ications in Psychology: Bulletin No. 53, Psychological Series No. 1.

Bryan, W. L. ....'92   *On the Development of Voluntary Motor Ability.* A. J. P., vol. 5, pp. 125-204.

Burk, C. F. ....'00   *The Collecting Instinct.* Ped. Sem., vol. 7, pp. 179-207.

Burk, F. L. ....'97   *Teasing and Bullying.* Ped. Sem., vol. 4, pp. 336-371.

Burk, F. L. ....'98   *From Fundamental to Accessory in the Development of the Nervous System and of Movements.* Ped. Sem., vol. 6, pp. 5-64.

Calkins, M. W. ......'01   *An Introduction to Psychology.*

Chamberlain, A. F. ....'00   *The Child. A Study in the Evolution of Man.*

Cleveland, A. A. ......'07   *The Psychology of Chess and of Learning to Play It.* A. J. P., vol. 18, pp. 269-308.

Colvin, S. S. ....'09   *Some Facts in Partial Justification of the So-called Dogma of Formal Discipline.* University of Illinois Bulletin, vol. 7, No. 26.

Cooley, C. H. ....'02   *Human Nature and the Social Order.*

Coover, J. E., and
Angell, F. ....'07   *General Practice Effect of Special Exercise.* A. J. P., vol. 18, pp. 327-340.

Cornman, O. P. ....'02   *Spelling in the Elementary School; An Experimental and Statistical Investigation.*

Courtis, S. A. ....'09   *Measurement of Growth and Efficiency in Arithmetic,* Elementary School Teacher, vol. 10, pp. 58-74, 177-199.

Courtis, S. A. .....'11,'12   *Report on the Courtis Tests in Arithmetic.* In the Interim Report of the Committee on School Inquiry of the Board of Estimate and Apportionment of the City of New York.

Dewey, J. ....'10   *How We Think.*

Earle, E. L. ....'03   *The Inheritance of the Ability to Learn to Spell.* Columbia Contributions to Phil., Psy., and Ed., vol. 11, No. 2, pp. 41-44.

Ebbinghaus, H. ......'85   *Ueber das Gedächtniss.*

Ebert E., and
Meumann, E. ....'05   *Ueber einige Grundfragen der Psychologie der Uebungsphänomene im Bereiche des Gedächtnisses.* Archiv für gesamte Psychologie, vol. 4, pp. 1-232.

Edinger, L. ....'96   *Vorlesungen über den Bau der Nervösen Centralorgane des Menschen und der Thiere.* Fifth edition.

Fay, E. A...........'98   *Marriages of the Deaf in America.*

Fracker, G. C.......'08   *On the Transference of Training in Memory.* Psychological Review Monograph Supplement, No. 38, pp. 56-102.

France, C. J., and
Kline, L. W..........'99   *The Psychology of Ownership.* Ped. Sem., vol. 6, pp. 421-470.

Friedrich, J. ....'97   *Untersuchungen über die Einflüsse der Arbeitsdauer und der Arbeitspausen auf die geistige Leistungsfähigkeit der Schulkinder.* Zeitschrift für Psychologie, vol. 13, pp. 1-53.

Galton, F. ....'69, '92   *Hereditary Genius: An Inquiry into its Laws and Consequences* (first edition '69, second edition '92). References are to second edition.

Galton, F. ....'83   *Inquiries into Human Faculty.* (References are to the edition published in Everyman's Library.)

Galton, F............'89   *Natural Inheritance.*

Gilbert, J. A..........'94   *Researches on the Mental and Physical Development of School Children.* Studies from the Yale Psychological Laboratory, vol. 2, pp. 40-100.

Guillet, C. ....'00   *Recapitulation and Education.* Ped. Sem., vol. 7, pp. 397-445.

Hahn, H. H., and
Thorndike, E. L......'14   *Some Results of Practice in Addition Under School Conditions.* Journal of Educational Psychology, vol. 5, No. 2.

426   BIBLIOGRAPHY

Hall, G. S............'04   Adolescence.
Heck, W. H. ....'09   Mental Discipline and Educational Values.
                            References are to the Second Edition, of 1911.
Heymans, G., and
Wiersma, E......'06 (a)   Beiträge zur speziellen Psychologie auf Grund
                            einer Massenuntersuchung. Zeitschrift für
                            Psychologie, vol. 42, pp. 81-127, 258-301.
Heymans, G., and
Wiersma, E......'06 (b)   Beiträge zur speziellen Psychologie auf Grund
                            einer Massenuntersuchung. Zeitschrift für
                            Psychologie, vol. 43, pp. 341-373.
Heymans, G., and
Wiersma, E. ....'07   Beiträge zur speziellen Psychologie auf Grund
                            einer Massenuntersuchung. Zeitschrift für
                            Psychologie, vol. 45, pp. 1-42.
Heymans, G., and
Wiersma, E. ....'08   Beiträge zur speziellen Psychologie auf Grund
                            einer Massenuntersuchung. Zeitschrift für
                            Psychologie, vol. 46, pp. 321-333.
Hill, L. B., and
Rejall, A. E., and
Thorndike, E. L.....'13   Practice in the Case of Typewriting. Ped.
                            Sem., vol. 20, pp. 516-529.
Hoch, A., and
Kraepelin, E. ......'95   Ueber die Wirkung der Theebestandtheile auf
                            körperliche und geistige Arbeit. Psycholog-
                            ische Arbeiten, vol. 1, pp. 378-488.
Hyde, W., and
Leuba, J. H..........'05   Studies from the Bryn Mawr College Psy-
                            chological Laboratory. An Experiment in
                            Learning to Make Hand Movements. Psy
                            Rev., vol. 12, pp. 351-369.

James, W. ....'93   Principles of Psychology.

Jennings, H. S........'06   Behavior of the Lower Organisms.

Johnston, J. B........'06   The Nervous System of Vertebrates.

Kirkpatrick, E. A.....'03   Fundamentals of Child Study.

Kirkpatrick, E. A.....'09   Genetic Psychology

Kölliker, A. ......'96, '02   *Handbuch der Gewebelehre des Menschen.* Sixth edition, vol. 2, and vol. 3. V. von Ebner is the responsible author of vol. 3, but I follow custom in using Kölliker's name in reference.

Kraepelin, E., and
Hoch, A. ....'95   *Ueber die Wirkung der Theebestandthiele auf körperliche und geistige Arbeit.* Psychologische Arbeiten, vol. 1, pp. 378-488.

Kraepelin, E., and
Rivers, W. H. R.....'96   *Ueber Ermüdung und Erholung.* Psychologische Arbeiten, vol. 1, pp. 627-678.

Ladd, G. T., and
Woodworth, R. S.....'11   *Elements of Physiological Psychology.*

v. Lenhossèk, M......'95   *Der Feinere Bau des Nervensystems.*

Leuba, J. H., and
Hyde, W. ....'05   *Studies from the Bryn Mawr College Psychological Laboratory. An Experiment in Learning to Make Hand Movements.* Psy. Rev., vol. 12, pp. 351-369.

Lindley, E. H........'00   *Ueber Arbeit und Ruhe.* Psychologische Arbeiten, vol. 3, pp. 482-534.

Mayo, M. J..........'13   *The Mental Capacity of the American Negro.* Archives of Psychology, No. 28.

McDougall, W. ......'08   *Social Psychology.*

Meumann, E. ....'07   *Vorlesungen zur Einführung in die experimentelle Pädagogik und ihre psychologischen Grundlagen.*

Meumann, E., and
Ebert, E. ....'05   *Ueber einige Grundfragen der Psychologie der Uebungsphänomene im Bereiche des Gedächtnisses.* Archiv für gesamte Psychologie, vol. 4, pp. 1-232.

Miesemer, K. ....'02   *Ueber psychische Wirkungen körperlichen und geistiger Arbeit.* Psychologische Arbeiten, vol. 4, pp. 375-434.

Oehrn, A. ....'95   *Experimentelle Studien zur Individual-psychologie.* Psychologische Arbeiten, vol. 1, pp. 92-151.

Ordahl, G. ....'08   *Rivalry: Its Genetic Development and Pedagogy.* Ped. Sem., vol. 15, pp. 492-549.

Pearson, K. ....'04   *On the Laws of Inheritance in Man, II. On the Inheritance of the Mental and Moral Characters in Man, etc.* Biometrika, vol. 3, Part II, pp. 131-190.

Radossawljewitsch, P. R.
.....................'07   *Das Behalten und Vergessen bei Kindern und Erwachsenen nach experimentellen Untersuchungen. (Das Fortschreiten des Vergessens mit der Zeit.)*

Rice, J. M. ....'97   *The Futility of the Spelling Grind.* The Forum, vol. 23, pp. 163-172 and 409-419.

Rivers, W. H. R., and
Kraepelin, E. ....'96   *Ueber Ermüdung und Erholung.* Psychologische Arbeiten, vol. 1, pp. 627-678.

Ruediger, W. C......'08   *The Principles of Education.*

Ruger, H. A.........'10   *The Psychology of Efficiency.* Archives of Psychology, No. 15.

Schneider, G. H......'80   *Der Thierische Wille.*

Schneider, G. H.......'82   *Der Menschliche Wille.*

Schuyler, W., and
Swift, E. J.........'07   *The Learning Process.* Psychological Bulletin, vol. 4, pp. 307-310.

Segal, J. ....'08   *Uber den Reproduktionstypus und das Reproduzieren von Vorstellungen.* Archiv für die gesamte Psychologie, vol. 12, pp. 124-235.

Shinn, M. W.....'93, '99   *Notes on the Development of a Child.* University of California Studies, Nos. 1-4. 1 and 2 appear under date of 1893; 3 and 4, under date of 1899.

Sikorski, J. ....'79   *Sur les effets de la lassitude provoquée par les travaux intellectuels chez enfants le l'âge scolaire.* Annales d'hygiene publique, vol. 2, pp. 458-464.

Spearman, C. ....'04 (b)   *"General Intelligence" Objectively Determined and Measured.* American Journal of Psychology, vol. 15, pp. 201-292.

Starch, D. ....'10   *A Demonstration of the Trial and Error Method of Learning.* Psychological Bulletin, vol. 7, pp. 20-23.

"   " ....'11   *Transfer of Training in Arithmetical Operations.* Journal of Educational Psychology, vol. 2, pp. 306-310.

"   " ....'12   *Periods of Work in Learning.* Journal of Educational Psychology, vol. 3, pp. 209-213.

Stern, W. ....'00   *Uber Psychologie der individuellen Differenzen.*

Stone, C. W.........'08   *Arithmetical Abilities and Some Factors Determining Them.* Columbia University Contributions to Education, Teachers College Series, No. 10.

Swift, E. J., and
Schuyler, W. ....'07   *The Learning Process.* Psychological Bulletin, vol. 4, pp. 307-310.

Swift, E. J ....'03   *Studies in the Psychology and Physiology of Learning.* A. J. P., vol. 14, pp. 201-251.

"   "   " ....'05   *Memory of a Complex Skillful Act.* A. J. P., vol. 16, pp. 131-133.

"   "   " ....'06   *Beginning a Language: A Contribution to the Psychology of Learning.* In "Studies in Philosophy and Psychology by Former Students of Charles Edward Garman," pp. 297-313.

"   "   " ....'10   *Relearning a Skillful Act: An Experimental Study in Neuro-Muscular Memory.* Psychological Bulletin, vol. 7, pp. 17-19.

Thorndike, E. L......'99   *The Instinctive Reactions of Young Chicks.* Psy. Rev., vol. 6, pp. 282-291.

"   "   " .....'00   *Mental Fatigue.* Psy. Rev., vol. 7, pp. 466-482 and 547-579.

"   "   " .....'05   *Measurements of Twins.* Archives of Philosophy, Psychology and Scientific Methods, No. 1.

"   "   " .....'06   *The Principles of Teaching: Based on Psychology.*

Thorndike, E. L......'07   *On the Function of Visual Images.* Journal of Phil., Psy. and Scientific Methods, vol. 4, pp. 324-327.

"   " ....'10   *Handwriting.* Teachers College Record, vol. 11, No. 2.

"   " ....'11   *Mental Fatigue.* Journal of Educational Psychology, vol. 2, pp. 61-80.

"   " ....'12   *The Curve of Work.* Psy. Rev., vol. 19, pp. 165-194.

Trettien, A. W.......'00   *Creeping and Walking.* A. J. P., vol. 12, pp. 1-57.

Van Gehuchten, A....'00   *Anatomie du système nerveux de l'homme.* Third edition.

Wells, F. L..........'12   *The Relation of Practice to Individual Differences.* A. J. P., vol. 23, pp. 75-88.

Weygandt, W........'97   *Ueber den Einfluss des Arbeitswechsels auf fortlaufende geistige Arbeit.* Psychologische Arbeiten, vol. 2, pp. 118-202.

Whitley, M. T.......'11   *An Empirical Study of Certain Tests for Individual Differences.* Archives of Psychology, No. 19.

Wiersma, H............   (See Heymans and Wiersma.)

Wimms, J. H........'07   *The Relative Effects of Fatigue and Practice Produced by Different Kinds of Mental Work.* British Journal of Psychology, vol. 2, pp. 153-195.

Woods, F. A........'06   *Mental and Moral Heredity in Royalty.*

Woodworth, R. S.....'03   *Le Mouvement.*

Woodworth, R. S., and
Ladd, G. T..........'11   *Elements of Physiological Psychology.*

Wright, W. R........'06   *Some Effects of Incentives on Work and Fatigue.* Psy. Rev., vol. 13, pp. 23-34.

Yoakum, C. S........'09   *An Experimental Study of Fatigue.* Psychological Review, Monograph Supplement No. 46.

INDEX

Abilities. *See* under separate headings

Ability, functions of, 181 f.; inheritance of, 360 ff.

Acceleration of improvement, 225

ACH, N., 145

ACHER, R. A., 19

Achievement, relative *versus* absolute, 367 f.

Acquired tendencies, 2

Acquisition, 17

Activities, sex differences in, 347 ff.

Activity, general mental, 64 f.; general physical, 66

Addition, amount and rate of improvement in, 190, 192 f.; of bonds as a factor in improvement, 202 ff.; of satisfyingness and annoyingness, 202 ff.; effect of different distributions of practice on, 207 f.; change of rate of improvement in, 226; permanence of improvement in, 250 f. *See* also Computation

Adjustment. *See* Set of the organism

Adornment, 63

Affection, 27 ff.

Age, changes in mental traits with, 369 ff.

AMBERG, E., 295

Amount and rate of improvement, 186 ff.; in typewriting 187, 189; in tossing balls, 188; in writing German script, 190; in substitution tests, 191; in shorthand, 191; in observing small visual details, 192; in addition, 192 f.; variation of, with individuals, 196 f.; of fatigue, 289 ff.

Analogy, response by, 135 f.; 148 f.

Analysis, 135 f., 138, 147 ff., 153 ff., 159

Anatomy of original tendencies, 84 ff.

Ancestry. *See* Inheritance

ANGELL, F., 243

ANGELL, J. R., 77, 276, 278

Anger, 23 ff.

Animal learning, 125 ff.

Animals, responses to, 18, 22

Annoyers, original, 50 ff.; explicable only by cerebral physiology, 53 ff.; in relation to readiness and unreadiness, 53 ff.; function of, in learning, 71 f.; 125 ff.

Annoyingness, addition and subtraction of, 202 ff., 210 ff.

Approval, responses to, 31, responses by, 32 f.

ARAI, T., 284 ff.

Arithmetic, order of formation of bonds in, 222 f.; permanence of improvement in, 250 f.; individual differences in, 332 ff. *See* also Addition, Computation, etc.

Arithmetical inductions, 159 f.

Arrangement of subject-matter, 219 ff.

Artistic instincts, 63

ASCHAFFENBURG, G., 200

Assertiveness, sex differences in, 347

Assimilation, 135 f., 148 ff.

Association, sex differences in, 345; inheritance of speed and control in, 365. *See* also Bonds and Connections

Associative learning, in man, 138 ff.; shifting, 136, 151 f.

Athleticism, sex differences in, 347

Attack, 23, 33 f., 47

Attention, 14 f., 23 ff.; to human beings, 30; to elements as an aid in analysis, 159 f.; as a condition of improvement, 214

Attention-getting, 30 f.

Attitude, functions of, 181. *See* also Set of the organism

Authority, misuse of, 39

BABBITT, E. H., 271

Babbling, 43, 59

BAGLEY, W. C., 146, 174

BARKER, L. F., 86, 88, 89, 90

BEAN, C. H., 245, 247

Behavior, defined, 2; of chicks, 125 ff.; of turtles, 128; of kittens, 129; of man in learning puzzles, 139 f.

BETTS, G. H., 262, 413 f.

BINET, A., 292, 309

Biting, 23

BOAS, F., 307

Bodily control, 15 ff.; 59 ff.

BOLTON, T. L., 299, 307 f., 313

Bonds, between situation and response, 5 ff., 125 ff.; arranged in series, 130 f.; with elements of situations, 134 f., 153 ff., 260; involving ideas, 140 f.; formation of, in man, 143 ff.; manipulation of, in analysis, 161 ff.; number of, in human learning, 173; the organization of, 176 ff., 243, 254 f.; order of formation of, 222 f.; interdependence of, 236 f.; addition and subtraction of, as elements in improvement, 202 ff.; selection and arrangement of, 219 ff.; number, difficulty and order of formation of, in relation to the form of the practice curve; 229 ff.: strengthening of, by inner

growth, 243; harmful, 245; weakening by disuse, 245 ff.; differences between, in respect to permanence, 251 ff.; facilitation and inhibition of, 259 ff.; opposite, 264 f.; in relation to mental discipline, 278 ff.

BOOK, W. F., 189, 212, 213, 228, 248 f., 253

BRYAN, W. L., 108

BÜHLER, K., 145

Bullying, 38 ff.

BURK, C. F., 109

BURK, F. L., 39, 104, 118

CALKINS, M. W., 77 f.

Calm, in relation to improvement, 214 ff.

Capacities, defined 4 f.; of sensitivity, 11 ff.; of bodily control, 15 ff., 59 ff.; productive of learning, 69 ff. *See* also Original tendencies

Catharsis, doctrine of, 119 f.

Cephalic index, inheritance of, 358

Chain-reactions, 55 f.

CHAMBERLAIN, A. F., 30

Changes, in the rate of improvement, 225 ff.; in addition, 226, 228; in telegraphy, 227; in substitution tests, 227; in typewriting, 229; general features of, 229; causes of, 229 ff.; in relation to the number and difficulty of formation and order of formation of bonds, 231 ff.; in relation to the potency of bonds, 235; in relation to changes in the learner's power, 235 f.; in relation to the correlations of bonds, 236 f.; in relation to re-learning and over-learning,

237 ff.; in the rate of fatigue, 294 ff.

Character, sex differences in, 347 ff.

Chicks, learning of, 125 ff.

Clasping, 28

Classification of individuals, 402-422, *passim*

CLEVELAND, A. A., 213

Climbing, 15

Clinging, 15, 22, 28

Clutching, 20, 22

Collecting, 20

COLVIN, S. S., 174, 276

Combat in rivalry, 25. *See* also Fighting

Combinations, of original tendencies, 9; of traits, 411 ff.

Comparison, as an aid to analysis, 159

Competing bonds, effect of, on permanence 257 f.

Computation, efficiency of, under continuous exercise, 284 ff.; early and late, in the school session, 308 ff.; individual differences in, 332 ff.; after equal increments of practice, 392 ff.

Concomitants, varying, 159 ff.

Conditions of improvement, 202 ff.

Conduction, readiness for, 53 ff.; physiology of, 98

Congruity between an organism's set and its response, 130

Connection-forming, 131, 138 ff.; and analysis, 161 ff.; and selective thinking, 169 ff.; complexity of results of, 175; essential in improvement, 202 f.; systematization of, by education, 223 f. *See* also Bonds

Connections. *See* Bonds

Connectors, 84

Conscientiousness, sex differences in, 347

Consciousness, in angry behavior, 25 f.

Constructiveness, 62 f.

Contempt, 31

Continuity of variations, 402 ff.

Control, mental, instinct of, 65.

Convergence, of stimuli, 92 f.

COOLEY, C. H., 38, 42

Cooing, 28

COOVER, J. E., 243

CORNMAN, O. P., 360, 390

Correlations of bonds, 236 ff. *See* also Facilitation and Inhibition

Counter-attack, 23

Counting letters, efficiency in, under continuous exercise, 290 f.

COURTIS, S. A., 332 f., 390

Courtship, 25

Crouching, 20 f.

Cruelty, 38 f.

Crying, 20, 59

Curiosity, 63 f.

Curves, of practice, 186 ff., 226 ff.; of work, 294 ff.; of satisfyingness, 301 ff.; of frequency, 338 ff.

Darkness and fear, 21

Darwin, C., 31

Deafness, inheritance of, 359

Defects in original nature, 120 ff.

Delayed original tendencies, 100 ff., 107 ff.

Deprivations due to mental work, 321 f.

Destructiveness, 62 f.

Deterioration of functions by disuse, 182, 243 ff.

Deviations. *See* Individual differences

DEWEY, J., 146, 214, 275

Dictation, 307

Differences. *See* Individual differences

Difficulty of formation of bonds, 232 ff.

Discipline, mental, 267 ff.

Discomfort. *See* Annoyers

Discrimination, by varying concomitants, 159 ff.

Display, 33

Dispositions. *See* Set of the organism

Distribution, of stimuli, 92 ff.; of practice, 205 ff., 293 f.; of amounts of mental traits, 337 ff., 402 ff.

Distributions, of children in respect to ability in arithmetic and progress through school, 337 ff.; corresponding to stated differences between groups, 343, 344; of whites and negroes in scholarship, 352, 408; of boys and girls in various traits, 405

Disuse, law of, 70; effects of, 243 ff.

Division, improvement in, 193, 207, 251

Domestic service and gregariousness, 30

DWIGHT, T., 272

EARLE, E. L., 359

Eating, 19

EBBINGHAUS, H., 245 f., 252

EBERT, E., 263

Economics, sex differences in scholarship in, 345

EDINGER, L., 88, 93

Effect, law of, 71, 125 ff., 165, 172

Effectors, 84

Efficiency, concept of, 182 ff.; measurement of, 183 ff.; means of increasing, 324 ff. *See* also Improvement and Fatigue.

Elements, of original tendencies, 9, 68; responses to, 134 f., 147 ff., 153 ff., 159 ff.; action of, in facilitation and inhibition, 260 ff.; spread of improvement by identical, 268 f., 274 ff.

Emotional excitement, in relation to improvement, 214 ff.

Emotions, sex differences in, 247 ff.

Emulation, 35 ff.

End spurt, 296 f.

English, sex differences in scholarship in, 345

Environment, coöperation of, with original nature, 2, 397 ff.; and sex differences, 340 f.; and family resemblances, 358, 360, 361, 363, 365 f.; and maturity, 370 f.; selective action of, 377 f.; and ability in spelling, 384 ff.; and the choice of a profession, 389 f.; method of action of the, 394 ff.; as a cause of multimodality, 407

Excess movements, 61 f.

Excitement, and improvement, 214 ff

Exercise, law of, 70, 161 ff.

Experimentation, instinct of, 65

Eye-color, inheritance of, 358

Eye-movements, 59 ff.

Eye-strain, and mental work, 324

Eyes, covering in fear, 20

Facilitation, 259 ff.

Faculties, alleged formation of connections by, 72 f.

Fallacy, of unfair selection, 377 f.

Fatigue, and improvement, 244; definitions of, 283; of a single function, 283 ff., 314 f.; amount and rate of, 289 ff.; measurement of, 290; changes in the rate of, 294 ff.; transfer of, 305 ff.; theories of, 314 ff.

FAY, E. A., 359

Fear, 20 ff.; gradual rise of, 110

Fighting instincts, 23 ff.

Fluctuations in improvement, 225 ff.; under continuous exercise, 295 ff.

Fondling, 28

Forgetting, rate of, 245 ff.; special protection against, 256 f. See also Permanence of improvement

FRACKER, G. C., 273

Fragments of original tendencies, action of, 9, 68

FRANCE, C. J., 119 f.

Frequency. See Distributions and Variability

Frequency of improvability, 193 ff.

FRIEDRICH, J., 308, 313

Functions, mental, defined, 176 f.; analysis of, 177 f.; characteristics of, 178 ff.; measurement of the efficiency of, 182 ff.; improvement of, 186 ff. See also Efficiency, Improvement, and Mental Discipline

GALTON, F., 356, 360 f., 382 f.

Genius, inheritance of, 360 f.

German script, improvement in writing, 190

GILBERT, J. A., 370, 375

Grasping, 17, 59

Gregariousness, 29 f.

GROSS, K., 65

Groups, measurement of differences between, 343 ff.

Growth. See Maturity.

GUILLET, C., 104 f., 117, 122

Habit-formation, in animals, 125 ff.; in man, 139 ff.

Habits, susceptibility of, to environmental influence, 401; relation of, to multimodality, 407. See also Bonds

HAHN, H. H., 193, 393

Hair-color, inheritance of, 358

HALL, G. S., 116, 117, 118, 119, 122

Handwriting, sex differences in, 347

Harmful bonds, formation of, 245, 263

Head, erection of, 33; lowering of, 33

Heart-beat, in fear, 20

HECK, W. H., 277 f.

HENRI, V., 309

Heredity. See Inheritance

HEYMANS, G., 347 ff.

Hiding, 22

History, sex differences in scholarship in, 345

Hitting, 23 ff.

Hoarding, 20

HOCH, A., 56

Hooting, 33

Hunting instincts, 18 f., 39, 47

HYDE, W., 190

Hygiene of mental work, 323 ff.

Ideals, in relation to mental discipline, 276, 277

Ideas, as terms in learning, 138

Identification of bonds, and improvement, 210 f.

Ideo-motor action, 75 ff.

Imagery, 412 ff.

Imitation, 40 ff.; alleged formation of connections by, 73 ff.

Immunization by early indulgence, 119 f.

Imperfection of instincts, 16

Improvability, frequency of, 193 ff.

Improvement, concept of, 182 ff.; amount and rate of, 186 ff.; frequency of, 193 ff.; rapidity of, 194 f.; individual differences in 196; limit of, 198 ff.; elements in, 202 f.; conditions of, 205 ff.; interest in, 212 ff.; changes in the rate of, 225 ff.; permanence of, 243 ff.; spread of, 259 ff.

Individual differences, 331 ff.; measurement of, 332 ff.; sex as a cause of, 340 ff.; remote ancestry as a cause of, 351 ff.; immediate ancestry as a cause of, 354 ff.; maturity as a cause of, 369 ff.; environment as a cause of, 376 ff.; effect of equalizing practice upon, 391 ff.; in single traits, 402 ff.; in combinations of traits, 411 ff.

Infallibility, doctrine of nature's, 116 ff.

Infants, responses to, 27 ff.

Influence of improvement in one function upon others, 259 ff.

Information, sex differences in, 345

Ingenuity, sex differences in, 345

Inheritance, from remote ancestry, 351 ff.; from near ancestry, 354 ff.; of physical traits, 358; of ability to learn to spell, 359 f.; of genius, 360 f.; of intellect, 361 ff.; and education, 367 f.

Inhibition, 259 f., 264 ff.

Initial spurt, 295 f.

Injury from mental work, 327 ff.

Inoculation, preventive mental, 119 f.

Instincts, defined, 4; imperfections of, 16; of food-getting, protection, flight and attack, 17 ff.; social, 27 ff.; of being satisfied and annoyed, 50 ff.; of vocalization, visual exploration and manipulation, 59 ff.; of curiosity and mental control, 63 ff.; of play, 66 ff.; productive of learning, 69 ff.; anatomy and physiology of, 84 ff.; order and dates of, 100 ff.; value and use of, 116 ff.; sex differences in, 350 f. *See* also Original tendencies

Intellect, sex differences in, 345 ff.; racial differences in, 351 ff.; inheritance of, 361 ff.; types of, 415 ff.

Intellectual instincts, 59 ff.

Interest, and improvement, 212 ff.; and fatigue, 325 f.

Interests, 50 ff., 111 ff., 347 ff.

Interference, 264 ff.; responses to, 23

Intervals between practice-periods, 205 ff.

Inventories of original tendencies, 11 ff.

Inverse correlations, 413, 418

JAMES, W., 18, 29, 75, 76, 77, 78, 80 f., 111 f., 114, 171

JENNINGS, H. S., 355

JOHNSTON, J. B., 92

Jumping, 15

Kicking, 23 f.

KIDD, D., 29

Kindliness, 38

KIRBY, T. J., 192 f., 196, 197, 207 f., 250 f.
KIRKPATRICK, E. A., 15, 63
Kittens, learning of, 129 f.
KLINE, L. W., 119 f.
KÖLLIKER, A., 85, 86, 88, 89
KRAEPELIN, E., 296, 299

LADD, G. T., 133
Language, original foundations of, 60
Languages, sex differences in scholarship in, 345
Laughter, 38, 47
Learning, original tendencies productive of, 69 ff.; by imitation, 73 ff.; by ideo-motor action, 75 ff.; physiology of, 98; of animals, 125 ff.; associative, 138 ff.; analytic and selective, 153 ff. *See* also Improvement
Leisure classes, and approval, 32
Length of practice-periods, 205 ff.
v. LENHOSSEK, M., 89, 99
LEUBA, J. H., 190
Lightning, and fear, 20 f.
Limit of improvement, 198 ff.
LINDLEY, E. H., 296, 299

MacCRACKEN, H. M., 272
McDOUGALL, W., 29 f., 45, 48, 75, 78
McMURRY, F. M., 146
MAGNEFF, N., 245, 248
Manipulation, 59 ff.
MARBE, K., 145
Marking tests, efficiency of, under continuous exercise, 290 f.; early and late, in the school session, 313 f.
Mastery, 33 ff.
Maternal instinct, 27 ff.

Mathematics, sex differences in scholarship in, 345
Maturity as a cause of individual differences, 369 ff.; and environmental influences, 370 f.
MAYO, M. J., 351 f.
Measurement, of the efficiency of mental functions, 183 ff.; of individual differences, 332 ff.; of group differences, 343 ff.; of resemblance, 357; of changes with age, 369 ff.
Memorizing, sex differences in, 345
Memory, 243 ff.; distribution of ability in, 405. *See* also Permanence of improvement
Mental discipline, 267 ff.; general rationale of, 278 ff.
Mental functions. *See* Functions
MESSER, A., 145
MEUMANN, E., 263, 413, 418 f.
MIESMER, K., 296, 299
Mirror-drawing, 140
Modifiability, of neurones, 98. *See* also Learning
Moral traits, sex differences in, 347 ff.
MORGAN, C. L., 270
MORRIS, J. H., 271
Motherly behavior, 27 ff.
Motives, original foundations of, 50 ff.
Motor ability, development of with age, 107 ff.; sex differences in, 345
Movements, original control of, 15 ff., 59 ff.
Multiple response, 6 ff., 56, 61, 132, 143 f.
Multiple-type theory, 404 ff., 415 ff.

Natural selection and the order of appearance of instincts, 105 ff.

Nature's infallibility, doctrine of, 116 ff.

Negative acceleration in improvement, 225

Neglect, transfer of, 279

Negritos, ability of, 353

Negroes, ability of, 351 f.

Nestling, 22

Neurones, action of, in satisfyingness and annoyingness, 53 ff.; structure of, 84 ff.; arrangement of, 87 ff.; sensitivity and conductivity of, 97; action of, in learning, 98

Nonsense syllables, rate of forgetting, 245 ff.

Novel data, responses to, 168 ff.

Nudging, 33

Number of bonds, in relation to the form of practice curves, 231

Nursing, 27 ff.

Obstacles, responses to, 23

OEHRN, A., 290, 295, 299

Opinions concerning mental discipline, 269 ff., 275 ff.

ORDAHL, G., 36 f.

Order, of appearance of delayed tendencies, 100 ff.; of disappearance of transitory tendencies, 100 ff.; of formation of bonds in learning, 219 ff., 232 ff.

Organization of bonds, 176 ff., 243, 254 ff.

Original tendencies, defined, 2; names for, 4 f.; components of, 5 ff.; action of, 9 ff.; to sensitivity, 11 ff.; to attentiveness, 14 f.; of gross bodily control, 15 ff.; of

food-getting, 17 ff.; to hunt, 18 f.; to collect and hoard, 20; to fear, 21 ff.; to fighting and anger, 23 ff.; to respond to the behavior of other human beings, 27 ff.; to be satisfied and annoyed, 50 ff.; to vocalization, visual exploration and manipulation, 59 ff.; to curiosity and mental control, 63 ff.; to play, 66 ff.; productive of learning, 69 ff.; anatomy and physiology of, 84 ff.; order and dates of, 100 ff.; value and use of, 116 ff.; defects in, 120 ff.

Over-learning, 237 f., 252

Ownership, 37

Pain, irrational response to, 24; and annoyingness, 51

Parabolic form of practice curves, 225

Partial activity, 134 f., 147 ff., 153 ff., 261

PAYNE, J., 270

PEARSON, K., 346 f., 358

Perception, sex differences in, 345; inheritance of ability in, 365 ff.; distribution of ability in, 405

Period-length, 205 ff.

Permanence of improvement, 243 ff.; in knowledge of nonsense series and poetry, 245 ff.; in tossing balls, 248; in typewriting, 249; in arithmetic, 250 f.; and over-learning, 252 f.; and the nature of the bonds concerned, 254 f.; and learning not to forget, 256; and competing bonds, 257 f.

Physiology of original tendencies, 84 ff.

Plateaus, and learning, 225
Play, 66 ff.
Pleasure, and satisfyingness, 51 ; at being a cause, 65
Poetry, rate of forgetting of, 248
Popularity, sex differences in, 347
Positive acceleration of improvement, 225
Possession, 17 f.
Potency of bonds, 235
Pouncing, 18
Practice, distribution of, 205 ff.; effect of, on individual differences, 391 ff. *See* also Improvement, Amount and rate of improvement, etc.
Problem-attitude, 214
Profession, choice of a, 389 f.
Protrusion of lips and tongue, 48
Psychological conditions of improvement, 208 ff.
Pugnacity. *See* Fighting
Pulling, 23, 38, 59
Purposive behavior, 171
Pushing, 23, 59
Puzzles, responses to, 139 f.

Race, and individual differences, 351 ; and multimodality, 408
RADOSSAWLJEWITSCH, P. R., 245 f., 247, 248, 252
Random activity, 6 f., 59 ff.
Rate, of improvement. *See* Amount and rate of fatigue, 294 ff.
Reaching, 17
Reaction-time, 345, 405
Reaction, varied. *See* Multiple response
Readiness, 53 ff., 244 f.
Reading, 220
Reasoning. *See* Selective thinking

Recapitulation theory, 100 ff.
Recreation, and gregariousness, 29 f.
Reflexes, 4
Reinforcement, 259 ff.
REJALL, A. E., 248 f.
Relearning, 237 f., 245 ff.
Rending, 47
Resemblances, measurement of, 357
Responses, 5 ff.; multiple, 6 ff., 56, 61, 132, 143 f.; to elements, 134 f., 147 ff., 159 ff.; to novel data, 162 ff., 168 ff.
Rest, 315
Restraint, escape from, 23
RICE, J. M., 360, 382, 384 ff., 390
Rivalry, 35 f.
RIVERS, W. H. R., 296, 299
ROARK, R. N., 270
ROWE, S. H., 275
Royal families, heredity in, 361 ff.
RUEDIGER, W. C., 276
RUGER, H. A., 139 f., 168, 209, 262, 263
Running, 15, 20

Satisfiers, original, 50 ff.; explanation of, 53 ff.; function of in learning, 71, 203 ff.; and mental work, 301 ff.
SCHNEIDER, G. H., 18, 104, 117, 118
Scholarship, sex differences in, 345; of whites and negroes, 351 f.
School work, and gregariousness, 30; and the approval-scorn series, 32; improvement in, 192 f., 207 f.; and fatigue, 307 ff.
SCHUYLER, W., 248, 253
Science, sex differences in scholarship in, 345
Scorn, responses to, 31 ; responses by, 32

Scratching, 24, 59
Screaming, 20
SEGAL, J., 413
Selection. *See* Natural selection,
  Analytic and Selective functions,
  and Selective
Selective, thinking, 138, 157 ff., 168
  ff., 345; fallacies, 377 f.
Self consciousness, sex differences
  in, 347
Sensory capacities, 11 ff., 97; sex
  differences in, 345
Set of the organism, 133 ff., 144 ff.
Sex, and individual differences, 340
  ff.; and multimodality, 407 f.
Sex differences, 340; in abilities,
  345 ff.; in character and interests,
  346 ff.
Sexes, differences in the training
  of the, 340 f.
Shifting, associative, 136, 151 f.
SHINN, M. W., 65
Shorthand, improvement in, 191
Shouting, 47, 59
Shoving, 33
Shyness, 347
SIKORSKI, J., 307, 309, 313
Similarity, association by, 171
Single-type theory, 410, 415 ff.
Situations, 5 ff.; activity of, 134, 281 f.
Skill, original foundations of, 15
  ff., 59 ff.
Smiling, 28, 31, 32, 38, 47
Sneering, 33
Social instincts, 27 ff.
Sounds, imitation of, 43 f.
Specialization, of bonds, in fear, 21
  f.; in fighting, 23 ff.; of mental
  functions, 274 ff.
Spelling, 345, 384 ff.
SPENCER, H., 61

Spread of improvement. *See* Men-
  tal discipline
Spurt, after fatigue and after dis-
  turbance, 297 f. *See* also Initial
  Spurt, End spurt, etc.
STARCH, D., 140, 191, 392 f.
Staring, 32
Starting, 20
Stature, inheritance of, 358
STERN, W., 420
Stiffening, 23
Strangeness, and fear, 20
Submission, 33 ff.
Substitution tests, 190, 191
Subtraction of bonds, as a factor in
  improvement, 202 f.
Sweating, 20
SWIFT, E. J., 191, 212, 213, 248 f.,
  253
Sympathy, 38
Synapses, 87 ff.

Tapping, 108 f., 345
Teasing, 38 ff.
Telegraphy, improvement in, 227
Temperament, sex differences in,
  347
Tension, and improvement, 214 ff.
Theories of work and fatigue, 314 ff.
Thinking. *See* Analysis, Selection,
  Bonds, etc.
THOMAS, C., 271
THORNDIKE, E. L., 277, 313, 365 f.,
  390, 393
Thunder, 20
Thwarting of original tendencies, 25
Tormenting, 38 ff.
Transfer of Improvement. *See*
  Mental discipline
Transitoriness of original tenden-
  cies, 100 ff., 111 ff.

TRETTIEN, A. W., 15
Turtles, learning of, 127 ff.
Twins, resemblances of, 365 f.; and the action of the environment, 367 f.
Types of intellect and character, 406 ff., 411 ff.
Type-setters, improvement of, 200 f.
Typewriting, improvement in, 187, 189, 228, 249 f., 252

Unreadiness of conduction units, 54 ff.
Use, law of, 70 f., 116 ff.
Utility theory of the order of original tendencies, 105 ff.

Value of original tendencies, 116 ff.
VAN GEHUCHTEN, 85, 89, 90, 91, 93, 94, 99
Variability, 332 ff.; methods of measuring, 337 ff., of individuals of the same sex and ancestry, 354 ff.; of germs from the same parents, 356 f.; of the same groups in different traits, 404 ff. See also Individual differences and Distributions
Varied reaction. See Multiple response
VEBLEN, T., 32
Visual exploration, 59 ff.

Vivacity, sex differences in, 347
Vocalization, 59 ff.
Voluntary thinking, 171 t.

Walking, 15
Wants, original foundations of, 50 ff.
Warming up, 298 f., 302
WASHBURN, M. F., 77
WATT, H. J., 145
WELLS, F. L., 228, 393
WEYGANDT, W., 296, 299
Whites and negroes compared in scholarship, 351 f.
WHITLEY, M. T., 192, 392
WIERSMA, H., 347 ff.
WILSON, W., 272
WIMMS, J. H., 299
WOODS, F. A., 361 ff.
WOODWORTH, R. S., 15, 133, 273
Work, mental, curve of, 294 ff.; definitions, 314 f.; mechanical and biological theories of, 317 ff.; prevention of injury from, 327 ff. See also Fatigue
Worry and improvement, 214 ff.
Writhing, 23
Writing, German script, 190; from dictation, 307, 308 f.

YERKES, R. M., 128
YOAKUM, C. S., 296